Supportive Care
for the Renal Patient

Supportive Care Series

Volumes in the series

Supportive Care for the Renal Patient

SECOND EDITION

Edited by

E Joanna Chambers

Edwina A Brown

Michael J Germain

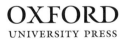

OXFORD
UNIVERSITY PRESS

OXFORD
UNIVERSITY PRESS

Great Clarendon Street, Oxford ox2 6DP

Oxford University Press is a department of the University of Oxford.
It furthers the University's objective of excellence in research, scholarship,
and education by publishing worldwide in

Oxford New York

Auckland Cape Town Dar es Salaam Hong Kong Karachi
Kuala Lumpur Madrid Melbourne Mexico City Nairobi
New Delhi Shanghai Taipei Toronto

With offices in

Argentina Austria Brazil Chile Czech Republic France Greece
Guatemala Hungary Italy Japan Poland Portugal Singapore
South Korea Switzerland Thailand Turkey Ukraine Vietnam

Oxford is a registered trade mark of Oxford University Press
in the UK and in certain other countries

Published in the United States
by Oxford University Press Inc., New York

British Library Cataloguing in Publication Data
Data available

Library of Congress Cataloging in Publication Data
Data available

Typeset in Minion by Glyph International, Banglore, India
Printed in Great Britain
on acid-free paper by the
MPG Books Group, Bodmin and King's Lynn

ISBN 978–0–19–956003–5

10 9 8 7 6 5 4 3 2 1

This book is dedicated to our patients and their families for all they teach us about courage in adversity and also to our colleagues for persisting in the pursuit of knowledge to help us care for people with advanced kidney disease as they approach the end of their lives.

Foreword

Many physicians do not find it easy to involve themselves in the management of the end of life. For physicians familiar with vigorous intervention in complex and acute illness, the argot of success is prolongation of life. Physicians may feel less secure in their practice when this goal recedes and the end of the patient's life is becoming inevitable. Is this a failure? Surely there are further strategies which will confound the inevitable? How can the physician trained to extend life communicate that this is no longer possible, and provide the best of care as life nears its end?

Renal physicians are not exempt from these difficulties, perhaps understandably so given that the specialty had its origins in the complex metabolic and haemodynamic challenge of the critically ill patient with acute kidney injury, and the immune compromised transplant recipient, and the technical demands of dialysis. But from another perspective, renal physicians should engage in supportive care with confidence since the element of our work complementary to acute and complex medicine is our commitment to the long term care of people with kidney disease whose life expectancy is cruelly diminished despite our many interventions.

As renal physicians we commit to the life long care of our patients, knowing that from the day they first walk into our clinic we are likely to have unrelenting involvement in their healthcare, supporting them with varying emphases throughout declining renal function and all aspects of renal replacement therapy to their death. We also know that for some older people especially that time may be all too short once kidney failure has supervened. This life long involvement is a special privilege for the renal physician, and with that privilege comes the responsibility to ensure that we support our patients as fully as possible to the end of their lives, to ensure that their lives end as well as they can; and to ensure that we understand and alleviate the symptoms and concerns of our patients as well in this last phase of their lives as we do in earlier phases. We must seek to understand and support all aspects of the patients concerns, being prepared to be at hand as patients we have often known for many years confront their own mortality.

The editors of this exemplary text book-Joanna Chambers, Edwina Brown, and Michael Germain-bring together a faculty of contributors who deliver highly informative and often wise advice about physical, psychological, spiritual, and organisational aspects of supportive care, including end of life care, in the contemporary practice of renal medicine. The text exudes the practical and common sense advice which assures the reader that its origins are rooted in practice not theory. It is realistic about the complexity of symptoms and complications which need to be analysed and managed. It emphasises the multidisciplinary approach which is the key to the best supportive care, both working together within the renal multiprofessional team, and also with other specialities, particularly palliative medicine.

I commend this book to all renal physicians whatever their vintage. For those embarking on a specialist career the clear understanding of supportive care provided here can help to build confidence in the management of this demanding aspect of our work. For those like me, who have been confronting these issues for many years, doing our best but conscious of the uncertainties, it is never too late to learn more, and the clear, practical and humane instruction this book contains will undoubtedly help to improve clinical care of all our patients.

Professor John Feehally

Consultant Nephrologist, University Hospitals of Leicester

Honorary Professor of Renal Medicine, University of Leicester

Secretary General & President Elect, International Society of Nephrology

October 2009

Series preface

Supportive care is the multidisciplinary holistic care of patients with chronic and life-limiting illnesses and their families – from the time around diagnosis, through treatments aimed at cure or prolonging life, and into the phase currently acknowledged as palliative care. It involves recognizing and caring for the side-effects of active therapies as well as patients' symptoms, co-morbidities, psychological, social, and spiritual concerns. It also values the role of family carers and helps them in supporting the patient, as well as attending to their own special needs. Supportive care is a domain of health-and social care that utilizes a network of professionals and voluntary carers in a 'virtual team'. It is increasingly recognized by healthcare providers and governments as a modern response to complex disease management, but so far it can lay claim to little dedicated literature.

This is therefore one volume in a unique new series of textbooks on supportive care, published by Oxford University Press which has already established itself as a leading publisher for palliative care. Unlike 'traditional' palliative care, which grew from the terminal care of cancer patients, supportive care is not restricted to dying patients and neither to cancer. Thus, this series covers the support of patients with a variety of long-term conditions, who are currently, largely managed by specialist and general teams in hospitals and by primary care teams in community settings. It will, therefore, provide a practical guide to the supportive care of the patient at all stages of the illness, providing up-to-date knowledge of the scientific basis of palliation and also practical guidance on delivering high-quality multidisciplinary care across healthcare sectors. The volumes – edited by acknowledged leaders in the specific fields discussed in each volume, – will bring together research, healthcare management, economics, and ethics through contributions from an international panel of experts of all disciplines. The underlying theme of all the books is the application of the latest evidence-based knowledge, in a humane way, for patients with advancing disease.

As Series Editor, I bring decades of research and clinical experience of acute medicine and palliative care. My work has spanned St Christopher's Hospice and the Leicestershire Hospice in England – both of which have been inspirational leaders of traditional palliative care; and the Academic Unit of Supportive Care at the University of Sheffield, England. I have advocated the supportive care approach to cancer and other chronic disease management and delighted to be collaborating on this series. I am committed to delivering high quality of end-of-life care when it is necessary, but constantly seeking to influence colleagues in all relevant healthcare disciplines to adopt the principles of modern supportive care to benefit a wider range of patients at earlier stages of illness. I aim, through this series, to inform and inspire other doctors, nurses, allied health professionals, pharmacists, social and spiritual care providers, and students, to improve the quality of living for all patients and families in their care.

Sam Hjelmeland Ahmedzai

Professor of Palliative Medicine

Academic Unit of Supportive Care

The University of Sheffield

Royal Hallamshire Hospital

Sheffield, UK

Preface

The first edition of this book was published just as there was increased recognition in the UK, US and elsewhere that renal replacement therapy (RRT) with dialysis or transplantation, though often miraculous and life extending, is also associated with significant morbidity and may not improve the quality of life of all who undertake it. We recognised then that extending life was not enough; and included chapters on pain and other symptom management as well as psychological and spiritual care; all are essential accompaniments to renal replacement therapy. These chapters are again included, and updated as further work has been done particularly on pain and symptom prevalence and its management.

Since 2004, there have been exciting developments both in the UK and US. In 2005 the UK's National Service Framework for renal diseases part 2 importantly recognised the importance of accurate, timely and sensitive information giving, as well as partnership with patients and palliative care to provide culturally appropriate end of life care. More recently in July 2008 the Department of Health published a National End of Life Strategy. Here the definition of End of Life (EOL) was extended to people with any condition from which they were not going to recover and in whom the prognosis was measured in weeks, months or possible a year or more and who had supportive care needs. Importantly the emphasis of this strategy is on all conditions, in all settings – bringing in chronic disease states such as advanced kidney disease, dementia and the frail elderly. Excellent care should not be confined to those cared for by hospice or palliative care services, but also at home, in hospital or care homes, depending on the person's wishes. The renal community have immediately responded to this with their own renal implementation document in June of this year; described in chapter 3 which spells out more specifically how this can be achieved and provides impetus for continuing to improve services.

In the US, this recognition of the need for supportive care led the Robert Wood Johnson Foundation to sponsor an End Stage Renal Disease (ESRD) working group to make recommendations which promote excellence and improved quality of life at the end of life for ESRD patients and their families through improving supportive care. Its recommendations published in 2003 resulted in a number of work products which included: a curriculum for nephrology trainees and the formation of a renal EOL coalition which aims to promote an effective interchange between patients, families, caregivers, funders and providers in support of integrated patient centered end of life care for ESRD patients; their increase in use of hospice demonstrates the greater recognition of EOL needs by the US nephrology community. In addition US and Canadian nephrologists have shown an increase in knowledge and an improvement in attitudes in a recent study. It is to be hoped that progress made in improving estimates of prognosis in the ESRD population, will help to identify those most in need. The Kidney End-of-Life Coalition (kidneyeol.org) is a multidisciplinary group of renal professionals and patients dedicated to improving end-of-life care for kidney patients

The Renal Physicians Association /American Society of Nephrology practice Guidelines described in chapters 3 and 5 are in the process of being updated and expanded to include stage 4 and 5 chronic kidney disease (CKD) patients. The process has led to debate as to for whom dialysis is the default or standard treatment on reaching stage 5 CKD and for whom it may neither improve quality or quantity of life.

These issues are addressed in the new chapters on the conservatively managed patient and the very elderly. In addition in several familiar chapters there has been a change of the emphasis not just to bring them up to date but to combine the academic with practical application to clinical practice. These include the chapters on advance care planning, quality of life and death and end of life care. The chapter on initiating and withdrawing dialysis is enlarged to include a section on communicating with the patient; again both academic and practical. The introductory chapters and that on the home dialysis patient have been revised.

We have continued with our thread of case history and ethical analysis; thus providing examples from practice and enabling the reader to follow possible thought processes through difficult decision making.

There is still work to be done to educate junior and senior doctors and other professionals about these aspects of care and to improve communication with patients and their families about end of life to ensure we offer optimum care. In order to improve care further research is needed to determine the ways such patients can be best supported

Team work has been essential in the production of this book and is essential to the care of all patients but kidney patients particularly. This book brings together many disciplines: medicine; renal, palliative and psychological; nursing, counsellors, chaplains, dieticians and psychologists and the teams of renal and palliative medicine. We need to work together with our patients and their families to provide the highest, most holistic care we are able; as the sum of our working is greater than the parts.

Joanna Chambers

Edwina Brown

Michael Germain

October 2009

Contents

Contributors

Dr David Ansell
UK Renal Registry,
Southmead Hospital,
Bristol, UK

Professor Edwina A Brown
Consultant Nephrologist,
Hammersmith Hospital,
London, UK

Dr Ira Byock
Professor of Anesthesiology and Community
& Family Medicine,
Dartmouth Medical School,
Lebanon, USA

Dr Fergus Caskey
Consultant Nephrologist
UK Renal Registry,
Southmead Hospital,
Bristol, UK

Dr E Joanna Chambers
Consultant in Palliative Medicine,
Southmead Hospital,
North Bristol Trust,
Bristol, UK

Dr Lewis M Cohen
Professor of Psychiatry,
Tufts University School of Medicine,
Baystate Medical Center,
Springfield, MA, USA

Dr Daniel Cukor
Assistant Professor of Psychiatry,
Associate Director, Anxiety Disorders Clinic,
SUNY Downstate Medical Center,
New York, USA

Canon Chris Davies
Head of Spiritual and Pastoral Care,
North Bristol and the University Hospitals,
Bristol NHS Trusts,
Southmead Hospital,
Bristol, UK

Dr Sara N Davison
Associate Professor,
University of Alberta,
Department of Medicine,
Division of Nephrology and Immunology,
Edmonton, Canada

Celia Eggeling
Lead for Psychosocial Care,
South West Thames Renal and
Transplantation Unit,
St.Helier Hospital,
Carshalton,
Surrey, UK

Eileen M Farrell
Yeshiva University - Albert Einstein College
of Medicine,
Ferkauf Graduate School of Psychology,
New York, USA

Professor Ken Farrington
Consultant Nephrologist,
Department of Nephrology,
Lister Hospital,
Stevenage, UK

Professor Terry Feest
Professor of Clinical Nephorlogy,
Department of Renal Medicine,
Southmead Hospital,
Bristol, UK

Dr Charles Ferro
Consultant Nephrologist,
University Hospital NHS Trust,
Edgbaston,
Birmingham, UK

Susan H Finkelstein
Hospital of St. Raphael,
Yale University,
Renal Research Institute,
New Haven,
Connecticut, USA

Dr Fredric O Finkelstein
Hospital of St. Raphael,
Yale University, Renal Research Institute,
New Haven, Connecticut, USA

Dr Michael Germain
Professor of Medicine,
Tufts University School of Medicine,
Baystate Medical Center,
Springfield, MA, USA

Dr Jean L Holley
Clinical Professor of Medicine,
University of Illinois,
Urbana-Champaign, USA

Helen Hurst
Peritoneal Dialysis Nurse Specialist,
Manchester Institute of Nephrology &
Transplantation, The Royal Infirmary,
Oxford Road, Manchester, UK

Dr Alastair Hutchison
Consultant Nephrologist,
Manchester Institute of Nephrology &
Transplantation, The Royal Infirmary,
Oxford Road, Manchester,UK

Lina Johansson
Research Dietician,
Imperial College Kidney and Transplant
Institute, Hammersmith Hospital,
London, UK

Dr Paul L Kimmel
Senior Advisor,
Division of Kidney Urologic and
Hematologic Diseases,
National Institute of Diabetes, Digestive
and Kidney Diseases,
National Institutes of Health,
Bethesda, MD;
Department of Medicine,
George Washington University,
Washington DC, USA

Dr Lionel U Mailloux
Clinical Professor of Medicine,
NYU School of Medicine, American Society
of Hypertension – Specialist in Clinical
Hypertension; Senior Attending in Medicine,
Nephrology, North Shore University Hospital
Port Washington, USA

Dr Alvin Moss
Professor of Medicine and Director,
Center for Health Ethics and Law,
Section of Nephrology,
Robert C. Byrd Health Sciences Center,
West Virginia University, USA

Dr Fliss Murtagh
Clinical Senior Lecturer
King's College London,
Department of Palliative Care,
Policy & Rehabilitation,
Weston Education Centre,
London, UK

Dr Tom Sensky
Professor of Psychological Medicine,
Imperial College London,
Claybrook Centre,
St Dunstan's Road, London, UK

Jane Seymour
Sue Ryder Care Professor of Palliative and
End of Life Studies,
University of Nottingham,
School of Nursing,
Queen's Medical Centre,
Nottingham, UK

Professor Neil Sheerin
Institute of Cellular Medicine,
Medical School,
Newcastle University,
Newcastle upon Tyne, UK

Maria Da Silva-Gane
Counsellor, Renal Unit,
Lister Hospital, Stevenage, UK

Dr S Risdale
UK Renal Registry,
Southmead Hospital, Bristol, UK

Dr Steven D Weisbord
Professor of Medicine,
Renal-Electrolyte Division,
Department of Medicine,
University of Pittsburgh School of Medicine,
Pittsburgh, USA

Abbreviations

ACP	advance care planning	h	hour(s)
AD	advance directive	H3G	hydromorphone-3-glucuronide
ADRT	advance decision to refuse treatment	Hb	haemoglobin
AIDS	acquired immune deficiency syndrome	HD	haemodialysis
APD	ambulatory peritoneal dialysis	HIV	human immunodeficiency virus
ADPKD	autosomal dominant polycystic kidney disease	HRQL	health-related quality of life
		5-HT3	5-hydroxytryptamine 3
ARF	acute renal failure	ICD	International Classification of Diseases
ASA	acetylsalicylic acid	IDDM	insulin-dependent diabetes mellitus
ASN	American Society of Nephrology	IM	intramuscular(ly)
B3G	buprenorphine-3-glucuronide	IOM	Institute of Medicine
b.d.	twice a day	IV	intravenous(ly)
BDI	Beck Depression Inventory	KDOQI	Kidney Disease Outcomes Quality Initiative
BUN	blood urea nitrogen		
CAPD	continuous ambulatory peritoneal dialysis	KDQOL	Kidney Disease Quality of Life Questionnaire
CCPD	continuous cycling peritoneal dialysis	LVEF	left ventricular ejection fraction
CKD	chronic kidney disease	M&M	morbidity and mortality
CMV	cytomegalovirus	M3G	morphine-3-glucuronide
CPAP	continuous positive airway pressure	M6G	morphine-6-glucuronide
CPR	cardiopulmonary resuscitation	MDRD	Modification of Diet in Renal Disease
CRF	chronic renal failure	MOAIs	monoamine oxidase inhibitors
CRN	community renal nurse	NCHSPCS	National Council for Hospice and Specialist Palliative Care Services
CVD	cardiovascular disease		
DSI	dialysis symptom index	NECOSAD	Netherlands Cooperative Study on Adequacy of Dialysis
ED	erectile dysfunction		
eGFR	estimated glomerular filtration rate	NHP	Nottingham Health Profile
EoL	end of life	NHS	[UK] National Health Service
ERA	European Renal Association	NICE	National Institute for Clinical Excellence
ESAS	Edmonton Assessment System		
ESF	established renal failure	NMDA	N-methyl-D-aspartate
ESRD	end-stage renal disease	NNT	number needed to treat
ESRF	end-stage renal failure	NTDS	North Thames Dialysis Study
GABA	gamma aminobutyric acid	PD	peritoneal dialysis
GAS	general adaptation syndrome	pmp	per million population
GFR	glomerular filtration rate	PMTs	pain measurement tools
GI	gastrointestinal	PO	by mouth (per os)
GM	glomerulonephritis	POLST	Physicians orders for life sustaining treatment

POS	Patient Outcome Scalev	SF-36	Medical Outcomes Study Short Form-36
PR	rectally (per rectum)		
prn	as needed	SIP	Sickness Impact Profile
PTH	parathyroid hormone	SSRIs	selective serotonin re-uptake inhibitors
PVD	peripheral vascular disease	STAI	State Trait Anxiety Inventory
QALY	quality adjusted life year	stat	immediately
q.h.s.	at bedtime	TCA	tricyclic antidepressants
q.o.d.	every other day	TENS	transcutaneous electric nerve stimulation
q.i.d.	four times a day		
RBC	red blood cell	t.i.d.	three times a day
rHuEpo	recombinant human erythropoietin	UK	United Kingdom
RLS	restless legs syndrome	USA	United States of America
RPA	Renal Physicians Association [of the USA]	USRDS	US Renal Data System
		WHO	World Health Organization
RPCI	Renal Palliative Care Initiative	WHOQOL	World Health Organization Quality of Life [Assessment]
RRT	renal replacement therapy		
SC	subcutaneous(ly)	WNERTA	Western New England Renal and Transplantation Associates
SCr	serum creatinine		

Introduction to ethical case analysis

Alvin Moss

In 2000 the Renal Physicians Association and the American Society of Nephrology published the clinical practice guideline *Shared decision-making in the appropriate initiation of and withdrawal from dialysis*. The guideline provides nine recommendations with regard to decision making about withholding or withdrawing dialysis and the care of patients who forgo dialysis. These guideline recommendations (see text below) and the process for ethical decision making described in the guideline (see Box) provide the basis for the ethical case analyses presented throughout this book. This guideline has been widely quoted in the nephrology and palliative care literature, and studies have documented the effectiveness of the guideline in patient care.[1,2] Nephrologists who are familiar with the guideline and report using it rate themselves as very well prepared to participate in decisions about withholding, starting, continuing, and stopping dialysis. These nephrologists are more likely to withdraw patients from dialysis, to use a time-limited trial of dialysis, and to refer dialysis patients to hospice than those who rate themselves as less prepared. The guideline recommends shared decision making which it defines as the process by which physicians and patients agree on a specific course of action based on a common understanding of the treatment goals and risks and benefits of the chosen course compared with reasonable alternatives. It acknowledges, however, that there are limits to the shared decision-making process that protect the rights of patients and the professional integrity of healthcare professionals. It states that the patient has the right to refuse dialysis even if the renal care team disagrees with the patient's decision and wants the patient to undergo dialysis. Similarly, the renal care team has the right to refuse to offer dialysis when the expected benefits do not justify the risks. In recent times, the most difficult ethical quandaries for nephrologists and palliative care clinicians have been how to address conflicts when the family of a dying dialysis patient who lacks decision-making capacity requests that 'everything possible be done' when the healthcare team believes that such treatment would be non-beneficial. The guideline provides recommendations for how to resolve such conflicts.

For further information, readers are referred to the Renal Physicians Association and the American Society of Nephrology clinical practice guideline *Shared decision-making in the appropriate initiation of and withdrawal from dialysis* (Washington, DC: Renal Physicians Association, February 2000). Throughout the ethical case analyses it is referred to as the RPA/ASN guideline.

RPA/ASN guideline recommendation summary

The following recommendations are based on the expert consensus opinion of the RPA/ASN Working Group. They developed *a priori* analytical frameworks with regard to decisions to withhold or withdraw dialysis in patients with acute kidney injury and end-stage renal disease (ESRD). Systematic literature reviews were conducted to address pre-specified questions derived from the frameworks. In most instances, the relevant evidence that was identified was contextual in nature and only provided indirect support to the recommendations. The research evidence, case and statutory law, and ethical principles were used by the Working Group in the formulation of their recommendations.

Recommendation 1: Shared decision making

A patient–physician relationship that promotes shared decision making is recommended for all patients with either acute renal failure (ARF) or ESRD. Participants in shared decision making should involve, at a minimum, the patient and the physician. If a patient lacks decision-making capacity, decisions should involve the legal agent. With the patient's consent, shared decision making may include family members or friends and other members of the renal care team.

Recommendation 2: Informed consent or refusal

Physicians should fully inform patients about their diagnosis, prognosis, and all treatment options, including: (1) available dialysis modalities, (2) not starting dialysis and continuing conservative management which should include end-of-life care, (3) a time-limited trial of dialysis, and (4) stopping dialysis and receiving end-of-life care. Choices among options should be made by patients or, if patients lack decision-making capacity, their designated legal agents. Their decisions should be informed and voluntary. The renal care team, in conjunction with the primary-care physician, should insure that the patient or legal agent understands the consequences of the decision.

Recommendation 3: Estimating prognosis

To facilitate informed decisions about starting dialysis for either ARF or ESRD, discussions should occur with the patient or legal agent about life expectancy and quality of life. Depending upon the circumstances (e.g. availability of nephrologists), a primary-care physician or nephrologist who is familiar with prognostic data should conduct these discussions. These discussions should be documented and dated. All patients requiring dialysis should have their chances for survival estimated, with the realization that the ability to predict survival in the individual patient is difficult and imprecise. The estimates should be discussed with the patient or legal agent, the patient's family, and amongst the medical team. For patients with ESRD, these discussions should occur as early as possible in the course of the patient's renal disease and continue as the renal disease progresses. For patients who experience major complications that may substantially reduce survival or quality of life, it is appropriate to discuss and/or reassess treatment goals, including consideration of withdrawing dialysis.

Recommendation 4: Conflict resolution

A systematic approach for conflict resolution is recommended if there is disagreement with regard to the benefits of dialysis between the patient or legal agent (and those supporting the patient's position) and a member(s) of the renal care team. Conflicts may also occur within the renal care team or between the renal care team and other healthcare providers. This approach should review the shared decision-making process for the following potential sources of conflict: (1) miscommunication or misunderstanding about prognosis, (2) intrapersonal or interpersonal issues, or (3) values. If dialysis is indicated emergently, it should be provided while pursuing conflict resolution, provided the patient or legal agent requests it.

Recommendation 5: Advance directives

The renal care team should attempt to obtain written advance directives from all dialysis patients. These advance directives should be honoured.

Recommendation 6: Withholding or withdrawing dialysis

It is appropriate to withhold or withdraw dialysis for patients with either ARF or ESRD in the following situations:

1 Patients with decision-making capacity – who being fully informed and making voluntary choices – refuse dialysis or request dialysis be discontinued.
2 Patients who no longer possess decision-making capacity who have previously indicated refusal of dialysis in an oral or written advance directive.
3 Patients who no longer possess decision-making capacity and whose properly appointed legal agents refuse dialysis or request that it be discontinued.
4 Patients with irreversible, profound neurological impairment such that they lack signs of thought, sensation, purposeful behaviour, and awareness of the self and environment.

Recommendation 7: Special patient groups

It is reasonable to consider not initiating or withdrawing dialysis for patients with ARF or ESRD who have a terminal illness from a non-renal cause or whose medical condition precludes the technical process of dialysis.

Recommendation 8: Time-limited trial of dialysis

For patients requiring dialysis, but who have an uncertain prognosis, or for whom a consensus cannot be reached about providing dialysis, nephrologists should consider offering a time-limited trial of dialysis.

Recommendation 9: Palliative care

All patients who decide to forgo dialysis or for whom such a decision is made should be treated with continued palliative care. With the patient's consent, persons with expertise in such care, such as hospice healthcare professionals, should be involved in managing the medical, psychosocial, and spiritual aspects of end-of-life care for these patients. Patients should be offered the option of dying where they prefer, including at home with hospice care. Bereavement support should be offered to patients' families.

The process of ethical decision making in patient care

1 Identify the ethical question(s).

2 Gather the medical, social, and all other facts relevant to the case.

3 Identify all relevant guidelines and values. Be sure to consider any distinctive values of the patient, family, physician, nurse, other healthcare professionals, or the healthcare institution.

4 Determine if there is a solution that respects all the relevant guidelines and values in the case; if there is, use it. If not, proceed to step 5.

5 Propose possible solutions to resolve the conflict(s) in values, or in other words, answer the question 'What could you do?'.

6 Evaluate the possible solutions for the particular case, determine which one is better, justify your choice, and respond to possible criticisms. In other words, answer the questions, 'What should you do?' and 'Why?'.

7 Determine what changes in policy, procedure, or practice could prevent such conflicts in the future.

The patient as person history

(from the Center for Health Ethics and Law, Robert C. Byrd Health Sciences Center of West Virginia University, Morgantown, WV, USA)

1 As you understand it, what is your medical problem?

2 How serious is your illness? What will happen if you are not treated?

3 What do you think caused your illness, and why did it start when it did?

4 Why are you being tested and treated as you are? Are there other choices of treatment besides the one you are receiving?

5 How has your illness affected you?

6 What is most important to you in receiving treatment for your illness?

7 What would you want to avoid in the treatment of your illness?

8 What is your understanding of the meaning of your illness? Is God or religion important to you as you face your illness?

9 What are your sources of strength? What role does faith play in your life?

10 How does faith influence your thinking about your illness?

11 Are there religious practices that are particularly meaningful to you?

12 Are there issues in your spiritual life that are troubling you now?

13 Would you like to talk with someone about these issues?

14 Help me understand how you see your family (and/or other significant social relationship)? What are your thoughts about their concerns or your concerns about them?

These questions are helpful in learning the patient's goals for treatment, in advance care planning, and in dealing with disruptive patients to learn their perspective.

Systematic evaluation of a patient or family request to stop dialysis

1 Determine the reasons or conditions underlying the patient/surrogate desires with regard to withdrawal of dialysis. Such assessment should include specific medical, physical, spiritual, and psychological issues, as well as interventions that could be appropriate. Some of the potentially treatable factors that might be included in the assessment are as follows:

  (a) Underlying medical disorders, including the prognosis for short- or long-term survival on dialysis.

  (b) Difficulties with dialysis treatments.

  (c) The patient's assessment of his/her quality of life and ability to function.

  (d) The patient's short- and long-terms goals.

  (e) The burden that costs of continued treatment/medications/diet/transportation may have on the patient/family/others.

  (f) The patient's psychological condition, including conditions/symptoms that may be caused by uraemia.

  (g) Undue influence or pressure from outside sources, including the patient's family.

  (h) Conflict between the patient and others.

  (i) Dissatisfaction with the dialysis modality, the time, or the setting of treatment.

2 If the patient wishes to withdraw from dialysis, did he/she consent to referral to a counseling professional (e.g. social worker, pastoral care, psychologist, psychiatrist)?

3 If the patient wishes to withdraw from dialysis, are there interventions that could alter the patient's circumstances which might result in him/her considering it reasonable to continue dialysis?

  (a) Describe possible interventions.

  (b) Does the patient desire the proposed intervention(s)?

4 In cases where the surrogate has made the decision to either continue or withdraw dialysis, has it been determined that the judgement of the surrogate is consistent with the stated desires of the patient?

5 Questions to consider when a patient asks to stop dialysis.

  (a) Is the patient's decision-making capacity diminished by depression, encephalopathy, or other disorder?

  (b) Why does the patient want to stop dialysis?

  (c) Are the patient's perceptions about the technical or quality-of-life aspects of dialysis accurate?

  (d) Does the patient really mean what he/she says or is the decision to stop dialysis made to get attention, help, or control?

  (e) Can any changes be made that might improve life on dialysis for the patient?

  (f) Would the patient be willing to continue dialysis while the factors responsible for the patient's request are addressed?

  (g) Has the patient discussed his/her desire to stop dialysis with significant others such as family, friends, or spiritual advisors? What do they think about the patient's request?

References

1 Davison SN, Jhangri GS, Holley JL, et al. (2006). Nephrologists' reported preparedness for end-of-life decision-making. *Clin J Am Soc Nephrol,* **1**, 1256–62.
2 Holley JL, Davison SN, Moss AH (2007). Nephrologists' changing practices in reported end-of-life decision-making. *Clin J Am Soc Neph*, **2**, 107–11.

Chapter 1

Changing patterns of renal replacement therapy

David Ansell, S Risdale, and Fergus Caskey

1.1 Introduction

End-stage renal disease (ESRD) is inevitably fatal unless treated by renal replacement therapy (RRT). Although George Hass undertook the first haemodialysis (HD) in a human in 1926, his patient died, and it was not until 1945 that the first successful HD was performed by Kolff for acute renal failure (ARF). It was only through the development of the arteriovenous shunt in the early 1960s that the outlook then also changed for patients with chronic renal failure (CRF).

Following the first partially successful renal transplant in 1950[1] and the first long-term survivor in 1954, the uptake of transplantation increased throughout the 1960s. Renal transplantation only became more successful once graft rejection could be effectively countered with the introduction of the effective immunosuppressant ciclosporin in 1983.

Although the first peritoneal dialysis (PD) was also performed in the human around 1926 by Georg Ganter through improvements in technology, it only became established as an important mode of therapy for chronic renal failure in the 1980s. The use of PD varies between countries and in developed countries the cost is lower than that of HD and there is no requirement for major infrastructure. In many developing countries with lower staffing costs and high 'disposables' costs, PD remains expensive. There has been a revolution in the care of patients with renal failure in these 50 years in all developed countries, with a continuing growth in the provision of RRT. This has come at considerable cost to healthcare systems as these treatments are expensive and have to be administered lifelong. In 2006 the US spent $33 billion on end-stage renal disease (ESRD) expenditure, while the UK estimate is about £1 billion.

In the decades up to 1990s there was considerable debate about the equity of provision of this high-cost technology which, at population level, only benefits a relatively small number of patients. Treatment in some countries, particularly tax-based systems such as the UK's National Health Services (NHS), was rationed, with care being restricted to younger, fitter patients. However, as technology and clinical expertise have advanced, it is now possible to treat older, sicker patients successfully. This success in treatment has led UK patients to dislike the use of the term 'End-Stage' Renal Failure/Disease and in the UK, the term Established Renal Failure (ERF) is now synonymous with ESRF/ESRD, which remains in common use around the world.

The debate about provision of RRT has widened to include not only concern about who is not being treated, but also consideration of formally not providing RRT to those likely to have a poor outcome on RRT. In parallel with this has been the development of alternative palliative models of care to dialysis. The great success of RRT has generated the new problem of caring for a very large and growing pool of patients on RRT and emphasized the public health importance of ESRD. Moreover, the significant and rising cost of RRT programmes make it a crucial issue for all healthcare systems.

This chapter outlines the scale of this growth in RRT and considers the implications for renal service provision.

1.2 Chronic kidney disease

Until recently, it was widely held that kidney disease affected only a very small proportion of the population. It is not feasible to accurately measure renal function outside of the research setting using inulin or iothalamate clearances, and additionally 24-h urine collections are often inaccurate due to incomplete collection. The identification of impaired renal function in epidemiological studies and clinical practice was therefore based on serum creatinine measurements, which took no account of differences in rates of creatinine generation specific to gender or age. As a result, marked renal impairment was often overlooked in poorly nourished, elderly females.

1.2.1 Estimating renal function

Although equations have been used in clinical practice for over 30 years to estimate kidney function from serum creatinine, these were not in widespread use[2] as they required additional factors such as patient weight. With the development of new equations to estimate kidney function – estimated glomerular filtration rate (eGFR) – from demographic and serum variables without requiring weight[3] it was possible to consider more widespread application. The National Kidney Federation then set up a working group to define and classify what they now called chronic kidney disease.[4] This led to the development of a global consensus on a simple definition of CKD – kidney damage or a GFR < 60 ml/min/1.73 m² for 3 months or more, irrespective of cause.[5] Kidney damage in many kidney diseases could be ascertained by the presence of proteinuria, defined as a urinary protein-to-creatinine ratio > 50 mg/mol in two of three spot urine specimens. The GFR could be estimated from calibrated serum creatinine using equations such as the Modification of Diet in Renal Disease (MDRD) Study equation[6] or the Cockcroft–Gault formula.

Severity of CKD was initially categorized according to the level of eGFR into one of five stages, with later revisions further dividing some stages and recognizing the prognostic importance of proteinuria (Table 1.1).

All the equations used to estimate kidney function are unreliable with an eGFR >60 and a decreasing GFR may also be a normal part of the ageing process. Possibly for these reasons, a cut-off

Table 1.1 Stages of CKD

Stage[a]	GFR (ml/min/1.73m²)	Description
1	≥ 90	Normal or increased GFR, with other evidence of kidney damage
2	60–89	Slight decrease in GFR, with other evidence of kidney damage
3A	45–59	Moderate decrease in GFR, with or without other evidence of
3B	30–44	kidney damage
4	15–29	Severe decrease in GFR, with or without other evidence of kidney damage
5	< 15	Established renal failure

[a] Use the suffix (p) to denote the presence of proteinuria when staging CKD (recommendation 1.2.1).
Source: Chronic kidney disease: early identification and management of chronic kidney disease in adults in primary and secondary care. London, National Institute for Health and Clinical Excellence, 2008.

of 60ml/min/1.73m^2 was applied for the diagnosis of CKD in the absence of evidence of kidney damage. Using this definition, it was estimated that 13% of the general population in the United States of America had CKD in the period 1999–2004, although less than 0.5% would have had stage 4 or 5 CKD.[7] Similar rates (16%) have been observed in the AusDiab study in Australia.

In the UK, data are only available from blood samples taken as part of routine clinical practice and identified either in laboratory or general practice databases. Such results must therefore be interpreted with some caution as they overlook individuals who avoid contact with the healthcare system unless it is essential. In addition, individuals with proteinuria but with an eGFR >60 are largely excluded from such studies. Despite this, UK rates of CKD of 10.6% for females and 5.6% for males do not seem dissimilar to those reported elsewhere.[8]

One of the major criticisms of using eGFR to diagnose CKD has been that it labels many elderly individuals – whose kidney function is decreasing as part of the normal ageing process – as having a 'disease'. This has been exemplified in a Dutch general-population cohort of 'healthy' individuals (i.e. no history of hypertension, diabetes, vascular disease, or kidney disease), in which the median GFR estimated using the MDRD equation decreased from 90–100 ml/min/1.73m^2 in the age range of 18–24 years to 60–65 ml/min/1.73m^2 in the age group of 85+ years.[9] As a result of this decrease, 42% and 44% of 'healthy' males and females over the age of 85 had a GFR of less than 60 ml/min/1.73m2 and would be labelled as having CKD stages 3–5 (Fig. 1.1).[9]

Much of the current literature talks about an epidemic of CKD.[10] The definition of an epidemic (from Greek *epi-* upon + *demos* people) is when new cases occur in a given human population, during a given period, at a rate that substantially exceeds what is 'expected', based on recent experience (the disease does not have to be communicable). Does CKD meet these criteria? It remains difficult to measure changes in historical prevalence rates of CKD in general populations and changes in incidence rates with time have not been measured, so a caution in the use of such phraseology is advised.

So what are the benefits of identifying individuals with reduced eGFR? Historically the answer to this question was simply to diagnose the cause of kidney disease, delay or halt progression to

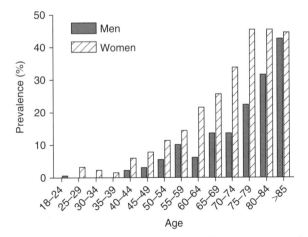

Fig. 1.1 Prevalence of CKD stages 3–5 (GFR: 60 ml/min/1.73m2) according to age in the non-diseased Caucasian Nijmegen Biomedical Study population. Black bars represent men and open bars women. Source: Wetzels JFM et al. (2007). Age- and gender-specific reference values of estimated GFR in Caucasians: The Nijmegen Biomedical Study. *Kidney Int*, **72**(5), 632–7, with Permission.

kidney failure, and, when necessary, to prepare for RRT. However, the cardiovascular risk associated with CKD – independent of traditional risk factors – has increasingly been recognized.[11] Indeed, data from a large Health Maintenance Organization in the USA has shown that individuals with an eGFR of 30–60 ml/min have a 5-year mortality risk of 24% compared with a 1% risk of receiving RRT in the same time interval.[12] As expected, the risk of requiring RRT was 20% higher amongst those with an a lower eGFR of 15–30 ml/min, but so was the risk of death (46%). [12] A diagnosis of CKD should therefore act as a flag for a high cardiovascular risk and lead to such patients' cardiovascular risk factors being appropriately managed.

1.3 Renal replacement therapy

1.3.1 Background

Most data on RRT have come from Renal Registries, which were established in many of the developed countries to monitor the patterns of this emerging technology. There are two widely used measures of RRT rates: incidence and prevalence. The incidence (or take-on) rates of RRT are 'new' cases started on RRT and reported per year per million population. These are influenced not only by the underlying incidence of ERF in the population, but also by levels of detection, referral, and acceptance onto RRT.

There are variations in the definition of a new case. For example, in many countries a new case is not included until after 90 days of treatment; this clearly excludes patients with established renal failure who die in the first 90 days and it underestimates incidence and workload for healthcare providers. However, ascertaining patients at day 0 is difficult. Some patients requiring HD may have acute renal failure; if those that die early are included, this may inflate estimates as some of these cases may have recovered renal function and not needed chronic HD. Some countries also include patients restarting dialysis after a failed renal transplant as 'new' patients. Such differences in definition need to be borne in mind when comparing rates.

Although RRT rates are not true epidemiological measures of the underlying rate of ERF in the population, they are widely available and are frequently used as proxy measures. To be diagnosed with ERF, a patient should have insufficient renal function to remain alive and well without RRT. The somewhat subjective nature of this definition is reflected by the considerable central and international variation in mean eGFR observed in patients commencing RRT. A more reproducible measure of RRT need is the number of patients with a GFR below 15 ml/min/1.73m^2 – stage 5 CKD – but as this represents only 0.2% of the general population,[13] large numbers of subjects would need to be screened to reliably determine an incidence rate. Alternative approaches to measuring the burden of renal disease in a population include use of mortality data, but these are unreliable because of significant under-ascertainment of renal disease on death certificates.[14] Moreover, the International Classification of Disease (ICD) coding does not reliably distinguish between acute and chronic forms of renal failure. Nor is it possible to use hospital-utilization data as these only relate to known treated cases; they overlook a large portion of RRT activity which is delivered to outpatients or to patients at home and they are limited by the shortcomings of the ICD coding discussed above.

This chapter utilizes Renal Registry data, based on the authors' experience in the UK and contrasted where appropriate with data from other developed countries.

1.3.2 Trends in incidence rates

In the UK the number and rate of patients accepted onto RRT has steadily increased over the last 25 years from 20 per million population in 1982 to 109 per million population. in 2007 (Fig. 1.2) with similar changes in other European countries The characteristics of the patients being treated have

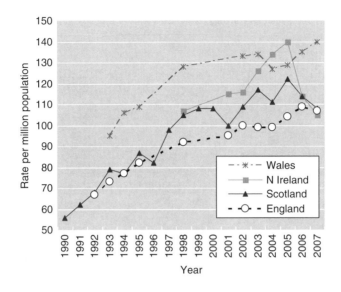

Fig. 1.2 RRT incident rates in the countries of the UK: 1990–2007.
Source: UK Renal Registry Report 2008.

changed dramatically in this time. In the early 1980s, RRT was restricted almost exclusively to those under 65, but 20 years later nearly half of all cases receiving RRT in the UK were over 65 (Fig. 1.3). Similar changes in the age of patients starting RRT have been reported in other European countries (Fig. 1.4). The UK age- and gender-specific patterns of RRT incidence in 2007 demonstrate higher rates in older ages and amongst males (Fig. 1.5). The interaction of factors that influence RRT rates is depicted in Fig. 1.6.

It is important to recognize the use of chronological age as a bar to treatment (Mignon 1993 OTN 504) is unethical, and in the UK the Department of Health has stated this to all Health Commissioners. Although older patients are likely to have a greater burden of co-morbidity and social problems, their relative quality-of-life gain is better than that of younger HD patients. One study found that the mental health-component score of the Short Form-36 (SF-36) was almost the same in elderly dialysis patients as in the age-specific general population.[15]

1.3.3 Cause of ERF

Establishing the cause of ERF can be difficult and coding systems vary between registries. Most European countries use the coding system of about 90 diagnostic categories established by the European Renal Association which has now been in place for over 30 years and is currently under major revision. Nevertheless, it is possible to discern a change in the pattern of causes of ERF over the last 25 years from Registry data. While rates of some primary renal diseases, such as glomerulonephritis, polycystic kidney disease, and pyelonephritis, have remained fairly constant, big increases have been seen in diabetic, hypertensive, and renovascular disease (Fig. 1.7).[16] In particular, diabetes mellitus has changed from being a rare cause of ERF (2%) to being the single commonest cause of ERF amongst those accepted (21% in the UK, 34% in Germany, France, and Canada, and 44% in the USA)[17] (Table 1.2). While the changing population demographics may have partly contributed to this shift, it is widely recognized that 25 years ago diabetes mellitus was often seen as a relative contraindication to being accepted onto RRT. The improved survival

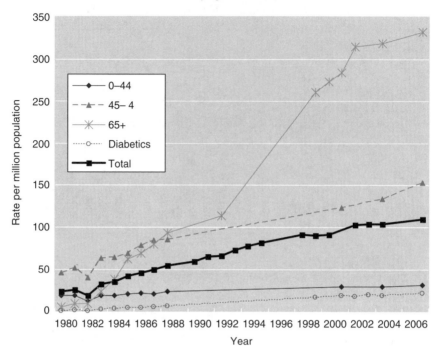

Fig. 1.3 Incidence rates for RRT in the UK from 1980 to 2007 by age and diabetes.
Source: UK Renal Registry unpublished data.

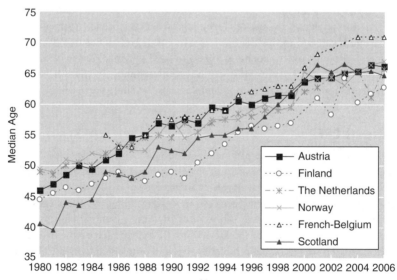

Fig. 1.4 Median age of patients starting RRT 1980–2006 from ERA-EDTA Registry.
Source: UK Renal Registry Report 2008.

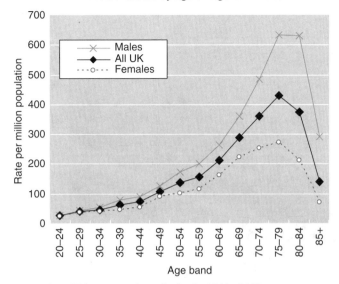

Incident rates by age and gender in 2007

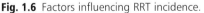

Fig. 1.5 Incidence rates for RRT by age and gender in the UK in 2007.
Source: UK Renal Registry Report 2008.

of patients with diabetes (and therefore reduced competing risk of death prior to reaching ERF) is also thought to have contributed to these changes.[18]

The current international differences in rates of ERF caused by diabetes, however, are likely to be due to differences in patterns of diabetes, especially Type 2, and the effectiveness of preventive health measures and variation in ascription (i.e. the proportion of patients with diabetic ERF that

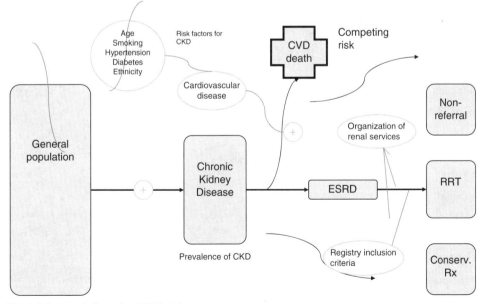

Fig. 1.6 Factors influencing RRT incidence.
Source: Caskey FJ et al. (2006). Exploring the differences in epidemiology of treated ESRD between Germany and England and Wales. *Am J Kidney Dis*, **47**(3), 445–54.

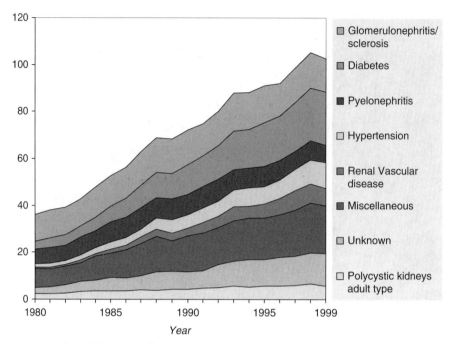

Fig. 1.7 Trends in incident rates of new acceptances by cause of established renal failure from European Renal Association Registry 1980–99.

Table 1.2 International rates of RRT incidence, prevalence, diabetic nephropathy and RRT modality

Country	Incidence (pmp)	Prevalence (pmp)	Diabetes %	In-centre HD* %	Home HD* %	PD* %	New transplants (pmp)
Australia	115	778	32.4	68.4	9.5	22	31.1
Bangladesh	9	92		99.6	0	0.4	0.3
Jalisco, Mexico	346	929	49.9	29.5	0	70.5	52.2
Malaysia	119	615	57.5	90	1.1	8.9	4.5
Norway	100	753	16.4	80.4	0.4	19.2	45.3
Romania	75	304	12.4	80.7	0	19.3	5.3
Russia	28	130	13.9	91	0	9	2.9
Spain	132	991	23.1	88.6	0.1	11.3	60.2
Taiwan	418	2226	42.4	92.4	0	7.6	
United Kingdom	110	759	21	78.8	2	19.1	36
United States	363	1641	44.3	91.1	0.7	9.4	60.3

*In-centre HD, Home HD and PD percentage are all for prevalent patients.

has been proven on biopsy). In the UK, e.g. 19% of patients accepted onto RRT have diabetes listed as the primary cause of ERF, but data on co-morbidity indicate that a further 7% of patients have diabetes that is not considered to have caused their ERF. Interestingly, rates of survival of these two patient groups are identical. Many countries do not specify whether or not 'diabetes' is limited to those who have diabetes as the cause of ERF.

Within the UK there is also variation in the incidence of RRT with higher rates in Wales, mostly due to the higher incidence of diabetic ERF and glomerulonephritis (GN) (Table 1.3).

1.3.4 Current international differences in incidence of RRT

There is substantial variation in the incidence rates with Taiwan having the highest rate, closely followed by the USA (Table 1.2). In Europe, the highest rate is seen in Germany (213 p.m.p. in 2006). In Eastern Europe, RRT programmes have developed rapidly since they became independent of the Soviet Union, with the Czech Republic and Hungary having RRT incidence rates of 173 p.m.p. and 159 p.m.p., respectively, in 2006.[17] How can these differences be explained?

An increasing number of nationally representative screening studies have been undertaken to establish the prevalence of CKD in countries around the world and the evidence suggests that, despite the variation in RRT incidence, there is little variation in the prevalence of CKD. One study has looked at the transition from CKD to ERF in an attempt to better understand this discrepancy and demonstrated that although the prevalence of CKD in Norway and the USA is comparable, the incidence of ERF in Norway is lower, suggesting greater progression to ERF in the USA.[19]

A true variation in the incidence of ERF therefore remains a possibility, but factors such as variation in competing risk (i.e. death from cardiovascular disease prior to reaching ERF), referral to a nephrologist, and acceptance onto RRT may also be important. One study comparing RRT incidence rates in the UK and Germany found that the higher rates in Germany could be largely explained by the higher rates of hypertensive and diabetic ERF,[20] but it also highlighted marked differences in organization and supply of renal services that may have been cause or effect.

Table 1.3 Primary Renal diagnosis: incidence rates p.m.p. by UK country

Diagnosis	England pmp	Northern Ireland pmp	Scotland	Wales	UK
Uncertain aetiology	25.2	17.1	14.8	40.3	24.8
Glomerulonephritis	10.2	8.5	10.3	17.1	10.5
Pyelonephritis	6.7	10.8	8.6	7.4	7.0
Diabetes	21.3	23.9	18.1	34.2	21.7
Polycystic kidney	6.5	10.8	10.3	7.4	7.0
Hypertension	5.9	7.4	2.7	7.0	5.7
Renovascular disease	6.6	10.8	11.5	10.7	7.3
Other	15.0	15.9	13.6	14.4	14.9
Data not available	10.8	0.0	18.3	1.0	10.6
All	108	105	108	140	110

Source: Ansell D, Feehally J, Fogarty D et al. UK Renal Registry Report 2008.

Perhaps linked to the availability of resources, earlier studies demonstrated differences in the attitudes of physician and nephrologists towards patient suitability for dialysis over the last two decades.[21–23] This is no longer considered to be a major reason for inter-country variation in RRT incidence rates.

Ethnicity is another key factor, and one that is likely to become increasingly important over the next decade. In the USA, black patients with hypertension or diabetes are 2–3 times more likely to develop ERF than their white counterparts;[24] rates 3–4 times higher than in the white population have been observed in blacks and Indo-Asians in the UK.[25] In the UK, the ethnic minority populations are younger than the white majority population, and this is reflected by a lower median age of incident ethnic minority RRT patients (57 years compared with 64 years for white incident patients). The maturation of these minority populations over the next two decades is likely to lead to a significant increase in demand for RRT.

1.4 Prevalence of renal replacement therapy

Prevalence rates, also called stock rates sometimes, are measures of the total number of patients on RRT at any time (usually at the year end) in a defined population per million. They indicate the healthcare burden and costs of an RRT programme.

As has already been described for RRT incidence, wide variation exists in RRT prevalence and RRT modality mix amongst countries (Table 1.2) with cultural acceptance of organ donation, the organization of cadaveric and live donation programmes, financial incentives for HD in certain healthcare systems and conversely for PD in others, clinician preferences, and historical precedent all contributing to each country's modality mix.

In the UK, the prevalence rate increased from only 27 p.m.p. in 1981 to 746 p.m.p. in 2007, with the annual increase in prevalence currently around 6%. This rise is due to a combination of the increase in incidence rates onto RRT, as outlined above, and improvements in patient survival on RRT as outlined below. In 2007 there were over 45 000 patients receiving dialysis treatment or living with a kidney transplant in the UK – 45% with a functioning renal transplant, 43% on in-centre HD and 11% on PD. In the last two decades the major absolute growth has been in the numbers of HD patients. The percentage of patients on PD is decreasing after the initial rapid rise at its introduction in the early 1980s from 16% up to 22% in 1990; it has now fallen to 10% of RRT patients (Fig. 1.8). Although the total numbers of patients on dialysis continues to rise, the total numbers on PD are in decline. The percentage on home HD has steadily fallen over the years from 24% of RRT patients in 1982 to 1% in 2007 accounting for 480 patients. The fall in these patients appears to have now plateaued.

Kidney transplantation is associated with better survival and quality of life for patients with ERF. Two countries that have been particularly successful at achieving high rates of kidney transplantation have done so by very different means – Spain instituted a systematic approach to cadaveric organ donation with an opt-out donation programme and Norway has the most active live donation programme. Despite a decrease in heart-beating deceased-donor kidney transplants, the organ donor rate in the UK has increased slightly in recent years as a result of expansion of the living kidney donor and non-heart-beating donor programmes. The percentage of RRT patients in the UK with a functioning renal transplant continues to decrease, but this reflects partly the disproportionate growth of the >75-age group on the dialysis programme.

Not everyone is suitable for a kidney transplant, The UK Renal Registry has shown that approximately 50% of the 35–44-year-old dialysis population are on the active transplant waiting list and this falls to 25% in the 55–64-year-old dialysis population.[26] A subsequent analysis looking at time-to-listing showed that only 45% of patients in the age group

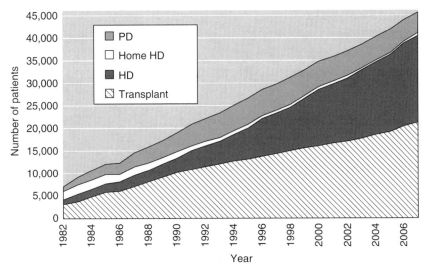

Fig. 1.8 Growth in UK prevalent patients by treatment modality at the end of each year 1982–2007. Source: UK Renal Registry Report 2008.

<65 years were activated on the transplant list within 1 year of starting RRT and 66% within 5 years.[27] Amongst patients who do receive a kidney transplant in the UK, the average waiting time is currently around 28 months.

1.5 Survival on renal replacement therapy

Much of the analysis of patient outcomes on RRT has come from Registry data rather than controlled trials comparing one treatment to another (e.g. poor phosphate control versus better phosphate control). This is very important as Registry data showing that a high serum phosphate is associated with poor survival does not demonstrate causality; i.e. lowering phosphate will improve survival even though this may be clinically plausible.

The key factors that are related to patient survival on RRT are listed below.

- **Sociodemographic**
  - Age – poorer survival with increasing age
  - Ethnic minority (blacks and South Asians have better survival than whites)
  - No difference in survival by gender, or socioeconomic status
- **Co-morbidity**
  - Cardiovascular disease, diabetes, malignancy, major organ system (e.g. respiratory). These factors have been incorporated into various developed scoring systems (Khan, Charlson, Lister, etc.).
  - The degree of independence as measures by the Karnofsky Performance Score is also predictive.
- **Primary renal disease**
  - Certain primary renal diseases have better survival, e.g. glomerulonephritis, polycystic kidney disease compared to systemic causes, e.g. diabetic nephropathy, renovascular disease.

◆ **Status at the start of RRT**
  • Nutritional status
  • Symptomatic with complications of ERF e.g. fluid overload
  • Vascular access using a non-tunnelled line catheter
  • Patients who present late are more likely to have several of these factors.
◆ **Care on RRT**
  • Dialysis adequacy
  • Control of anaemia
  • Control of serum phosphate
  • Management of cardiovascular disease

Compared with the general population, patients with ERF have a considerably higher risk of death (Fig. 5.2 , Chapter 5), although the relative risk declines with age. There is also significant inter-country variation in mortality in patients with ERF. A wide-ranging and influential study in the 1980s demonstrated that mortality in such patients was lower in Japan than in Europe, and that mortality in Europe was lower than in the USA.[28] A case-mix adjusted follow-up study restricted to Europe and the USA confirmed these disparities in survival although an attenuation in the effect was observed.[29]

Registry data on survival are also available and are used for both central and international comparisons. Adjustment for case-mix requires survival to be stratified by modality, age, and cause of ERF (i.e. diabetic or non-diabetic). Table 1.4 shows the differences in case-mix of incident RRT patients from different national registries.

Table 1.4 Summary of co-morbidity of incident RRT patients in selected national renal registries

	National registries			
	ANZDATA	**USRDS**	**UK RR**	**Necosad 2**
Study period	2003	1995–2003	1999–2003	1997–2000
Number of patients	1953	696 043	15 197*	1041
Ischaemic heart disease incl. MI	30.5%	23.8%	24.7%	11.1%
Cerebrovascular disease	11.0%	9.0%	11.7%	7.2%
Peripheral vascular disease	19.0%	14.3%	14.2%	13.0%
COPD	12.0%	7.1%	7.7%	7.2%
Diabetes**	35.0%	41.2%	18.8%	19.5%
Malignancy	not collected	5.3%	11.5%	10.1%
Smoking	11.0%	5.2%	18.4%	not collected
Congestive cardiac failure	not collected	32.0%	not collected	12.3%
Patients with no co-morbidity at start of RRT***	39.0%	9.4%	38.7%	not collected

Notes: *Comprehensive co-morbidity information was only available in 5916 patients.
**Countries may sometimes include those patients who were diabetic not as a primary cause of renal failure in this total.
***US data includes hypertension (74%) and also congestive cardiac failure as a co-morbidity. COPD: chronic obstructive pulmonary disease.

Data from countries that collect data from all RRT patients from day zero has consistently shown that half of all deaths in the first year occur between day 0 and day 90. This is potentially important in making decisions about commencing RRT. There is apparent variation in early mortality amongst centres and countries. Differences in the timing of reporting of patients with acute or acute-on-chronic renal failure to registries may account for much of this quoted variation in 1-year survival. To overcome this, most registries quote first-year survival starting from day 90 to 1 year +90.

The UK has shown improvement in the survival of dialysis patients over the past 10 years,[30] and the survival of renal transplant recipients has also improved significantly.[31] In the UK, e.g. 1-year age-adjusted survival of all patients commencing RRT has improved from 85.8% in 1999 to 89.1% in 2006. The 1-year prevalent dialysis-survival has also improved from 82.8% in 1997 to 88.6% in 2007. Similarly, the USA – which began with higher mortality rates in the 1980s – saw a marked reduction in first-year mortality on dialysis during the early 1990s, which paralleled national-level improvements in dialysis adequacy.

The prognosis for some patients on RRT remains poor. For example, a patient over 75 would have a 63% chance of surviving for 1 year after commencing RRT and a 34% chance of remaining alive 3 years after commencing RRT (Fig. 5.1, Chapter 5). In addition, there are important differences in relative risk for ERF patients compared with their general-population counterparts. Older patients with diabetes have considerably lower survival rates than younger patients, but the impact of diabetes on their relative risk of death, compared to younger patients, is much less (Fig . 1.9). Such data, which are published annually by the UK Renal Registry, may be helpful for patients and their families when making difficult decisions about the propriety of commencing RRT.

1.6 **Causes of death**

Cardiovascular events dominate as the cause of death for patients with ERF in all countries[31] reflecting a complex interrelationship between CKD and cardiovascular disease, although it should be noted that cardiovascular disease is also a major cause of death within the general population. Renal impairment leads to secondary hypertension, abnormal lipid profiles, arterial wall damage, and adversely alters other cardiovascular disease risk factors (e.g. homocysteine and fibrinogen levels). Some factors, such as smoking, and diseases, such as diabetes, are important risk factors for both conditions. The UK Renal Registry data show that smoking remains as common in the RRT population as the general population.

A significant proportion of patients choose to withdraw from dialysis, although for cultural reasons these rates vary considerably between countries. Data on withdrawal from dialysis, however, are often not reliably collected by registries. The UK Renal Registry has found that 12% of deaths on dialysis are ascribed to withdrawal and this was significantly higher in the first year of RRT at 16%.[30] There was also a difference by age – withdrawal accounted for 19% of deaths in those in the age group >65 on dialysis compared with 8% in those <65 (Table 1.5). In the ERA, withdrawal was coded less frequently at under 5%; it is not clear whether this represents a true difference or under-recording.[31]

With the increasing acceptance of older, more co-morbid patients onto RRT programmes, the number of such patients is likely to increase further. In Australia, 33% of deaths in dialysis-dependent patients in 2006 were ascribed to withdrawal, mostly in older age groups. This contrasts with the 14% of deaths due to withdrawal from RRT for the period 1983–92.[32]

It is impossible to predict the survival of individual patients and also how they will adapt to treatment, so some nephrologists have suggested a 'trial of dialysis' except in cases with severe dementia or advanced malignancy.[33] Others think that a trial is poor clinical practice.

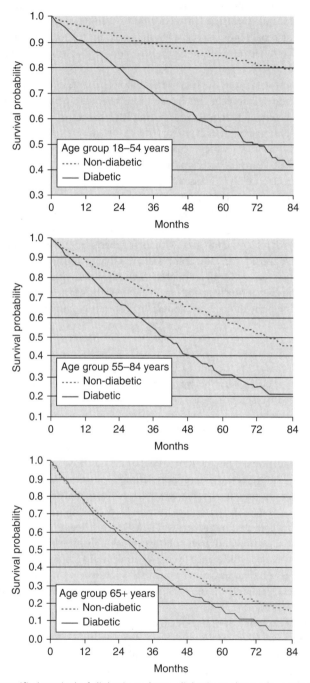

Fig. 1.9 Age-stratified survival of diabetic and non-diabetic nephropathy patients on RRT after 90 days.
Source: UK Renal Registry Report 2005.

Table 1.5 Cause of death by age in 1 year after 90 days for UK incident patients, 2000–06

Cause of death	All age groups		<65 years		≥65 years	
	Number of deaths	%	Number of deaths	%	Number of deaths	%
Cardiac disease	534	25	165	27	369	24
Cerebrovascular disease	137	6	36	6	101	7
Infection	400	19	114	19	286	19
Malignancy	213	10	79	13	134	9
Treatment withdrawal	344	16	51	8	293	19
Other	373	17	109	18	264	17
Uncertain	153	7	56	9	97	6
Total	**2154**		**610**		**1544**	
No cause-of-death data	2578		730		1848	

Source: Ansell D, Tomson C et al. UK Renal Registry Report 2008.

Consequently, withdrawal from RRT will remain an important and increasing cause of death which has considerable implications for supportive terminal care of such patients and their families. However, some patients who are referred for RRT may be considered unsuitable for RRT due to poor prognosis and/or associated problems, and this number is likely to increase over time. There is a challenge to develop alternative models of supportive care to sustain such patients and their families.

1.7 Late presentation (referral) for renal replacement therapy

A major and enduring problem is that 25% of all patients commencing RRT are presented to the renal unit within 3 months of their first treatment.[34] This late presentation may be a consequence of the patient's disease (unavoidable) or of late referral from another clinician. Late referral for RRT impacts on pre-ESRD care, affects selection of dialysis modality, vascular access, and also has economic implications. Patients presenting late generally fare less well, as they are more likely to be in a sub-optimal clinical state at the start (e.g. lower haemoglobin and albumin) and tend to have more temporary access, longer initial hospitalization, and a higher early mortality.[30] One study showed that whilst a proportion are unavoidable (e.g. late presenters with no prior symptoms or signs of CRF, or irreversible acute renal failure), around 50% are potentially avoidable due most frequently to having had documented rising creatinine levels for several years.[35] In the UK, the CKD Quality Outcomes Framework for primary-care physicians may improve these late-referral rates.

1.8 Future demand for renal replacement therapy

As a result of the ageing population – the effects of which are going to be most marked in ethnic minority and indigenous populations – the increasing rates of type 2 diabetes, and the improvements in RRT survival, the number of patients on RRT looks set to continue to rise in most countries. Indeed, modelling exercises in the UK suggests that there will be substantial growth in the RRT numbers in the medium term, with a steady state not being reached for at least 25 years.[36] The UK Registry data have shown a year-on-year 6% rise in prevalence over the last 10 years. The rate of this rise varies between RRT modalities, with HD rates increasing by 8% annually. All renal units remain in a perpetual state of expansion requiring annual funding increases beyond just inflation. Similar projections have been made for populations in Europe, Asia-Pacific, and North America.

1.9 **Conclusion**

There has been a continuing and substantial growth in the incidence and prevalence of RRT in all developed countries, although there are substantial inter-country variations. Increasing numbers of patients with ERF are elderly and have a greater co-morbid burden, yet patients are now living longer on RRT. Early referral of patients with CKD allows patients to be fully informed about RRT so they can make an informed decision about whether to embark on treatment or not.

The predominant mode of RRT for elderly, frail patients is likely to continue to be HD, irrespective of the success of efforts to enhance live and cadaveric kidney transplant programmes. As conservative care becomes an increasingly accepted treatment option, our new challenge as healthcare professionals is to support our patients and their carers and provide them with high-quality care, tailored to their individual wishes, as they live with renal failure .

References

1 Lawler R (1950). *JAMA*, **844**.

2 Cockcroft DW and Gault MH (1976). Prediction of creatinine clearance from serum creatinine. *Nephron*, **16**(1), 31–41.

3 Levey AS, Bosch JP, Lewis JB et al. (1999). A more accurate method to estimate glomerular filtration rate from serum creatinine: a new prediction equation. Modification of Diet in Renal Disease Study Group. *Ann Intern Med*, **130**(6): 461–70.

4 K/DOQI Clinical Practice Guidelines for Chronic Kidney Disease: Evaluation, Classification, and Stratification, Part 4 (2002). Definition and classification of stages of chronic kidney disease. *Am J Kid Dis*, **39**(2), S46–S75.

5 Levey AS et al. (2005). Definition and classification of chronic kidney disease: a position statement from Kidney Disease: Improving Global Outcomes (KDIGO). *Kidney Int*, **67**(6), 2089–100.

6 Levey AS, Kusek JW, Beck GJ (2000). A simplified equation to predict glomerular filtration rate from serum creatinine. *J Am Soc Nephrol*, **11**, 155A.

7 Coresh J et al. (2007). Prevalence of chronic kidney disease in the United States. *JAMA*, **298**(17), 2038–47.

8 Stevens PE et al. (2007). Chronic kidney disease management in the United Kingdom: NEOERICA project results. *Kidney Int*, **72**(1), 92–9.

9 Wetzels JFM et al. (2007). Age- and gender-specific reference values of estimated GFR in Caucasians: The Nijmegen Biomedical Study. *Kidney Int*, **72**(5), 632–7.

10 Coresh J, Stevens LA, Levey AS (2002). Chronic kidney disease is common: what do we do next? *Nephrol Dial Transplant*, **23**(4), 1122–5.

11 Muntner P et al. (2002). Renal Insufficiency and Subsequent Death Resulting from Cardiovascular Disease in the United States. *J Am Soc Nephrol*, **13**(3), 745–53.

12 Keith DS et al. (2004). Longitudinal follow-up and outcomes among a population with chronic kidney disease in a large managed care organization. *Arch Intern Med*, 2 **164**(6), 659–63.

13 Coresh J et al. (2003). Prevalence of chronic kidney disease and decreased kidney function in the adult US population: Third National Health and Nutrition Examination Survey. *Am J Kidney Dis*, **41**(1), 1–12.

14 Goldacre MJ (1993). Cause-specific mortality: understanding uncertain tips of the disease iceberg. *J Epidemiol Community Health*, **47**(6), 491–6.

15 Lamping DL et al. (2000). Clinical outcomes, quality of life, and costs in the North Thames Dialysis Study of elderly people on dialysis: a prospective cohort study. *Lancet*, **356**(9241), 1543–50.

16 Stewart JH et al. (2006). The enigma of hypertensive ESRD: observations on incidence and trends in 18 European, Canadian, and Asian-Pacific populations, 1998 to 2002. *Am J Kidney Dis*, **48**(2), 183–91.

17 U.S. Renal Data System (2008). 2008 Annual Data Report: Atlas of End-Stage Renal Disease in the United States. *National Institute of Diabetes and Digestive and Kidney Diseases.*

18 Ritz E, Lippert J, Keller C (1995). Hypertension, cardiovascular complications and survival in diabetic patients on maintenance haemodialysis. *Nephrol Dial Transplant*, **10 Suppl 7**, 43–6.

19 Hallan SI et al. (2006). International comparison of the relationship of chronic kidney disease prevalence and ESRD risk. *J Am Soc Nephrol*, **17**(8), 2275–84.

20 Caskey FJ et al. (2006). Exploring the differences in epidemiology of treated ESRD between Germany and England and Wales. *Am J Kidney Dis*, **47**(3), 445–54.

21 Challah S et al. (1984). Negative selection of patients for dialysis and transplantation in the United Kingdom. *Br Med J*, **288**(6424), 1119–22.

22 Parry RG et al.(1996). Referral of elderly patients with severe renal failure: questionnaire survey of physicians. *Br Med J*, **313**(7055), 466.

23 McKenzie JK et al. (1998). Dialysis decision making in Canada, the United Kingdom, and the United States. *Am J Kidney Dis*, **31**(1), 12–8.

24 Xue JL et al. (2007). Longitudinal study of racial and ethnic differences in developing end-stage renal disease among aged medicare beneficiaries. *J Am Soc Nephrol*, **18**(4), 1299–306.

25 Roderick PJ et al. (1996). The need and demand for renal replacement therapy in ethnic minorities in England. *J Epidemiol Commun Health*, **50**(3), 334–9.

26 Ansell D, Feest T (2000). *UK Renal Registry Report 2000,* Chapter 20. UK Renal Registry: Bristol.

27 Ansell D et al. (2005). *UK Renal Registry Report 2005*, Chapter 5. Bristol.

28 Held PJ et al. (1990). Five-year survival for end-stage renal disease patients in the United States, Europe, and Japan, 1982 to 1987. *Am J Kidney Dis*, **15**(5), 451–7.

29 Marcelli D et al. (1996). ESRD patient mortality with adjustment for comorbid conditions in Lombardy (Italy) versus the United States. *Kidney Int*, **50**(3), 1013–18.

30 Ansell D et al. (2008). *UK Renal Registry Report 2008*. Bristol.

31 van Dijk PCW et al. (2001). Renal replacement therapy in Europe: the results of a collaborative effort by the ERA-EDTA registry and six national or regional registries. *Nephrol. Dial. Transplant*, **16**(6), 1120–9.

32 Disney AP (1995). Demography and survival of patients receiving treatment for chronic renal failure in Australia and New Zealand: report on dialysis and renal transplantation treat. *Am J Kid Disease*, **25**(1), 165–75.

33 Mignon F et al. (1993). Worldwide demographics and future trends of the management of renal failure in the elderly. *Kidney Int Suppl*, **41**, S18–26.

34 Ansell D et al. (2007). *UK Renal Registry Report 2007*. UK Renal Registry, Bristol, UK.

35 Roderick P et al. (2002). Late referral for end-stage renal disease: a region-wide survey in the south west of England. *Nephrol Dial Transplant*, **17**(7), 1252–9.

36 Roderick P et al. (2004). Simulation model of renal replacement therapy: predicting future demand in England. *Nephrol Dial Transplant*, **19**(3), 692–701.

Chapter 2

The concept of supportive care for the renal patient

E Joanna Chambers and Edwina A Brown

The utility of living consists not in the length of days, but in the use of time: a man may have lived long, and yet lived but little.
Montaigne, 1533–92

2.1 Introduction

End-stage renal disease (ESRD) presents many challenges to the patients – who experience and suffer from it – and the healthcare professionals who care for them. Its chronicity and the morbidity associated with it – which often includes difficult and intractable symptoms – make palliative and supportive care natural accompaniments to its management. The team-based approach to the care of patients with ESRD makes it ideally suited to incorporate palliative and supportive care. Programmes for the management of ESRD should include a supportive care plan as well as routine prevention, diagnosis, renal replacement therapy (RRT), and transplantation.

2.2 The development of palliative care

In 1990 the World Health Organization (WHO) defined palliative care (see also Appendix 1) as:

> The active total care of patients whose disease is not responsive to curative treatment. Control of pain, of other symptoms, and of psychological, social and spiritual problems is paramount. The goal of palliative care is achievement of the best quality of life for patients and their families. Many aspects of palliative care are also applicable earlier in the course of the illness in conjunction with anticancer treatment.[1]

World Health Organization (1990)

Although this definition applied primarily to patients with cancer it is equally appropriate for people with other chronic diseases, in particular ESRD. It significantly highlights that palliative care has applications early in the course of an illness and looks at the needs of the whole person in the context of his or her social situation. Many subsequent definitions have built on this concept of addressing patient symptoms as well as psychosocial and spiritual needs in addition to disease-directed therapy in chronic and life-limiting illnesses. This distinction with regard to the broad clinical applicability and appropriateness of palliative care is important, because supportive and palliative care can then be seen as care that goes alongside 'active' or aggressive therapies such as dialysis. Ahmedzai and Walsh[2] have further developed this model in relation to cancer (Fig. 2.1) where patient- and family-directed care are integrated with disease-directed care, e.g. chemotherapy.

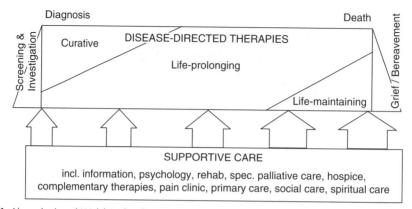

Fig. 2.1 Ahmedazi and Walsh's development of the model of supportive care[2].

It is applicable to most chronic diseases including ESRD, where it demonstrates the importance of dialysis or transplantation whilst recognizing the role of the multi-professional renal team and that many other specialties are needed to support the patient and family such that, whatever the disease trajectory seen in patients with ESRD – and they are varied – supportive care is provided where needed throughout the illness that will last for the rest of the patient's life.

Hospice care in the United Kingdom (UK) was developed for the care of the dying – almost exclusively for those dying of cancer – because of the visible suffering of people with cancer and the low importance given to symptom-control and psychosocial support for those who were terminally ill. Palliative care has moved from being synonymous with hospice care to being part of mainstream medical care and an adjunct to care within many disciplines, and thus not reserved for the last days and weeks of life. The role of the hospice has changed from a place where people die, to being part of a larger supportive care strategy which includes: refuge for good symptom-control or respite-care, outreach and support to people in their own homes, as well as excellent terminal care within the hospice or at home through 'Hospice at Home' programmes and bereavement support. In order to qualify for hospice care in the United States (US) the attending physician and hospice medical director need to certify that the patient has 6 months or less to live if the disease takes its normal course. This care may be through support of the patient in his or her own home or in a hospice. Increasing numbers of patients who cease dialysis access this care. Those who continue to dialyse may receive services under both the ESRD benefit and the hospice benefit if their terminal condition is not related to ESRD.

2.3 Supportive, palliative, and end-of-life care

The palliative and supportive care philosophy is patient centred, focussing on the wishes and goals of the individual, and should be part of all medical care. However, it has been shown, in studies of people approaching the end of their lives, how there can be conflict over the goals of care amongst clinician and patient or family. Cure and restoration of function are unspoken goals of medical and nursing care. When professionals recognise those goals are no longer achievable, communication is essential to prevent conflict over futility and to allow the patient and their family to make decisions about their own care based on a true picture of the situation. It is helpful to consider the words of Joseph Fins in *A palliative ethic of care*: "Instead of: letting available technology drive the goals of care, let the goals of care drive the therapy".[3] Thus, whilst dialysis may technically be possible for the patient with multiple co-morbidities and diminishing quality of life, it may not be the kind of care they would choose if they had full understanding of their prognosis with dialysis. Equally, the patient who wishes to continue dialysis in the face of increasing co-morbidity and dependence must be supported in his or her decision with ongoing communication about the risks and benefits to the patient.

There is considerable overlap between the meaning of palliative care and supportive care. Many mainstream treatments palliate rather than cure the clinical condition, e.g. coronary artery bypass surgery, dialysis or insulin therapy for diabetes; this in no way reduces their importance or effectiveness. Palliative care may, however, be the sole focus of care when disease-modifying therapy is stopped, or, as seen increasingly in the UK, it is applied alongside disease-modifying treatments such as chemotherapy and radiotherapy. Hence, it overlaps with supportive care or rather is a part of it.

'Supportive care' is defined in the UK as care that "…helps the patient and their family to cope with their condition and treatment of it – from pre-diagnosis, through the process of diagnosis and treatment, to cure, continuing illness or death and into bereavement. It helps the patient to maximise the benefits of treatment and to live as well as possible with the effects of the disease. It is given equal priority alongside diagnosis and treatment" (National Council for Palliative Care (NCPC) 2006)[4]. 'Palliative care' resides within this as seen from the National Institute for Clinical Excellence (NICE) definition of palliative care as: "…the active holistic care of patients with advanced progressive illness. Management of pain and other symptoms and provision of psychological, social and spiritual support is paramount. The goal of palliative care is achievement of the best quality of life for patients and their families. Many aspects of palliative care are also applicable earlier in the course of the illness in conjunction with other treatments".[5]

In addition, when, in 2008, the Department of Health published a Strategy for End of Life Care[6] in the UK, the definition of end-of-life care was broadened considerably to include: "care that helps all those with advanced progressive incurable illness to live as well as possible until they die". It refers to patients living with the condition from which they may die in weeks, months, or years. It emphasizes that it refers to all conditions, i.e. cancer, organ failure, frail elderly, dementia, etc., in all settings. This strategy is particularly helpful in that it encourages the recognition of those likely to die in the next few months or year. It also promotes open and honest communication and the coordination of care with the right levels of support being available quickly and simply for patients and carers whatever the setting or diagnosis with care of the family carers after death being included.

2.4 **The need for supportive care for the renal patient**

2.4.1 **The needs of the patients**

ESRD is increasingly a disease of the elderly (see Chapter 14). The UK Renal Registry shows that the median age of patients starting dialysis has been fairly stable at around 65 years over the last few years,[9] although the number of 'old elderly' patients is increasing. In the US, the number of octogenarians and nonagenarians starting dialysis increased from 7054 persons in 1996 to 13 577 persons in 2003; after allowing for population growth, this represents a 57% increase in the rate of those starting dialysis in this age group.[10] In France, in 2005, almost 40% of patients starting dialysis were over the age of 75.[11]

2.4.2 **Failure of current practice**

Medical education tends to focus on the diagnosis and treatment of specific conditions, although the potential of mortality and predictors of poor outcomes may be part of the educational process, the actual features leading up to death and 'how the person dies' are not focused upon. It is therefore not surprising that doctors are often overoptimistic about the potential outcomes of their treatment. Furthermore, management of acute intercurrent illness tends to focus on the acute problem and may not consider where the current situation fits into the total disease trajectory of the patient. Death and dying, therefore, are often seen as a failure of management rather than the inevitable irreversibility of the clinical situation. Recognizing the end of life would allow a positive approach to enable a patient to have a good-quality death. A recent survey of American and Canadian nephrologists[12] showed that nephrologists who had been in practice longer and who were caring for larger numbers of patients were more prepared to make end-of-life decisions. Interestingly, a study looking at burnout amongst oncologists has shown that physicians who viewed end-of-life care as an important role reported increased job satisfaction; physicians who primarily described a biomedical role reported a more distant relationship with the patient and a sense of failure at not being able to alter the course of the disease.[13]

Most nephrologists have not been trained to initiate discussions about end-of-life management, advance care planning, or dialysis withdrawal. Such discussions are time consuming and do not fit into current working practices with the increasing use of shift patterns by trainees and 'week on the wards' by senior doctors. There is also a fear that having frank discussions with patients about treatment outcomes destroys hope and that patients do not want to know the truth about their shortened life expectancy. Evidence is growing, though, that this is not true.[14] Davison and Simpson also concluded from a study interviewing patients that facilitated advance care planning through the provision of timely appropriate information can positively enhance rather than diminish patients' hope.[15] This is also true for relatives; a large study of relatives of patients in intensive care units (ICUs)[16] has shown that most next of kin of critically ill patients do not view withholding prognostic information as an acceptable way to maintain hope, as timely discussions about prognosis help families begin to prepare for the patient's death.

Belief patterns of healthcare workers also affect attitudes with regard to end-of-life decisions. This has been extensively studied in the intensive care setting. The End-of-Life Practices in European Intensive Care Units (ETHICUS) study showed that the choice of limiting therapy rather than continuing life-sustaining therapy was related to geographical region and physician religion as well as various patient factors.[17] In the absence of focussed end-of-life training, physicians will be unable to surmount their own belief system to be able to understand the beliefs and deliver the wishes of the patients and their families.

2.5 Supportive care in nephrology practice

In the last few years, it has been increasingly recognized that supportive care should be integral to renal care.[18,19] There is, however, wide variation in the practice and extent of supportive care amongst renal units both in the UK[20] and in the US. The use of different terminology can also confound comparison. The morbidity and mortality described above inform us that the need for supportive care in nephrology is as strong, if not stronger, within renal medicine as in cancer and that what is needed in practice are good models of care which can be used and adapted to local situations, but that all renal teams should have an explicit supportive care strategy.

2.5.1 Good practice

One way to ensure all renal patients receive the supportive care they need is to build in regular reviews of symptoms and psychological and social concerns. The frequency and depth will vary according to the person's circumstances at the time, in particular, how well they are both physically psychologically and in their functioning. Trained members of the renal team could carry this out, with review by the multidisciplinary team at the normal meetings, with referral to other services as needed. Information is accumulating from studies to help guide clinicians to concentrate on those most at risk.[21–23]

2.5.2 Haemodialysis patients

These patients represent a large and well-defined group of renal patients with dialysis most commonly within either a main renal unit or a satellite unit. Many patients are elderly with multiple co-morbidities. They are a very symptomatic group with the severity and persistence of multiple symptoms affecting their quality of life.[24] Patients with co-morbidities such as diabetes or peripheral vascular disease have their kidney function replaced by dialysis, but this does not prevent the progression of their underlying condition and the development of complications; thus, although dialysis supports life, its quality may diminish as symptom burden and dependence increase.

Delivery of dialysis also frequently becomes more difficult as patients near the end of life. Increase in patient dependence not only means that patients usually require hospital transport to and from the dialysis unit, but also may make the patient unsuitable for dialysis in their local satellite unit so that they then have to be transported longer distances to a more intensively staffed unit. Haemodynamic instability becomes more marked as patients near the end of life, with a higher risk of cardiac arrhythmias and hypotension during the dialysis session. Vascular access also often becomes problematic with poor cardiac function and higher risk of infection resulting in catheter and fistula loss.

Recognition of these various issues has led to the development of supportive and palliative care programmes alongside dialysis for these patient such as that at Alberta where a multiprofessional team is involved in the provision of symptom assessment and management, with the possibility of advance care planning and review of goals of care as needed.[19]

2.5.3 Peritoneal dialysis patients

These patients also have the burden of problems relating to peritoneal dialysis (PD) in addition to those of renal failure and their other illnesses. The ability to carry out PD depends on both cognitive and motor ability. Therefore, in most countries, older and more frail patients are placed on haemodialysis (HD) unless there are carers (usually family members) available to help with the PD. Similarly, PD patients are often transferred to HD when they are no longer able to perform the technique themselves. In France, there has been an infrastructure of private community nurses for many years providing assistance with PD; as a result, older, more frail patients are preferentially offered PD rather than HD.[25] Assisted PD is also now being developed in other countries.[26–28]

Peritoneal dialysis does enable patients to be cared for at home as they approach the end of life. Gradual withdrawal from PD is often less of an emotional challenge than the 'all-or-nothing' withdrawal of HD. Both patients and their carers will need a supportive network, particularly as the patient becomes more frail.

2.5.4 Conservatively managed patients

Conservatively managed patients or those who choose maximum medical management without dialysis are described in detail in Chapter 13. We know that patients in this group can have a major symptom burden which goes alongside declining performance status and increasing dependence. In the UK, such a patient should be registered as having palliative care needs by primary care so that the primary care team can have a regular review with relevant members providing appropriate pharmacological, practical, and social support. If admitted to the hospital in an emergency, documentation as to their previous decisions concerning dialysis should be readily available to medical practitioners where it can be reviewed and reassessed. Such patients may be helped by having as a key worker either a renal practitioner or someone from primary care who can access other expertise as and when required for the patient whilst keeping an overview of the situation. The expertise of the renal physician will be needed to ensure optimal management of anaemia, hypertension, etc., and their input can be tailored to the patient's clinical requirements.

2.5.5 Patients who choose to stop dialysis

Such patients represent a special situation; the time leading up to a decision is often one of deterioration in physical status and functioning which may be associated with intense dialogue amongst the renal team members and the patient and family as they come to this often painful decision. Support from within the regular team members will include nursing staff and counsellors. Where symptoms are difficult to control, palliative care team members may contribute. If discussions have taken place well in advance of the decision, plans for care can have been formulated and acted upon. Where such advance care planning has not taken place, urgent discussion will be needed to determine the person's preferred priorities of care, and rapid arrangements should be made where possible. Here, supportive, palliative, and terminal care is combined in the final care of the patient till death and for the family following death.

2.5.6 Failing transplant – not for dialysis

It is rare for patients with a failing transplant not to return to dialysis and/or go back on to the transplant waiting list. However, some transplant patients will have been on dialysis previously and may have exhausted options for vascular access or may have had such a poor quality of life that they do not want to return to it. Patients will also be older than when first on dialysis with the associated problems of ageing and may therefore opt for conservative care. Management of such patients is similar to that of conservative care (Section 2.5.4).

2.5.7 Complex hospitalized patients

There are always patients on the renal wards who have had extended hospital stays with repeated complications related to their renal disease or co-morbidity. This is not surprising as the co-existence of dialysis complicates management. As an example, a common scenario involves a patient admitted with a stroke; rehabilitation is slow because dialysis has to be fitted into the week's routine and the patient tires easily, nutrition becomes impaired, and the patient's resistance to infection decreases with resultant chest infection or vascular access-related infection. Management of such patients is then frequently handed from one team of doctors to another. The obvious communication problems that may then ensue can be helped by one physician remaining in overall charge – ideally the physician who also looks after the patient whilst an outpatient in the dialysis unit. Overall deterioration can otherwise be missed as the healthcare team focus on the here and now and not how current events fit into the larger picture. For such patients, it is important to have frequent communication with the patient and their family to keep them informed about any changes and to give a realistic prognosis. It is essential that the details of such meetings are recorded so that different members of the team can give a consistent picture. A realistic approach to the clinical course and recognition that the patient is dying will enable appropriate planning with the patient and family about withholding or withdrawing treatment, if there is no improvement in the patient's condition, or, in the event of loss of capacity, as wished by the patient if an advance decision to refuse treatment exists. The family can also be prepared for the inevitable outcome and thereby improve the likelihood of a 'good-quality' death.

2.6 **The needs of patients, carers, and families**

Central to the provision of good supportive care is the understanding of what patients and families see as important. Studies that look at their preferences for end-of-life care[29] can be extrapolated in some areas to supportive care. Of a total of 44 possible attributes of quality end-of-life care, 26 (60%) were reported as important by patients, relatives, and physicians; these included: preparation for end-of-life care, achieving a sense of completion, saying goodbye, and treatment preferences.[30] Without good communication skills and advance care planning many of these will not be achievable, thus emphasizing the importance of supportive care early in the illness. In addition, items rated more important by patients than the physician included: being mentally aware, having funeral arrangements in place, not feeling a burden, feeling life was complete, and coming to peace with God. This argues for earlier discussions with patients about prognosis to enable tasks to be achieved, particularly as the incidence of cognitive impairment is high in patient with renal disease and increases as death approaches and, if present, would preclude the satisfactory completion of tasks. Davison's study on hope and advance care planning importantly has shown that "facilitating advance care planning through the provision of timely appropriate information can positively enhance rather than diminish patients' hope".[15]

Focus groups of dialysis patients, family members, bereaved family members, and medical healthcare professionals conducted by the US Renal Supportive Care Team[31] identified the following priorities: education of patient and families about the disease process; open communication; ongoing support amongst patients, families, and staff; continuity of care, pain control, and assistance with advance care planning when looking at how to promote improved palliative care for ESRD.

Unfortunately, evaluation of care of the dying through interviewing of bereaved relatives indicate that there are many unmet needs of people dying, particularly for those dying in institutions.[32] Through its integration of the needs of the family with that of patients, at least one study has shown improved satisfaction for carers in the realm of emotional and spiritual support in patients in a palliative care programme compared with those receiving usual care.[33]

Much is expected of family carers; most give willingly from love of the ill person; however, they too experience a whole range of emotions including depression and feelings of isolation which impact on their well-being.[34] In order to support the increasing number of people who express a preference to die at home, carers' needs must be assessed and addressed. For the carer of someone with ESRD, the caring role may last many years with gradually increasing dependency.

2.7 **Barriers to good practice**

The key to high-quality supportive care at the end of life is good communication with realistic outcomes amongst patients, their family, and healthcare teams. The difficulties that doctors face in such practice have already been discussed in Section 2.4.2. The failure to do so is illustrated by the ETHICATT study[35] in which responses to a questionnaire by physicians and nurses working in ICUs, patients who survived ICU, and families of ICU patients were compared. Quality of life was more important for physicians and nurses than patients and families; more medical professionals wanted fewer ICU treatments and would prefer care at home or in a hospice for a terminal illness than patients and families wanted. This suggests that professionals are aware of the realistic outcomes of ICU treatments but have not communicated this with patients.

Barriers to good practice can be institutional, clinician related, or come from patients and their families themselves when they do not wish to engage in discussions about prognosis and the future. Institutional failures relate to the climate of clinical practice where success is measured in cure or survival rates – as is appropriate for much of medicine – but if this is at the expense of quality of care for those whose diseases are not curable, this will result in less optimal care for them. Medical students are not, on the whole, taught about how someone dies of the illness under study (and hence how they could be cared for) but only of those aspects of care which relate to cure. Many of the failures in practice described in Section 2.4.2 become barriers to good practice and perpetuate less than optimal care.

Patient and family barriers to achieving good practice should not be underplayed. Even into the early 20th century, most people from early childhood would have encountered a close family member dying. This is no longer true in advanced economies, which are now facing the increasing social burden of an ageing population. Expectations are, therefore, to live into one's 80s and 90s and even beyond without the realization that this is often accompanied by the burden of chronic disease and diminishing quality of life. Medical television serials and stories in the media often suggest that modern medicine achieves miracles; thus, it is not surprising that patients have unrealistic expectations, or find it difficult to face the reality of outcomes from treatment.

A major barrier that is often not talked about is the religious and cultural beliefs of doctors, nurses, and patients. The impact of the physician's religion on end-of-life management was illustrated by the ETHICUS study,[17] as discussed in Section 2.4.2. Healthcare workers and patients come from many cultural and religious backgrounds. This is particularly true for patients with kidney disease which is more common in many ethnic groups than in the white population. Thus, in many UK and US units there are a disproportionately high number of patients from varying ethnic groups, many of whom are recent immigrants and do not speak English – an added barrier to good communication and education.

Most physicians are not familiar with the perspectives of different religions on end-of-life decisions. Patients themselves may or may not adhere to the views of their own religion and often have varying interpretations depending on cultural beliefs. As pointed out in a useful review of the views of major religions by Bülow et al.[36] even clear-cut statements are not necessarily accepted culturally. As an example, although according to Islamic law one is allowed to abstain from overzealous treatment, the frequency of withdrawing of treatment and do-not-resuscitate orders varies in different Muslim countries depending on local cultural differences. It is, therefore, not surprising that religious and cultural beliefs can easily lead to clashes between patients and their families and healthcare professionals, making it difficult to achieve good end-of-life care for an individual patient by the standards of Western medical practice.

2.8 Education

All healthcare professionals are exposed to dying patients, so all should receive appropriate education about end of life early in their training and then continuously during their years of practice. The General Medical Council (GMC) document 'Tomorrow's doctors' is clear that palliative care, including care of the terminally ill, is an integral part of the undergraduate curriculum for UK medical students.[37] The extent of this varies considerably amongst medical schools. Palliative care is now part of the curriculum for renal trainees in the UK and US, but in most centres, there is no official training as such, and attending relevant courses is seen as less important than attending a course, e.g. on glomerulonephritis. Experience from the US suggests that teaching to general medical trainees, often in the form of case scenarios with discussion, does not appear to be particularly effective.[38] The strategy that is being discussed in the UK is for renal centres to develop a medical lead in palliative care; such an individual will have to do some formal training in palliative care medicine.

2.9 **Conclusion**

The practice of high-quality supportive care is essential to achieve good-quality care for those approaching the end of their life, and for their carers, so as to enable those who so wish to prepare for their death. Education of both public and healthcare professionals will provide a greater openness with better understanding of people's needs and therefore a stronger basis for improving care. This in turn can lead to a greater chance of achievement of an individual's preferred priorities of care. Such achievements are contingent on good communication between patients, families, and their healthcare team and within the healthcare team. The delivery of supportive care depends upon the recognition that the individual is approaching the end of his or her life. Sensitive communication with patients and families, which can encourage and support advance care planning whilst providing appropriate symptom control, can enable them to make decisions about their end-of-life care and to take control. Realistically, choices depend on facilities and support available in their place of choice, most frequently the community, so that not only can patients and families can choose where to die – in hospital, hospice, or at home – but this can be achieved for a greater number.

Case Study

JJ was first noted to have impaired renal function at the age of 19 and started dialysis when he was 31. His first transplant was at age 33 but lasted only 2.5 years; a second transplant at 37 failed immediately. In total, he spent 19 years on HD, including home HD for 14 years and peritoneal dialysis for 3 years.

Complications of renal failure included: tertiary hyperparathyroidism requiring parathyroidectomy at age 35; aluminium overload requiring chelation therapy; mitral and aortic valve calcification; calcific uraemic arteriolopathy (calciphylaxis) resulting in painful skin necrosis; and dialysis-related amyloidosis, causing bilateral carpal tunnel syndrome requiring surgical release; worsening shoulder stiffness; and uraemic pruritus refractory to emollients, antihistamines, activated charcoal, ultraviolet light, and naltrexone. At age 46, JJ underwent right hemicolectomy for ischaemic ulceration of the caecum. Ischaemic heart disease developed and required angioplasty to a heavily calcified left anterior descending coronary artery. Psoriasis caused severe fissuring of the soles of the feet and required additional treatment. Erectile impotence developed. Severe agitated depression was an intermittent problem.

In the last year of his life JJ developed discitis with severe pain managed by an implanted intrathecal morphine pump. At the same time, the first ischaemic ulcer appeared on his foot. Following an unsuccessful attempt to perform an arterial bypass, he underwent a below-knee amputation of the right leg, followed 3 weeks later by a below-knee amputation of the left leg further followed by above-knee amputation on the right leg because of ischaemic problems in the right stump. An extensive sacral sore kept him in hospital for the next 3 months, towards the end of which he developed gangrene of his fourth finger which had to be amputated, followed by further gangrene of the right stump. At this point, after protracted discussions with his nephrologist about the limited options available, JJ chose to stop dialysis and return home to die.

Until the last year of his life, most of which was spent in hospital, JJ continued to contribute to the running of the family business. In that year he experienced an increasing burden of losses, both social and physical. He had experienced unpleasant symptoms for many years and severe pain from many sources in the last year. He experienced moments of sheer hell such as when he experienced major hallucinations from opioid toxicity or contemplated never leaving hospital again. At other times, he demonstrated extraordinary resilience and spirit, illustrated by seeing him after both legs had been amputated, sitting in the sun, lifting his head from a Harry Potter book and smiling wryly.

JJ's nephrologist coordinated his care throughout, but many others supported him and his wife, including the palliative care team. He also spent two valuable periods of care in the hospice, which gave him and his team respite whilst he had the opportunity to explore some of his feelings of hopelessness. Pain control in the last year was complex needing frequent review with contributions to his renal team both from a pain anaesthetist and the palliative care team. When the decision to stop dialysis and go home was taken, the palliative care nurse who had known him for the last year was able to liaise and set up the necessary services to enable this to happen rapidly.

Ethical analysis

JJ's dialysis-related amyloidosis, uraemic pruritus, premature atherosclerosis, and resultant depression are all tragic markers of our inadequacies in managing dialysis patients in previous decades. JJ experienced unpleasant symptoms for many years and severe pain from many sources in the last year. Nonetheless, JJ was a long-term survivor on RRT.

Competence is one of the key ethical responsibilities of clinicians. JJ received competent care in several important respects. First, JJ was able to continue working and contribute to the running of his family business up until the last year of his life. Only a small percentage of dialysis patients continue to work. Being able to dialyse at home for 17 of his 19 years on dialysis facilitated his continued employment. Second, JJ was cared for by a team. We now understand that a team approach is the best way to care for patients who are chronically ill. Third, a palliative care approach, including the involvement of a pain specialist and hospice, was instituted in the final year of JJ's life. He had the opportunity to explore the meaning of his life and to deal with his feelings of hopelessness. Because of the involvement of the palliative care team, a smooth transition to hospice care at home occurred. The patient and his wife received the psychosocial and spiritual support that they needed in the patient's final weeks.

This case applies a number of the recommendations in the Renal Physicians Association and the American Society of Nephrology's clinical practice guideline, *Shared Decision-making in the Appropriate Initiation of and Withdrawal from Dialysis*.[18] The case described shared decision making amongst the nephrologist, the patient, and his wife. The decision to withdraw from dialysis was made by JJ, who had decision-making capacity, was fully informed, and was making a voluntary decision (recommendations 1 and 2). The patient received palliative care that included pain and symptom management and psychosocial and spiritual support (recommendation 9). In this case, there is no mention of advance care planning. It was foreseeable that he might lose decision-making capacity and that medical decisions might need to be made for him by someone else. Advance care planning to identify the person that JJ would have preferred to make decisions for him when he lost decision-making capacity and his preferences for end-of-life care should have been conducted (recommendation 5). One of the fortunate aspects of this case is that our thinking with regard to withdrawal from dialysis has progressed. When JJ started dialysis, decisions to stop dialysis were problematic. Now we have an understanding of the ethical and legal principles that should govern a decision to stop dialysis. Ethically and legally, patients with decision-making capacity have a right to accept or refuse life-sustaining treatment such as dialysis; nephrologists have found it helpful to review this systematically (see the Introduction). In JJ's case, as in others, if no reversible factors are found to improve the patient's satisfaction with life on dialysis and if the patient is making an informed and voluntary decision that is not hindered by a major depression, encephalopathy, or other major mental disorder, the nephrologist is obligated to honour the patient's informed refusal of continued dialysis (recommendation 2).

Overall, JJ's life was prolonged for more than 21 years by RRT. From a medical and ethical perspective, he received the best care that was possible at the time. Fortunately, advances have been made in our ability to manage the complications of ESRD. As ESRD patients live longer with chronic illness, the ethical dimensions of their care – shared decision making, informed consent, estimating and communicating prognosis, and advance care planning – will remain critically important to ensure quality care at the end of their lives.

Appendix 1: Completion of WHO definition of 1990[1]

Palliative care:

◆ Affirms life and regards dying as a normal process.

◆ Neither hastens nor postpones death.

◆ Provides relief from pain and other symptoms.

◆ Integrates the psychological and spiritual aspects of patient care.

◆ Offers a support system to help patients live as actively as possible until death.

◆ Offers a support system to help the family cope during the patient's illness and in their own environment.

Appendix 2: NCPC: continued description of Supportive Care[4]

Supportive care should be fully integrated with diagnosis and treatment and encompasses:

◆ Self-help and support

◆ User involvement

◆ Information giving

◆ Psychological support

◆ Symptom control

◆ Social support

◆ Rehabilitation

◆ Complementary therapies

◆ Spiritual support

◆ End-of-life and bereavement care

References

1 World health Organisation (1990). *Cancer Pain relief and Palliative Care,* Technical Report Series 804. Geneva: World Health organisation.

2 Ahmedzai S, Walsh D (2000). Palliative medicine and modern cancer care. *Semin Oncol,* **27**,1–6.

3 Fins J (2005). *A palliative ethic of care: clinical wisdom at life's end.* Sudbury, MA: Jones & Bartlett Publishers.

4 The National Council for Palliative Care. http://www.ncpc.org.uk/palliative_care.html. Accessed Jan 20 2009.

5 National Institute for Clinical Excellence. http://www.nice.org.uk/nicemedia/pdf/csgspmanual.pdf. Accessed Jan 20 2009.

6 Department of Health (2008). End of Life Strategy – promoting high quality care for all adults at the end of life.

7 Coresh J, Astor BC, Greene T, et al. (2003). Prevalence of chronic kidney disease and decreased kidney function in the adult US population: Third National Health and Nutrition Examination Survey. *Am J Kid Dis,* **41**, 1–12.

8 Carter JL, O'Riordan SE, Eaglestone GL, et al. (2008). Chronic kidney disease prevalence in a UK residential care home population. *Nephrol Dialy Transplant,* **23**, 1257–64.

9 The Renal Association, UK Renal Registry Report 2007.

10 Kurella M, Covinsky KE, Collins AJ, et al. (2007). Octogenarians and nonagenarians starting dialysis in the United States. *Ann Intern Med,* **146**, 177–183.

11 REIN Registry 2005 Annual report. Available at: http://www.agence-biomedecine.fr/fr/experts/greffes-organes-rein.asp REIN Registry 2005 Annual report. Available at: http://www.agence-biomedecine.fr/fr/experts/greffes-organes-rein.asp.

12 Davison SN, Jhangri GS, Holley JL, et al. (2006). Nephrologists' Reported Preparedness for End-of-Life Decision-Making. *Clin J Am Soc Nephrol*, **1**, 1256–62.

13 Jackson VA, Mack J, Matsuyama R, et al. (2008). A qualitative study of oncologists' approaches to end-of life care. *J Pall Med*, **11**, 893–906.

14 Stainhauser (2008). Do preparation and end of life completion discussions improve functioning and quality of life in seriously ill patients? Pilot RCT *Pall Med*, **11**, 1234–40.

15 Davison SN, Simpson C (2006). Hope and advance care planning in patients with end stage renal disease: qualitative interview study. *Brit Med J*, **333**, 886–91.

16 Apatira L, Boyd EA, Malvar G, et al. (2008). Hope, truth and preparing for death: perspectives of surrogate decision makers. *Ann Int Med*, **149**, 861–8.

17 Sprung CL, Cohen SL, Sjokvist P, et al. for the Ethicus Study Group (2003). End-of-life practices in European intensive care units. *JAMA*, **290**, 790–7.

18 Levy J, Chambers EJ, Brown EA (2004). Supportive care for the renal patient. *Nephrol Dialy Transplant*, **19**, 1357–60.

19 Fainsinger RL, Davison SN, Brennis C (2003). A supportive care model for dialysis patients. *Pall Med*, **17**, 81–2.

20 Gunda S, Thomas M, Smith S (2005). National survey of palliative care in end-stage renal disease in the UK. *Nephrol DialyTransplant*, **20**, 392–5.

21 Couchoud C, Labeeuw M, Moranne O, et al. (2009). A clinical score to predict 6-month prognosis in elderly patients starting dialysis for end-stage renal disease. *Nephrol Dialy Transplant*, **24**(5): 1553–61.

22 Wong CF, McCarthy M, Howse ML (2007). Factors affecting survival in advanced chronic kidney disease patients who choose not to receive dialysis. *Ren Fail*, **29**(6), 653–9.

23 Chanda SM, Schulz J, Lawrence C, et al. (1999). Is there a rationale for rationing chronic dialysis? A hospital based cohort Study of factors affecting survival and morbidity. *BMJ*, **318**, 217–23.

24 Weisbord SD, Fried LF, Arnold RM, et al. (2005). Prevalence, severity and importance of physical and emotional symptoms in chronic haemodialysis patients. *J Am Soc Neprol*, **16**, 2487–94.

25 Verger C, Ryckelynck JP, Duman M, et al. (2006). French peritoneal dialysis registry (RDPLF): Outline and main results. *Kidney Int*, **70**, S12–S20.

26 Povlsen JV, Ivarsen P (2005). Assisted automated peritoneal dialysis (AAPD) for the functionally dependent and elderly patient. *Perit Dial Int*, **25**, Suppl 3, S60–S63.

27 Brown EA, Dratwa M, Povlsen JV (2007). Assisted peritoneal dialysis: an evolving dialysis modality. *Nephrol Dial Transplant*, **22**, 3091–2.

28 Oliver MJ, Quinn RR, Richardson EP, et al. (2007). Home care assistance and the utilization of peritoneal dialysis. *Kidney Int*, **71**, 673–8.

29 Steinhauser KE, Clipp EC, McNeilly M, et al. (2000). In search of a good death: observations of patients, families, and providers. *Ann Intern Med*, **132**, 825–32.

30 Steinhauser KE, Christakis NA, Clipp EC, et al. (2000). Factors considered important at the end of life by patients, family, physicians, and other care providers. *JAMA*, **284**, 2476–82.

31 Berzoff J, Swantkowski J, Cohen LM (2008) Developing a renal supportive care team from the voices of patients, families, and palliative care staff. *Palliat Support Care*, **6**, 133–9.

32 Teno JM, Clarridge BR, Casey V, et al. (2008). Family perspectives on end-of-life care at the last place of care. *JAMA*, **291**(1), 88–93.

33 Gelfman LP, Meier DP, Morrison RS (2008). Does palliative care improve quality? A survey of bereaved family members. *J Pall Med*, **36**(1), 22–8.

34 Riley J, Fenton G (2007). A terminal diagnosis: the carers' perspective. *Couns Psychother Res*, **7**(2), 86–91.

35 Sprung CL, Carmel S, Sjokvist P, et al. for the ETHICATT Study Group (2007). Attitudes of European physicians, nurses, patients, and families regarding end-of-life decisions: the ETHICATT study. *Intensive Care Med*, **33**, 104–110.

36 Bülow HH, Sprung CL, Reinhart K, et al. (2008). The world's major religions' points of view on end-of-life decisions in the intensive care unit. *Intensive Care Med*, **34**, 423–30.

37 General Medical Council. http://www.gmc-uk.org/education/undergraduate/GMC_tomorrows_ doctors.pdf. Accessed Jan 20 2009.

38 Fischer SM, Gozansky WS, Kutner JS, et al. (2003). Palliative care education; an intervention to improve medical residents' knowledge and attitudes. *J Pall Med*, 3: 391–9.

Chapter 3

Planning a renal palliative care programme and its components

Maria Da Silva-Gane and Lewis M Cohen

3.1 Introduction

This chapter describes the changes that have evolved in the United Kingdom (UK) and the United States (US) in the area of renal supportive and palliative care by providing an overview of strategy developments and clinical demonstration projects.

3.2 Background

In the UK and the US, end-stage renal disease (ESRD) has become a geriatric disorder, and the demographics reveal a robust increase in numbers and severity of co-morbid illnesses. Consequently, it should come as no surprise that the annual mortality rate is greater than 20%, which is higher than that of many cancers.[1–4]

Renal units are aware that ESRD patients may withdraw from renal replacement treatment either through their own choice or by a decision made by caregivers. In the New England region of the US, four-in-ten deaths are now preceded by discontinuation of dialysis.[5,6] There is also an increasing recognition amongst nephrologists that initiating dialysis in patients with multiple co-morbidities and those who are elderly and have diminished activities of daily living may not improve survival.[7–9] In the UK more than in the US, this recognition has led to conservative management programmes – the care of patients following a decision to withhold dialysis. Neither the UK nor the US tracks the number of patients entering conservative management programmes, but in one unit about 20% of the ESRD population was satisfactorily managed without initiating dialysis.[7]

3.3 Strategic developments in the United Kingdom

Since 2004, there have been several initiatives to increase the support for patients with long-term conditions and to develop skills amongst healthcare professionals.[10] This includes the introduction of specialist nurses in the community whose role includes a focus of working with patients who have chronic and progressive conditions with the aim of prevention of repeated hospital admissions as well as supporting patients to make choices about their future care. This may include end-of-life (EoL) planning.[11]

3.3.1 Patients in their end-of-life modules

The National Service Framework (NSF) for Renal Services in England[12] and the Renal NSF for Wales[13] both identified three groups of patients in their EoL modules. These were patients who decide not to undergo dialysis treatment, those who choose to withdraw from dialysis after a period of treatment, and those who are coming to the end of their lives whilst continuing dialysis. The quality requirement in the NSF for Renal Services in England states that:

> People with established renal failure receive timely evaluation of their prognosis, information about the choices available to them, and those near to end of life a jointly agreed palliative care plan, built around their individual needs and preferences.

Both of the NSFs also highlight markers of good practice which include:

- Access to a multi-skilled renal team with expertise in communication, shared decision-making, and symptom management.
- Prognostic assessment.
- Timely information about the choices available to them and a palliative care plan.
- Ongoing medical treatment.
- Dignity in death, and where possible to die in their preferred place of care.
- Culturally appropriate bereavement support.

3.3.2 The End of Life Strategy for England

The End of Life Strategy for England[14] promotes high-quality care for adults at the end of their life. One of the major developments in the strategy is that it is not disease specific. The Scottish Partnership for Palliative Care in Palliative and End of Life Care in Scotland: the case for a cohesive approach[15] similarly highlights the need to ensure the delivery of a high-quality palliative care service for all patients with a progressive chronic condition. The key elements of the above EoL strategies are:

- Active and ongoing communication as the EoL approaches.
- Assessment, care planning, and review.
- Coordination of care for individual patients.
- Delivery of high-quality services in different settings.
- Care in the last days in life.
- Care after death.

3.3.3 Established end-of-life tools

Established EoL tools are mentioned both in EoL Strategy/policy documents. These are: The Gold Standards Framework (GSF),[16,17] the Preferred Priorities for Care (PPC),[18] and the Liverpool Care Pathway (LCP).[19] All of them aim at facilitating assessments, providing symptom amelioration, and attending to EoL needs in collaboration with patients, families, and health and social care agencies. Whilst these tools were initially developed for cancer care, the EoL Strategy documents stress the propriety of transferring and applying the tools in supporting patients with any progressive chronic disease that is life limiting, including ESRD.

The Gold Standards Framework is a framework of strategies and tools designed to help primary care teams improve the organization and quality of care for patients in the last year of life. The basis of the GSF is to encourage and enable the primary care teams to enhance knowledge and understanding of palliative care. It highlights the importance of effective communication, co-ordination, and continuity of care for the patient and family in the community.[17]

The Preferred Priorities for Care is a patient-held document designed to facilitate, capture, and record the discussions amongst doctors, nurses, others professionals, and patients with regard to their preferences and priorities for treatment and management of their condition including their

EoL care. The PPC initiative seeks to offer patients informed choice about palliative care and the manner and place of their care at the end of life.[18]

The Liverpool Care Pathway is an integrated-care pathway that was developed to bring the best of hospice and EoL care into hospitals and other settings. It is designed for patients who are in the final days and hours of life. It facilitates effective communication within the multidisciplinary team and with the patient and family, anticipatory planning, including psychosocial and spiritual needs, and appropriate symptom control and bereavement care.[19]

3.3.4 Access to care

The importance for all patients, irrespective of the type of life-limiting disease, to have access to care based on the principles of palliative care has led to the development of a Framework for Implementation of End of Life Care in Advanced Kidney Disease in England.[20] This framework combines the previously mentioned elements of good practice into a disease-specific strategy that aims to support renal patients and the professionals involved in their care.

3.4 Demonstration projects in the United States and United Kingdom

The US was early in recognizing the value of infusing the care of renal patients with the advances offered by palliative medicine. It boldly acknowledged the wisdom of treatment trials and withdrawal of dialysis.[21] Whilst there are still some UK centres that do not have conservative or supportive care provision,[22] there has been an increase in recent years in the number of renal units that have developed a supportive and palliative care programme. Such a provision aims to ensure that support commences from time of recognition that the patient has supportive care needs, and increases as the disease progresses. There is evidence that the sooner supportive care begins the better the quality of life that can be achieved.[7] It has also been recognized that families require supportive care throughout the illness progression.[22]

3.4.1 Lister Hospital

In the UK, many nephrology teams have forged partnerships with palliative care teams and hospices in their locality to improve supportive care to their patients. The renal team at Lister Hospital – a regional unit providing services to the population of Hertfordshire and Bedfordshire – first developed a conservative management programme in 1996.

The development of a conservative management pathway came about from an increasing awareness of a subgroup of patients with a high level of dependency and co-morbidities who often fared poorly on dialysis.[7] The conservative management approach is part of the philosophy of the wider nephrology team who are keen to continue to develop a supportive care approach.

Crucial to the initial and ongoing development of the conservative management programme has been the close and collaborative working relationships amongst the renal team and other medical teams, both within the hospital and in the wider community. This includes specialist-palliative care teams, as well as incorporating new developments, and ensuring that innovations such as the GSF and PPC become embedded in the service. The use of the LCP on the renal ward has been introduced to ensure that patients, both conservatively managed and those withdrawing from dialysis, receive appropriate EoL care.

Patients referred from primary or secondary care are first assessed medically. They are then referred to the renal liaison team which has nursing, social work, and counselling skills. This team manages and oversees conservative management and pre-dialysis patients including discussing treatment options that are available for the patient. There is at least one visit to the patient's home to enable a more relaxed and unhurried discussion; it also allows other family members to be present. Discussions are continued in the outpatient clinic by the nephrologists and a decision is reached between the team and patient for the most appropriate care pathway. This is not a one-time decision but a process – some patients are able to make a clear informed decision in a relatively short time scale, some require more time and reflection, whilst others do not wish to be overly involved in the process and defer decisions to either the family or the clinical team.

Once a decision for a conservative management pathway has been established, patients continue to attend the nephrology clinic to ensure optimal medical, social, and psychological management. The renal liaison team maintains contact with the patient and family in the clinic, at home, and through telephone contact. These enable ongoing discussions about medical management, disease progression, psychological care, social issues, palliative care treatment options, and personal goals/objectives. Referrals to other agencies and specialist teams are made in consultation with the patient. Regular multi-professional review meetings – led by a consultant nephrologist – are held fortnightly, providing an opportunity for ongoing holistic review. Recommendations are made – e.g. to contact the general practitioner to request that the patient be included on their GSF support register, or to give feedback on the outcome of referrals made to specialist palliative care teams or that the focus needs to move to EoL care. Ongoing reviews are crucial to enable flexible care planning that meets patient and family needs and to ensure timely referrals, collaboration, and to aid good communication with the community and specialist-care teams.

Bereavement support is an important element – for the patient to be reassured that continued support will be available to the family and for the family to feel that the supportive care does not vanish at a crucial time. Bereavement support is available from the renal team or, if preferred, from the hospice or specialist community bereavement services.

Over 250 patients have followed the conservative management pathway and have been supported until the end of their life; 60% have remained and died in their own home, 5% have entered a hospice for their EoL care; whilst 35% have died in hospital. Although, at times, a lack of resources may culminate in a hospital admission for EoL care, it is – for some patients and family – a chosen option and in such circumstances should not be seen as a failure.

In common with many nephrology services in the UK, the Lister team has explored how best to support patients on chronic dialysis who are facing an accumulation of medical complications, and for whom options for effective intervention may have become limited. Patients, families, and staff at this time must make difficult choices that affect the length and the quality of life.

Such patients need advance care planning for their future treatment and this will include EoL care. The team felt that there was a need to have a more consistent and proactive approach to support patients and staff to facilitate communication and care planning. To address this, a 'Cause for Concern' (CfC) support pathway has been developed for patients identified as either not coping on dialysis and/or as approaching the end of their life.

A CfC integrated-care pathway, incorporating the established end of life tools was devised by a steering group drawn from the multi-professional team. A medical and non-medical lead was agreed upon, and a link nurse was identified in each clinical area. Link nurses are crucial as they have regular contact with, and are aware of changes impacting on, their patients. There are several referral routes for the CfC; these include the patient or family raising a concern, a member of their community team; GP, community nurse, social worker, or any member of the renal team.

Once a cause for concern has been identified, the next step is for a clinic appointment with a consultant nephrologist. This initial discussion will include the reason for the concern, an understanding of the current medical situation, a realistic prognosis, and establishing the aims and goals of the patient. These discussions are usually followed up by a home visit to review or to further the discussions that have already been initiated. The outcome is agreed and documented, any referrals required are actioned and the renal multidisciplinary and community teams are made aware of the care plan. The care plan may be for a planned withdrawal from the dialysis programme or for an agreed approach, should there be further medical complications or deterioration. The care plans are reviewed monthly to ensure that they are still appropriate and continue to meet the needs of the patient.

3.4.2 Barts and The London National Health Services (NHS) Trust's Renal Supportive Care Service

The renal team at Barts and The London NHS Trust has developed a Renal Supportive Care Service (RSCS) which offers a palliative care pathway for patients with progressive, chronic kidney disease treated without dialysis and dialysis patients who are considering withdrawal from treatment. The team consists of clinical nurse specialists, a consultant nephrologist, and professionals from other disciplines.

Once a decision has been made not to begin dialysis, the nephrologist refers the patient to the RSCS. Contact is made by the team with the patient or care-giver within 3 months of referral, but patients can be seen earlier depending on clinical need. An appointment is offered to discuss diagnosis, treatment decisions, treatment management, and treatment goals; this is regularly reviewed and followed up within 3 months in clinic or at the patient's home. The team makes necessary referrals to other disciplines and agencies. Ongoing discussions include use of the PPC. Regular contact is maintained with the general practitioner and the specialists.

In the 4 years of the project there has been an increase in referrals, home visits, and home and hospice deaths.[23] Bereavement support is being provided.

3.4.3 The Baystate Renal Palliative Care Initiative

In 1986, American nephrologists began to openly write about and discuss the practice of dialysis termination.[24] This was followed by the development of guidelines for the initiation and withdrawal of dialysis.[25] (See Chapter 5 for guidelines). In 1998, Baystate Health System and the Western New England Renal and Transplant Associates began the Renal Palliative Care Initiative (RPCI).[26] The collaborators in this demonstration project believed that EoL care should not be limited to cancer, acquired immune deficiency syndrome, and hospice populations, but that the focus should be broadened to include the numerous, chronic, end-stage organ disorders, including ESRD. The Initiative has been successful in developing multiple, innovative practice interventions, and along with other dialysis facilities throughout the country the palliative medicine approach and practices are now being actively encouraged by organizations such as the American Society of Nephrology and the Renal Physicians Association.[27]

The Baystate Health System is a not-for-profit provider of a broad range of regional health services in the Connecticut River Valley Region of the US. It includes the Baystate Medical Center – a tertiary-care and teaching hospital of Tufts University School of Medicine – as well as several small community hospitals. The RPCI consists of the dialysis and transplantation services that are based at those hospitals, as well as at nine free-standing dialysis clinics in the region. The RPCI dialysis facilities are chiefly situated in Western Massachusetts, but are also located in Connecticut and New Hampshire. They are owned by Fresenius Medical Care, Inc. – the largest proprietary chain of dialysis clinics in the US. Clinical care is directed by the physicians of the Western New England Renal and Transplantation Associates.

Naturally, not all of the interventions that were implemented by the RPCI a decade ago have continued to be used actively.[28] The ones that appear to be standing the test of time include:

3.4.3.1 Treatment protocols

Treatment protocols to address common ESRD symptoms and terminal care situations, e.g. facilitating referral to hospice, or the treatment of pruritus. The protocols are available at all dialysis nursing stations and the hospital renal unit. The protocols offer an opportunity for consistent care, and can be updated as new techniques are recognized.

3.4.3.2 Annual renal memorial services

These have been especially well received, and they are attended each year by substantial numbers of families, loved-ones, staff, and active patients. The renal memorial service organizing committee consists of social workers, nurses, chaplains, and families, and it meets regularly throughout the year. The services of remembrance require the participation and contributions of the greater community, and they epitomize the belief that post-death care should be essential to the practice of dialysis. Evidence is accumulating that these moving events are helping to change the culture of dialysis and transplantation and to make dialysis staff more appreciative of EoL issues. Educational manuals and videotapes describing the annual renal memorial services have disseminated this intervention to programmes throughout the country.

3.4.3.3 Bereavement support

Support is being offered to families, friends, and staff. Several different approaches to notify people from the dialysis clinics about the deaths are being tried, e.g. displaying the newspaper obituaries near the nursing stations. Letters of condolence are being sent out by the nephrologists and/or social workers to families.

3.4.3.4 Renal supportive care teams

These include palliative medicine consultants and hospice staff and have recently been studied at three of the dialysis facilities to determine if the hospice referral rates can be increased. The hypothesis is that greater familiarity and interaction between healthcare professionals from these two specialties will lead to more integrative services. In the US, unfortunately there are financial and regulatory barriers that interfere with many ESRD patients obtaining hospice care. Nevertheless, RPCI research has found a moderately significant increase in the hospice referrals and management of dying dialysis patients from the intervention clinics as compared to the control clinics.

The Baystate RPCI originally evolved from a series of EoL investigatory studies.[29] Most of its current activities continue to be focussed on promoting these research investigations. They include an exploration of prognostic models and also a protocol to improve communication amongst staff, patients, and families.

3.5 Summary

Both the US and the UK are actively trying to address the challenges posed by an ESRD population that continues to grow, age, have multiple co-morbidities, increased severity of symptoms, and elevated mortality rates. Both countries are trying to change nephrology's long-standing denial of these issues,[30] and both have turned to the burgeoning field of palliative medicine for answers. The US was the first to openly examine the options of limited trials of dialysis, treatment withdrawal, and symptom-amelioration protocols, whilst the UK has more recently been actively investigating dialysis withholding and the institution of conservative management programmes. All of these efforts need to continue.

The major barrier towards instituting a renal supportive and palliative care model is the already impressive staff workload and expense of operating dialysis facilities. Nephrologists, dialysis and transplant personnel all work together in highly organized, efficient, and demanding environments. At times, it seems unimaginable that staff can reasonably add new tasks to their existing clinical responsibilities. However, the demonstration programmes in the US and UK are discovering daily that the satisfaction of learning new ways to manage symptoms and attend to EoL issues outweighs all additional burdens. In addition, management for patients who choose not to dialyse will take place largely in primary care and thus release the renal team to concentrate theirs skills in the hospital.

Case Study: Withdrawal from haemodialysis

Mr A aged 84, married for 54 years, had three children and six grandchildren. A retired engineer, creativity was important to him so he pursued hobbies of painting and pottery and took an art degree in his retirement.

He commenced haemodialysis (HD) at 74 following a second nephrectomy for renal cancer. The initial adjustment to dialysis was difficult but he settled on dialysis with support from the renal team. Four years later he was diagnosed with Parkinson's disease and this and his general health deteriorated over the next 3 years. Support to help with personal care was declined. They continued to manage well for the following 2 years.

At a regular HD clinic, Mr A commented that he was finding HD difficult to tolerate; it was suggested dialysis might be reduced to twice weekly and Mr A wondered whether it was appropriate for him to continue with treatment. Following discussion with the nephrologists he was referred to the renal counsellor for follow-up.

At a home visit the main issues were:

- His deteriorating physical state.
- Increased difficulty with HD.
- Spending most of the time in bed.
- Inability to pursue creative hobbies.
- Loss of quality of life.

His main concerns in stopping dialysis were;

- How much time he would have after stopping dialysis
- What his death would be like
- Would it be considered suicide
- Support for his wife after his death
- How to tell his children and grandchildren of his wishes

Mrs A was fully supportive of her husband's desire to cease HD; but over the following 3 months the discussions, both at home and in the clinic were continued to ensure that all his issues were discussed in the depth he required and at his pace. He continued thrice weekly dialysis; made a do not resuscitate order and accepted the following referrals:

- Help with personal care and aids and adaptations
- General practitioner (GP) and district nurse support
- Hospice referral.

During ongoing discussions with the renal team (including a family meeting), it became clear that Mr A needed 'permission' from the nephrologist to stop dialysis and when offered the theoretical possibility of the doctor suggesting dialysis was not benefiting him; he said he would "be relieved".

With further deterioration, the option of a plan to stop dialysis was taken by the nephrologist. Mr A responded with relief and his family were fully supportive. The relevant agencies were informed and a date decided on for his last dialysis, with discussion as to how he wished to handle it.

He chose to have his last weekend at home with a family meal and then to go into the local hospice where he died 4 days later. Mrs A received bereavement support which was also offered to the rest of the family.

Ethical case analysis

One might wonder why it took 3 months to honour Mr. A's desire to stop dialysis. Mr. A's quality of life had become unsatisfactory to him and continuing dialysis was difficult. His wife was understanding and 'fully supportive' of his desire to stop. It appears that Mr. A wanted his nephrologist to become reconciled to the patient's stopping of dialysis and give permission before Mr. A felt comfortable in stopping. Fortunately, this need was identified and communicated to his nephrologist. The nephrologist took the cue and suggested to Mr. A that it was time to stop. Withdrawal of dialysis with hospice referral seems to have proceeded smoothly thereafter. The solution to preventing delays in honouring patients' wishes and prolonging suffering, as occurred in the case of Mr. A, is to have established palliative care protocols in dialysis units. In such protocols the renal supportive care team would routinely (1) invite failing patients to discuss their goals and preferences for treatment and (2) ensure that the remainder of the renal care team is aware of the patient's wishes and is willing to respect them. The RPA/ASN guideline recommendation #9 endorsed this approach. This chapter describes models for how it can be accomplished.

References

1 Ansell D, Feehally J, Feest TG, et al. (2007). *The Tenth Annual Report of the UK renal Registry*. Bristol: UK Renal Registry.

2 Lamping DL, Constantinovici N, Roderick P, et al. (2000). Clinical outcomes, quality of life, and costs in the North Thames Dialysis Study of elderly people on dialysis: a prospective cohort study. *Lancet*, **356**(9241), 1543–50.

3 Chandna SM, Shultz J, Lawrence C, et al. (1999). Is there a rationale for rationing chronic dialysis? A hospital based cohort study of factors affecting survival and morbidity. *Brit Med J*, **318** (7178), 217–23.

4 Cohen LM, Moss AH, Weisbord SD, et al. (2006). Renal palliative care. *J Pall Med*, **9**(4), 977–92.

5 U.S. Renal Data System (2008). USRDS Annual Data Report: Atlas of Chronic Kidney Disease and End-Stage Renal Disease in the United States. Bethesda, MD: National Institute of Diabetes and Digestive and Kidney Diseases, National Institutes of Health.

6 Murtagh F, Cohen LM, Germain MJ (2007). Dialysis discontinuation: quo vadis? *Adv Chr Kid Dis*, **14**(4), 379–401.

7 Smith C, Da Silva-Gane M, Chandna S, et al. (2003). Choosing not to dialyse: evaluation of planned non-dialytic management in a cohort of patients with end stage renal failure. *Nephrol Clin Pract*, **9**(2), 40–6.

8 Murtagh FE, Marsh JE, Donohoe P, et al. (2007). Dialysis or not? A comparative survival study of patients over 75 years with chronic kidney disease stage 5. *Nephrol Dial Transplant*, **22**(7),1955–62.

9 Chesser A (2005). Palliative care in renal disease. In Faull C, Carter Y, Daniels L (eds) *Handbook of palliative care*, 2nd ed. Oxford: Blackwell Publishing.

10 Department of Health (2004). *The NHS Improvement Plan*. London: Department of Health.

11 Department of Health (2005). *Supporting people with long term conditions: liberating the talents of nurses who care for people with long term conditions*. London: Department of Health.

12 Department of Health (2005). *National Service framework for renal services – Part two: chronic kidney disease, acute renal failure and end of life care.* London: Department of Health.

13 Welsh Assembly Government (2007). *Designed to Tackle Renal Disease in Wales: A Policy Statement and National Service Framework (NSF).* Cardiff: Welsh Assembly Government.

14 Department of Health (2008). *End of Life Strategy – promoting high quality care for all adults at the end of life.* London: Department of Health.

15 Scottish Partnership for Palliative Care (2007). *Palliative and end of life care in Scotland: the case for a cohesive approach.* Edinburgh.

16 Thomas K (2003). *Caring for the dying at home: companions on the journey.* Abingdon, Oxon: Radcliffe Medical Press.

17 Gold Standards Framework (2006). http://www.goldstandardsframework.nhs.uk/gp_contract.php.

18 Preferred Priorities for Care (2007). http://www.endoflifecareforadults.nhs.uk/eolc/CS310.htm.

19 The Marie Curie Palliative Care Institute Liverpool (2008). The Liverpool Pathway for the dying patient: http://www.mcpcil.org.uk/liverpool_care_pathway.

20 NHS Kidney Care (2009). *End of life care in advanced kidney disease: a framework for implementation.*

21 Cohen LM, Germain MJ (2003). Palliative and supportive care. In Brady HR, Wilcox CS (eds) *Therapy in nephrology and hypertension: a companion to Brenner and Rector's the kidney,* pp. 753–6, 2nd ed. London: Elsevier.

22 Noble H, Kelly D (2006). Supportive and palliative care in end stage renal failure: the need for further research. *Int J Pall Nurs,* **12**(8), 362–4, 366–7.

23 Noble H, Chesser A (2009). Moving forward: advancing renal supportive and end of life care. *Brit J Ren Med,* **14**(2), 18–21.

24 Neu S, Kjellstrand CM (1986). Stopping long-term dialysis: an empirical study of withdrawal of life-supporting treatment. *N Engl J Med,* **314**(1), 14–20.

25 Renal Physicians Association and American Society of Nephrology (2000). *Shared decision-making in the appropriate initiation of and withdrawal from dialysis.* Guideline number 2. Washington, DC: RPA.

26 Poppel DM, Cohen LM, Germain MJ (2003). The Renal Palliative Care Initiative. *J Pall Med,* **6**(2), 321–6.

27 Poppel D, Cohen LM (2003). Renal disease. In Taylor GJ, Kurent JE (eds) *A clinician's guide to palliative care,* pp. 90–103. Malden, MA: Blackwell Publishing.

28 Germain M, Cohen LM (2005). Nephrology. In Kuebler KK, Davis MP, Moore CD (eds) *Palliative practices: an interdisciplinary approach,* pp. 181–95. St. Louis, MO: Elsevier Mosby.

29 Cohen LM (2004). Planning of a renal palliative care program and its components. In Chambers EJ, Germain MJ, Brown EA (eds) *Supportive care for the renal patient,* pp. 27–34. London: Oxford University Press.

30 Cohen LM, McCue JD, Germain M, Woods A (1997). Denying the dying: Advance directives and dialysis discontinuation. *Psychosomatics,* **38**(1), 27–34.

Chapter 4

Advance care planning in patients with end-stage renal disease

Sara N Davison, Jean L Holley, and Jane Seymour

4.1 Introduction

Despite continuing technological improvements, more than 83 000 patients who need long-term dialysis die each year in North America with an annual unadjusted mortality rate of 20–25%.[1,2] Advances in dialysis care have blurred the boundaries between life-sustaining and palliative treatments and have challenged our expectations about how these patients die.[3] Most will live for many years with a progressive decline in functional status and a substantial burden of suffering. [4–6] Often, patients, family, and care-providers are unable to identify a phase in which the patient is clearly recognized as dying. Appropriate palliative care is, therefore, often delayed or not initiated and, as a result, the quality of the dying experience for patients with end-stage renal disease (ESRD) is suboptimal.[7–11] Approximately 20–25% of deaths amongst dialysis patients occur after a decision to discontinue dialysis.[1,2] Comprehensive care of ESRD patients, therefore, requires expertise not only in the medical and technical aspects of dialysis but also in palliative care, including advance care planning (ACP).[3]

This chapter explores the purpose and use of advance directives (ADs) and ACP within the context of ESRD. We discuss the empirical evidence about the degree to which ADs and ACP have met their intended goals, interventions to enhance the use and value of ADs and ACP, and new research that helps define how to initiate and facilitate effective ACP for patients with ESRD.

4.2 Definitions of advance directives and advance care planning

The traditional focus of planning for future end-of-life (EoL) care has been the completion of written ADs, which are legal documents with powers and requirements that vary widely from jurisdiction to jurisdiction and which tend to focus on the documentation of limited treatment options.[12–14] ADs are generally of two types: instructional (e.g. personal directive, living will) and proxy (e.g. durable power of attorney for healthcare). Instructional directives specify patients' medical care preferences whilst proxy directives appoint another person to act as a surrogate decision-maker. In the UK, since the passage of the Mental Capacity Act 2005[15] the following terms, which supercede the terms living wills or advance directives, are used:

- *An advance statement* (a statement of wishes and preferences).
- *An advance decision to refuse treatment (ADRT)* (a specific refusal of treatment in a predefined potential future situation). This only comes into force if the person loses capacity.
- *The appointment of a personal welfare lasting Power of Attorney (LPA)*, who can only act when the patients lacks capacity to make the required decision.

Table 4.1 Goals of advance care planning in end-stage renal disease [76]

1 Enhance patient and family understanding about illness and end-of-life issues including prognosis and likely outcomes of alternative plans of care.[3]
2 Define the patient's key priorities in end-of-life care and develop a care plan that addresses these issues.[16]
3 Enhance patient autonomy by shaping future clinical care to fit the patient's preferences and values.
4 Improve the process of healthcare decision-making generally, including patient and family satisfaction.[16]
5 Specify a proxy for future medical decision-making.
6 Help the proxy understand their role in future medical decision-making.
7 Promote shared understanding of relevant values and preferences amongst the patient, proxy, and healthcare providers.
8 Help patients find hope and meaning in life and help them achieve a sense of spiritual peace. [13,17]
9 Explore ways to ease emotional and financial burdens borne by patients and families.[13,16]
10 Strengthen relationships with loved ones.[13,16]

Central to end-of-life decision-making is the discussion of clinical circumstances and prognosis, and the understanding of patients' values and goals within this clinical context. ACP is a process that involves ongoing reflection, understanding, discussion, and communication amongst a patient, their family, and healthcare staff for the purpose of clarifying values, treatment preferences, and goals for EoL care.[16,17] ACP emphasizes not only decisions about whether to use a treatment but also practical arrangements, and includes attention to ethical, psychosocial, and spiritual issues which relate to starting, withholding, and stopping treatments such as dialysis.[10,16,17,18] Although often encouraged, ADs are only one optional component within the broader range of ACP. The goals of ACP in ESRD are outlined in Table 4.1.

4.3 **The ethics of advance care planning**

ACP is grounded in the ethical principles of patient autonomy and respect for persons. Patient autonomy implies that every person has the right to self-determination with the view that the patient is usually the best person to make healthcare decisions for themself. Medical ethics, law, and professional policy require that medical professionals not only refrain from carrying out unwanted interventions by obtaining patients' consent for medical procedures but that they also promote patients' ability to make informed decisions.[19,20] When an intervention will not achieve the patient's goals, care should shift to other treatments including palliative care.

Patients without capacity have the same rights to self-determination and respect for persons as patients with capacity. Part of the vision of ACP is to extend patients' control over their medical care at a time when they are not able to voice their preferences by permitting surrogates to make decisions that the patient would have made for himself or herself.[21] The surrogate decision-maker, therefore, should be the person with the best knowledge of the patient's specific wishes, or of the patient's values and beliefs, as they pertain to the present situation. When the patient's wishes, values, or beliefs are not clear or known, the surrogate should make decisions in the best interest of the patient. In the UK, only someone with a personal welfare LPA can make decisions for the patient who has lost capacity. However, health professionals must make a decision in the patient's 'best interests' taking into account views expressed by the patient in any advance statements and those of close family and carers.

Cultural values play an important role in ACP and the usefulness of ACP is not limited to those who value individualism. The grounding ethical principle of respect for persons mandates that ACP extend to those whose cultural values emphasize interdependence and the well-being of the family or community as a whole.

4.4 Limitations of advance directives: why they do not work

Historically, the value of an AD was felt to lie in the preservation of patient autonomy via communication to physicians of patients' preferences for future care in the event of incapacity. However, ADs have failed to promote incapacitated patients' autonomy as they do not appear to drive EoL care.[22,23] ADs have failed to improve surrogate decision-makers' knowledge of patients' values and preferences for EoL care[24,25] and have failed to enhance communication between patients and physicians about EoL care.[25,26] Most importantly, ADs have failed to improve the quality of EoL care.[27] The well-known *Study to Understand Prognoses and Preferences for Outcomes and Risks of Treatments* (SUPPORT) study found that the completion of AD forms which were made available to patients' physicians had no impact on the incidence or timing of 'do-not-resuscitate' orders, or on the doctors' reported knowledge of patients' preferences.[25]

Many of the limitations of ADs (Table 4.2) stem from the fact that the completion of an AD in no way ensures that the discussion of patients' values in the context of their clinical circumstances has occurred. Autonomy requires that individuals critically assess their own values and preferences. Not everyone has well-formed preferences about future care prior to being asked. Moreover, all potential future clinical circumstances cannot be anticipated; there is often insufficient knowledge to permit decision-making within the context of individual patients' goals, values, and culture. Effective ACP, therefore, must incorporate an individual's core values within the context of their illness.

However, the value of ACP extends beyond promoting patient autonomy in the event of future incapacitation (Table 4.1). There is a compelling need for ESRD patients to think about the future direction of their medical care even if they should remain competent. In a medical crisis, patients may be emotionally incapable of objectively weighing the benefits and burdens of treatment options and may defer decision-making to their physician or family members. The focus at such

Table 4.2 Limitations of advance directives

1 AD documents provide guidance for only a limited set of future medical possibilities.

2 Preferences for life-sustaining treatment appear to depend on the context in which they are made. [145]

3 Some patients have limited desire to exert specific control over end-of-life medical decision-making and would prefer instead to leave future specific decisions to their families or physicians.[83,91,146]

4 Proxy decision-makers may have difficulty interpreting and converting patients' documented treatment preferences into clinical decisions.[64,147]

5 Healthcare providers do not consistently follow ADs.

6 Patients have difficulty predicting their future treatment preferences.[22]

7 Expressed preferences may be subjugated to physician influence concerning the clinical appropriateness of life-sustaining treatment.[148–150]

8 Healthcare providers may be unaware of the existence of an AD.

9 The AD may not be available to clinicians or the proxy when needed.

times is typically short-term rather than long-term prognosis and there is often insufficient time or knowledge to consider the natural history of the patient's underlying disease or the effect of the interaction of multiple co-morbidities.[28] Finally, it takes time for patients to grasp and process the significance of their illness and prognosis and to be able to incorporate this knowledge into meaningful choices for care.

4.5 The current state of advance care planning in end-stage renal disease

Although most dialysis patients support the idea of ACP, not all patients will wish to complete an AD. Only 6–51% of dialysis patients complete ADs, and there are no data indicating how many patients undergo the full process of ACP.[29–31] Dialysis patients' ADs tend to outline limited treatment options and do not typically discuss or consider withdrawal of dialysis.[32,33] Most chronic dialysis patients report never having discussed with their nephrologist or family the circumstances in which dialysis treatment should be discontinued.[31] In fact, dialysis patients often do not know that they have the option to withdraw from dialysis.[32] They typically do not view themselves as having a terminal illness, and many mistakenly assume they can be kept alive indefinitely on dialysis.[31–33] Issues relating to death and dying are commonly avoided until late in the illness when patients may no longer be competent to make decisions for themselves. The majority of patients lack decision-making capacity at the time the decision to withdraw dialysis is made.[34]

Cardiopulmonary resuscitation (CPR) rarely extends survival for dialysis patients.[35–37] Unfortunately, most dialysis patients have poor knowledge of their chance of survival following CPR and, as a result, relatively few dialysis patients choose a 'do-not-resuscitate' order.[38,39]

4.5.1 Clinical correlates of advance directives in end-stage renal disease

Within the context of ESRD, being male, having a higher level of education, a poorer perceived health-related quality of life, and being approached in hospital (i.e. in a context in which ADs are potentially seen by patients as being more relevant) are factors associated with completing an AD.[31,40] Most patients who ultimately make the decision to stop dialysis do not seem to be influenced by major depression or suicidal ideation.[41] Duration of dialysis ≥4 years and prior experience with CPR increase the probability of refusing CPR by 12 times.[42] Up to 83% of ESRD patients request that physicians periodically check with them to determine if their EoL-care preferences have changed.[42]

4.5.2 How end-of-life decisions are currently being made

Most dialysis patients do not have ADs and do not discuss circumstances in which they would no longer wish dialysis to be continued. Despite this, the second leading cause of death for chronic dialysis patients is withdrawal from dialysis and, at the time the decision is made to withdraw dialysis, the majority of patients are no longer competent or involved in the decision-making. Together, these facts are not conducive for quality EoL care. Unfortunately, surrogates often lack knowledge of patients' values and preferences for EoL care, including patients' valuations of various heath states.[43,44] Neither family members nor physicians are accurate in their predictions of patients' desires about life-sustaining treatments, including wishes for ongoing dialysis. (24;45) Spouses consistently overestimate patients' desires to continue dialysis across hypothetical health conditions.[46] For example, in a Japanese study of 398 pairs of dialysis patients and a family member, only 50% of family members correctly predicted the patient's current preference for CPR, 44% their wish for dialysis in a severely demented state, and 47% their wish for dialysis if they had terminal cancer. The corresponding figures for physicians were 44%, 47%, and 43%.[47]

Although little is known about how EoL discussions are handled between nephrologists and ESRD patients, the general literature illustrates that the majority of EoL discussions do not provide essential information to inform care at the end of life. Physicians tend to do most of the talking. They focus on pejorative descriptions of life-sustaining treatments rather than desired outcomes and fail to articulate a set of positive treatment objectives to frame the discussion of forgoing life-sustaining treatment.[48–51] Prognosis, spirituality, religion, and what dying may be like is often not addressed.[52] Patients' values are rarely explored and discussions do not distinguish amongst treatments patients may want to forgo now versus treatment they would want to forgo if they were to become worse (e.g. comatose).[48–50]

4.6 Barriers to effective advance care planning

Patient- and physician-related barriers to effective ACP in ESRD are outlined in Table 4.3. Patients' psychosocial adjustment substantially impacts the quality of an illness experience. [17,53–55] Coping strategies and concepts such as 'hope' and 'denial' affect overall psychosocial adjustment.[56] Since the majority of dialysis patients appear to either deny or be unaware of possible imminent death, it is believed that denial-like coping mechanisms may be used commonly to adapt to life on dialysis.[31–33,57–60] While denial may be an effective coping mechanism early in the illness-trajectory when the diagnosis is overwhelming and there has been insufficient time to adapt, ongoing denial may present a barrier to effective ACP. Most dialysis patients are uncomfortable initiating EoL care discussions despite having strong EoL care preferences and a

Table 4.3 Barriers to effective advance care planning and advance directive completion

Patient-Related Barriers

1 Inadequate knowledge about ACP and how to complete an AD.[151]
2 Perception that ACP and ADs are difficult to facilitate and/or execute.
3 Perception that even if completed, AD statements will not be followed by clinicians.
4 Reluctance to broach the issue of 'death' and end-of-life planning.
5 Belief that it is the physician's responsibility to initiate end-of-life discussions.
6 Lack of insight into health status and prognosis and a false sense that ACP is not relevant for their care.[22,151]
7 View that ACP is unnecessary because one's family or provider will 'know' what to do.

Physician-Related Barriers

8 Lack of training and comfort with end-of-life decision-making.[151,152]
9 Lack of familiarity with suitable alternatives to aggressive treatment.[153]
10 Belief that ACP discussions are not needed.[153]
11 Belief that patients and families do not want these discussions.[153]
12 Concern that discussing end-of-life issues while embarking on a life-sustaining therapy such as dialysis may destroy hope.[151]
13 Time constraints.[151]
14 Postponing end-of-life discussions until patients are too ill to fully participate in the discussions.[89]

desire to talk about these issues. They trust that their healthcare providers will initiate these discussions when they become relevant to their care.[16] Unfortunately, many healthcare providers are unwilling to initiate these discussions in a timely manner.[63]

4.6.1 Stability of patients' end-of-life preferences

The stability of patients' preferences for EoL care is unclear. The phenomenon of 'response shift' in which patients facing declining health status 'downsize' their perceptions of what is a reasonable quality of life, may lead to fundamental changes in medical decision-making.[64]

Data specific to the stability of ESRD patients' EoL preferences are not available. Several studies of elderly or chronically ill patients demonstrated modest stability in preferences over periods of up to 2 years[51,63–65] while others found patients' preferences change during the progression of an illness, thus necessitating ongoing discussion and updating of preferences.[66,67] The manner in which treatment information is presented, the course of disease progression, and patient characteristics can all influence patient decision-making[68] and the stability of preferences for EoL care.[21,63,69–73] Change in cognitive status appears to be particularly important in predicting a change in EoL-care preferences.[66,68,69,74] However, in patients ≥65 years of age, most (85%) who had chosen to forego life-sustaining treatments maintain that choice 2 years later.[75] In addition, patients with a living will are less likely to change their wishes (14% vs. 41%).[75]

4.7 New approaches to facilitate advance care planning in end-stage renal disease

Physicians have typically borne the responsibility of initiating and facilitating ACP with patients and their families. However, unlike other interventions, there are no standards of care about when to initiate or how to conduct these discussions. ESRD patients' perspectives of the salient elements of ACP discussions and their preferences with regard to how ACP should be facilitated by the healthcare team have recently been explored.[1.6,76]

4.7.1 When to initiate advance care planning

It needs to be recognized that a certain proportion of dialysis patients have minimal co-morbidity and/or are eligible to receive a kidney transplant, which, if obtained, would substantially change their quality of life and mortality risk. Not all of these patients would benefit as greatly from ACP and they are likely to be less interested in participating in it. Unfortunately, there are no data in ESRD to clearly identify which patients would most benefit from ACP.

The pattern of rapid functional decline that occurs in the last 3 months of life for most cancer patients is generally recognized by patients, family, and healthcare providers as the beginning of the dying process.[74,77,78] Thus, discussions with regard to the appropriateness of treatment options during this time are held with the recognition that death is approaching. In contrast, ESRD is characterized by progressive physical decline that is often protracted over years and punctuated by episodes of life-threatening exacerbations and complications. ESRD patients, their families, and physicians are more likely to have difficulty recognizing when such a patient is dying, and by implication, when EoL decision-making should occur. ACP is, therefore, best initiated early with ongoing communication and re-evaluation throughout the illness trajectory. [3] Sentinel events (hospitalizations, acute illnesses, etc.) present opportunities to engage in ACP. Answering no to a simple 'surprise question' ("Would you be surprised if this patient died within the next 6 months or 1 year?") should prompt nephrologists and dialysis-care-unit team members to initiate ACP discussions.[79,80] Ideally these discussions should be part of the educational process that occurs when patients are presented with dialysis options.[16]

Given that the majority of patients lack decision-making capacity at the time the decision to withdraw dialysis is made,[34] ACP should occur earlier in the illness while comprehension and decision-making capacity are preserved.

Patients are less concerned than physicians that EoL-care discussions will damage hope.[81] Many dialysis patients have already considered EoL options[17,81,82] and welcome the opportunity to engage in these discussions with their physician.[49,81] In one study, the vast majority of dialysis patients (97%) wanted to be given life-expectancy information, and for the physician to do so without having to be prompted.[83] These findings parallel those of other elderly or chronically ill patients. Ninety-three percent of surrogate decision-makers of incapacitated patients in intensive care units (ICUs) felt that avoiding discussions about prognosis was an unacceptable way to maintain hope and that these discussions were essential to allow family members to prepare emotionally and logistically for the possibility of a patient's death.[84] In a study of primary-care patients, most felt that EoL discussions should occur at an earlier time – earlier in the natural history of disease when the patient is healthy, and earlier in the patient–physician relationship than did primary-care physicians.[85] Physicians need to be aware, however, that not all patients are ready to engage in ACP. In the SUPPORT study,[86] 707 of 1832 seriously ill patients did not wish to discuss their preferences for resuscitation. These patients perceived they had better prognosis than patients who wished to discuss their resuscitation preferences. Patients' reluctance to discuss EoL issues may reflect a perception that these issues are not yet relevant to their care.

4.7.2 Who all to involve in advance care planning

ESRD patients feel their nephrologists are responsible for initiating and facilitating ACP, mainly because physicians are seen as the primary source of information central to this process.[16] This is similar to primary care and elderly patients who agree that it is the physician's responsibility to initiate these discussions and typically respond favourably to physician-initiated EoL discussions, even in the context of routine clinic visits.[85,87–89] However, not all patients want to talk extensively with their physicians about ACP. Some ESRD patients view conversations with their loved ones as the most valuable piece of ACP.[16,69] One study showed that 50% of chronic dialysis patients discussed their preferences for EoL care with family members compared to 6% of patients with their physicians ($p < 0.001$) and that more patients wanted to include family members in future discussions than physicians (91% vs. 36%; $p < 0.001$).[90] ESRD patients are also comfortable with legislation in North America that grants their family leeway in EoL decision-making in the event of their own incapacity.[90,91] In a study of 150 dialysis patients, 42% indicated they wanted their surrogates to have leeway to override their ADs.[68,82] Health professionals, therefore, must be prepared to initiate EoL conversations and then step back while these conversations proceed outside of the patient–health professional relationship. However, as outlined below, research in ESRD clearly supports a role for physicians much greater than merely introducing the topic and encouraging patients to discuss the salient issues with their families. There will be dialysis patients who require more active engagement with their healthcare providers to help them reflect on and work through EoL issues.[16] Social workers or spiritual counselors may be particularly helpful in these cases.

4.7.3 Information-giving during the advance-care-planning process

Dialysis patients experience substantial fear and uncertainty about their future which they often do not disclose to their healthcare providers.[16] Clear, honest discussions about prognosis and future care have been shown to be a critical element of the ACP process for patients with ESRD. Such discussions promote self-reliance, alleviate fear and uncertainty, help prepare for the future, including death, and give dialysis patients the knowledge to make decisions compatible with their values and beliefs.[16] This process of information-giving was also seen as key to building trusting relationships with the nephrology team. Varying amounts of time are required for this process to be effective and some patients will choose not to participate.

Physicians typically do not provide the information that patients believe is fundamental to EoL discussions (see Section 4.5.2). Dialysis patients want straightforward and honest discussions on expected outcomes of EoL care rather than on technical processes.[81] Patients require information about how medical interventions will impact their daily lives and help them achieve personal goals.[16] Health states and severity of illness influence EoL preferences far more than treatment descriptions.[92] These findings are consistent with a study that showed that the majority of elderly patients who initially opted for CPR decided to forego CPR after learning the probability of survival following CPR.[68]

The framing of EoL discussions will have a substantial impact on the decisions patients and surrogates make. It has been suggested that for patients with an extremely poor prognosis, such as end-stage dementia – where it has been documented that the majority of patients would not prefer to receive CPR, that the default approach should be flipped so that resuscitation would routinely be withheld unless the patient or surrogate specifically requested otherwise.[91] Whilst this is a contentious issue for policy implementation, it may offer an alternative clinical approach for patients who are clearly dying and would benefit from a transition to a more palliative approach to care. Potential advantages include minimizing the guilt-laden process of withholding or withdrawing life-prolonging treatments experienced by surrogates while preserving clinical care that is consistent with the preferences of most patients (while still allowing for the minority's preferences).

4.7.4 How to facilitate advance care planning

Table 4.4 highlights some of the necessary steps for facilitating effective ACP.

4.7.4.1 Patient participation

Attention to patient participation is central to facilitated ACP and focusses on a sixfold process as outlined in Table 4.4.[76] Depression, denial, or cognitive dysfunction may prevent meaningful participation in ACP. Unfortunately, there is little consensus or clinically relevant empirical data about how to assess a patient's understanding of specific treatment decisions.[94] Effective ACP may be jeopardized due to patients' lack of interest or their perception that their opinions or wishes are either unimportant or will not alter the EoL care they will receive. Determining the 'perception of potential benefits' of ACP for individual patients is perhaps the most under recognized aspect of patient participation and potentially the most crucial. Dialysis patients identify ACP as an important part of medical care if they understand how the process benefits them; they are less likely to engage actively in a process from which no benefit is perceived.[16] The patient's vantage point and agenda need to be the focus for initiating ACP.[16,17] ACP facilitators must also identify the patient's support system and the resources required by and available to individual patients to enable them to effectively participate in ACP. Lastly, determining who patients want to involve in this process will help define the roles of various healthcare providers such as nephrologists, social workers, and nurses.

4.7.4.2 Decision-making and defining priorities for goals of care

(i) **Understanding illness:** In order to plan effectively for EoL care, patients and/or families need to understand how illness and various treatment options will affect them in their daily lives (Table 4.4). Encouraging individuals to describe their illness beliefs along five dimensions (identity,

Table 4.4 Key elements to facilitate effective advance care planning in end-stage renal disease

Patient participation

1 Determine the patient's *ability* to be involved in ACP

2 Determine the patient's interest in participating in ACP

3 Determine the patient's *perception* of level of control and power

4 Determine the patient's *perception of potential benefits* of participation in ACP

5 Determine the patient's *resources* to participate in ACP

6 Identify *whom* the patient wishes to engage in ACP

Decision-making and defining priorities for goals of care

1 Measure *understanding* of illness

2 Determine *how* patients expect to make decisions

3 Determine *expectations* regarding outcomes of end-of-life care

4 Determine patient *values* that drive end-of-life preferences

Patient–physician relationship

1 Use of lay language to promote understanding

2 Empathetic listening

3 Affirm patients' self-worth

4 Maintain trust, honesty, promise keeping, confidentiality, and caring

Documentation

1 Easily identifiable

2 Travel with the patient across healthcare settings so it is available for all professional care-givers involved in the care of the patient.

Quality improvement

cause, time-line, consequences, and cure/control) can highlight existing beliefs that are barriers to effective coping. Information can then be presented in a highly contextual manner to influence, replace, or modify existing beliefs.[95,96] Although physicians should avoid depriving their patients of hope, an unrealistic appraisal of a patient's health status, or no appraisal at all, may result in burdensome treatment that will not achieve the patient's goals. A recent study affirms the necessity of providing truthful prognostic information to designated decision-makers and that such information does not destroy hope.[17] Throughout this process, patients need to be assured that they will not be abandoned and that every effort will be made to support their goals of care. These goals of care – within the context of a solid knowledge of their illness – are used as guidelines to delineate a specific plan of treatment when faced with the need for specific decision-making.[28]

(ii) How patients expect decisions to be made: It is important to determine the role the patient wants in decision-making and to ensure that the ACP process supports the patient's preferred decision-making methods. Some patients prefer to make their own decisions while others may rely more extensively on family or healthcare professionals: in such cases, education may need to focus more heavily on surrogate decision-makers. The degree of authority the patient wants the surrogate to have must be communicated to the surrogate in order to increase the surrogate's confidence in decisions that might have to be made at a future time. The locus of decision-making may shift as events occur, resulting in stress for families. Even for patients who wish to maintain control over decisions, identifying individuals they perceive to be important and clearly defining their roles (e.g. whether they provide information, opinion, support, pressure) for the patient will be helpful. Many of these patients still expect health professionals to guide them through the ACP process. Perceiving the full burden of decision-making to be entirely theirs often leads to feelings of isolation and uncertainty.[16] Some dialysis patients have reported family as a barrier to ACP; they fear that family may be upset by the process of ACP or uncomfortable with the topic. These patients expressed feelings of isolation and hopelessness when they were not able to honestly and openly discuss their hopes and fears for the future with loved ones.[16] Facilitators need to provide a platform in which to engage family in these conversations in a supportive environment.

(iii) Expectations for end-of-life care: ACP facilitators ought to explore patients' and surrogates' expectations for both outcomes of care and the role they expect care providers to fill. This affords an opportunity to re-examine the understanding of their illness and explore unrealistic expectations or misconceptions. It also allows for an exploration of goals of care. It is clear that EoL-care goals reflect expectations which must be balanced with adequate knowledge. Identifying discordance between patient and care-provider expectations allows an opportunity for re-alignment of expectations and goals of care and helps minimize future conflict surrounding EoL decisions.

(iv) Values that drive end-of-life preferences: If knowledge is one major driver of patients' EoL preferences, values is the other. The questions asked in the process of facilitated ACP should be designed to help the patient explore what they guard most closely and rely upon most heavily. This will be discovery for some and patients will have to work with the healthcare team to discover how their values shape their goals for care. One approach is to ground the conversation in people's lives. An example of this would be to review how past difficult events in their lives have been managed, why those particular events held importance, who were the recurrent players in these events and why. To keep these discussions outcome-focussed, disease-specific scenarios addressing unique health states the patient may experience and the related treatment choices can be used. The decisions related to each of these scenarios reflect the patient's perception of what living well means and can provide the basis for a surrogate's decision if needed in the future.[95] Decisions will typically be based on the prioritization of goals such as maximizing comfort, maintaining function, and prolonging life. Through these discussions, patients and their surrogates come to understand what is truly important to the patient and to understand their choices in new ways. Potential questions that can help explore the various aspects of facilitated ACP are outlined in Table 4.5.

4.7.4.3 Communication skills and the patient–physician relationship

Language is a powerful tool in facilitated ACP: medical jargon has the potential to cause confusion and misunderstanding. Dialysis patients clearly appreciate staff that are comfortable in discussing EoL issues.[16] Dialysis patients do not view facilitated ACP as merely an information-giving session or as a way of providing solutions to all their EoL concerns. They stress the importance and acknowledge the therapeutic benefit of empathetic listening and view facilitated ACP as an opportunity to build trusting relationships with the healthcare team. Interviewing skills that focus on empathy and strong reflective listening can be taught.[97–100] The self-worth of patients is affirmed when healthcare professionals reassure patients about the appropriateness of their EoL preferences and commend them for their efforts in their ongoing self-care.[16]

4.4.4.4 Documentation and quality improvement

Documentation of ACP is important to communicate key issues and specific treatment decisions that may arise from the process. Those who are involved in ACP discussions with patients and

Table 4.5 Advance care planning approach for patients with end-stage renal disease[76]

1. Participation: Provides a measure of **ability** to be involved in ACP; **interest** in participating; **perception** of level of control/power; **perceived benefits** of participation, and **resources** to participate.

Prompts	Follow-Up
ABILITY Clinically assess cognitive capacity to participate in ACP	Many dialysis patient have cognitive impairment and assessing cognitive capacity is especially important prior to conducting ACP.[1] Psychiatric assessment may be required "Are you depressed/anxious?"
INTEREST "Do you think it is important to participate actively in decisions that affect you? Your end-of-life care?" "Do you spend time thinking about your health and your future?"	"YES": probe reasons why: indicates **perceived benefits** "NO": probe reasons why • Depression, denial, lack of trust, need for privacy etc • Other possible barriers: see **perception, resources,** and **perceived benefits** • Are there individuals they discuss health issues with? May indicate those with whom decision making may be shared and a potential surrogate decision-maker.
PERCEPTION (control/power) "Do you think that your health providers want to know what you think about end-of-life care?" "Do you think sharing your preferences makes a difference to the care you receive?" "Do you have enough information to participate?"	"YES" indicates perception of personal importance in participation in the ACP process. "NO" indicates barriers that need to be addressed for effective ACP. • Symptoms of depression negatively affect perception of control
PERCEIVED BENEFITS "What benefits do you expect from ACP? For yourself? For others?" "What concerns you the most about end-of-life care? About dying?"	This helps determine patient-specific value in ACP. Examples: • Avoid pain and suffering • Avoid prolongation of dying • Avoid specific health states such as coma, severe dementia or technologies such as ventilation, admission to the intensive care unit etc.... • Relieve burden on loved ones • Maintain control, dignity • Strengthen relationships with loved ones

(Continued)

Table 4.5 (continued) Advance care planning approach for patients with end-stage renal disease[76]

Prompts	Follow-Up
RESOURCES **Personal (Internal):** "What experience do you have in making health-related choices?" (For self or others) "What decisions should be made alone? With others?" "Generally, do you have difficulty or feel anxious making tough decisions?" **External:** "How would you go about gathering information to make a decision about your care or treatment?" "Are there challenges or people in your day-to-day life that interfere with or limit your choices?"	Follow-up questions should assess: **Personal:** • Language barriers; literary barriers • Social isolation • Religious or Spiritual Issues • Cultural issues (language, education, beliefs) • Others (e.g. conflicting care-giving responsibilities, co-morbidities (esp. psychiatric) **External:** • Access to information/advice • Social support • Support groups • Accommodation • Care-giver Stress/Support • Home Care Involvement • Financial Status/Concerns • Family: family dynamics; concern for survivors • Legal issues • Transportation; geographic barriers • Others?

2. Patient Decision Making & Defining Priorities for Goals of Care: Determine **understanding** of current situation; **how** patients expect to make decisions ("Locus of Control"); **expectations** for various outcomes; and **values** as they relate to desirability and importance of certain outcomes.

Prompt	Follow-Up
UNDERSTANDING Have patient review current health status including: • mental health • overall health related quality of life Have patients review their understanding of: • current treatment and its purpose • treatment options: include options of no dialysis; trials of dialysis; when to stop dialysis • Prognosis Assess family perceptions where possible • note any gaps between family's and patient's responses	• Investigate sources of information • Query extent of communication between patient and physician – i.e. "Have you communicated current concerns to your physician" • Assist patient to develop a list of questions and to develop a plan to obtain answers if indicated • Facilitate discussion of prognostic information with their physician • Provide clarification, corrections, additional information if requested and/or if indicated • To test understanding, it is useful to ask patients "How serious is your illness?"
LOCUS OF CONTROL "How do you make medical (end-of-life) decisions? – i.e. alone or consider the opinions of others, or let others make decisions for you?" "Are there people you want involved in making end-of-life decisions?"	"Have you thought about whom you would want to be with you if you became very ill for a period of time?" "If someone had to make a decision on your behalf, who would be the best person for that job? Why?" "Who's likely to be there?" "Are there people you would not want to be present? Why?"
EXPECTATIONS "Ideally, what would you like your current treatment to achieve?" "Realistically, what do you expect it to achieve?" "Have you set goals for yourself with respect to • Your health? • Your family? • Your job? • Other?	"What do you expect of your health care providers: Availability? Information provision? Participation in decision- making?" • Review personal and external resources that could be employed to support desired out-come (see 1. **Participation**, "**Resources**" section) • Determine what care plan would support those goals.

(Continued)

Table 4.5 (continued) Advance care planning approach for patients with end-stage renal disease[76]

PROMPT	FOLLOW-UP
VALUES "How have you dealt with loss/death in the past?" • "What do you wish had been different?" • "What was OK for them, but would not be OK for you? "What do you miss most about being well?" "How do you want to live when you may be very ill and may not recover?" "If you become very ill, what parts of your life are most important for you to protect – e.g. memory, physical ability, relationships, etc.?" "What would be intolerable to endure toward the end of life?" "Are there certain treatments that you think you would never want?" Why?" "What's most important to your treatment of your illness" "What do you think your family/loved ones would want for you?" Do you anticipate disagreements? What? Between whom? Why?"	"Have you made specific decisions that relate to the care you want at the end of your life?" • If patient is on or considering dialysis, is there a point at which he/she would want it to be stopped? When? Why? Case-specific scenarios can be used: • "If you had a serious complication such as a stroke or heart attack resulting in a prolonged hospital stay and many medical interventions with a less than 5% chance of survival, what would you do?" • "If you had a serious complication and a good chance of survival but were faced with permanent disabilities (unable to speak, walk or know who you are) that would require 24 hour nursing care, what would you want?" • "If you have a sudden event that causes you heart and breathing to stop and your chance for survival is low, what would you do?" Have they discussed this with anyone else?

families should familiarize themselves with facility/programme policies and guidelines that may limit the scope of their involvement in the actual drafting of ADs. The initiation of a new ACP programme should be accompanied by a comprehensive evaluation process that can guide future programme enhancement.

4.7.4.5 Conflict resolution

Conflicts around EoL decisions often occur in the setting of poor provider–patient communication and lack of ACP. Conflicts typically arise from inadequate knowledge or misunderstandings/disagreements about fundamental values and are a source of substantial distress for healthcare providers, patients, and families.[101] When disagreements persist, a negotiated solution should be sought. If necessary, seek the services of someone trained in conflict mediation such as a clinical bioethicist, social worker, or psychologist.[101]

4.8 Cultural differences that influence advance care planning

Some research suggests that ADs are not compatible with the cultural traditions of some patients. [22,102] Several dimensions involved in EoL care vary culturally; these include: concept of autonomy, decision-making models, communication of bad news, and attitudes towards ACP and EoL care.[103]

4.8.1 Cultural differences in autonomy and decision-making models

The concept of autonomy best highlights the contrast between Western and many non-Western cultures. Many non-Western cultures, such as traditional Chinese culture, view the person as a 'relational-self' – a self for whom social relationships, rather than individualism, provide the basis for moral judgements.[104] In a similar manner, Hindu and Sikh bioethics is primarily duty based; the person is seen as intimately integrated with family, community, and environment. [105] From these perspectives, an insistence on self-determination erodes the value placed on personal interconnectedness, challenging the assumption that the patient is best suited to make his or her own medical decisions. Different views of autonomy result in substantial differences in decision-making models in which the family may function as both the collective decision-maker and the conduit for moral and social norms.[103] The North American Aboriginal concept of autonomy includes respect for interpersonal relationships and non-interference[106] where persuading, or even advising in some cases, is 'undesirable behaviour'.[107] Yet despite the importance of non-interference, the value placed on interpersonal relationships results in most Aboriginal patients preferring that family be intimately involved in EoL decision-making. [106,108] Korean Americans and Mexican Americans also tend to operate within a more family-centred model of decision-making compared to European Americans and Blacks. Consequently, healthcare providers must recognize that many patients, particularly from non-Western cultures, may prefer that family or community drive decision-making and co-ordinate future patient care, even when the patient is competent.[103]

4.8.2 Cultural issues relating to communication of bad news

Some Aboriginal and Asian cultures prohibit explicit references to dying based on an interpretative framework in which language has the capacity to create reality.[109] Positive thinking is felt to promote health while truth-telling (of bad news) is viewed as disrespectful as it could shorten the life of the patient. This can make it difficult to discuss survival and natural history of the illness directly with the patient. Healthcare providers need to understand that, in some contexts, it may be appropriate for family to communicate prognostic information and manage most of the ACP discussions, allowing them to balance hope with the 'bad news'.

4.8.3 Cultural differences in attitudes to advance care planning and end-of-life care

Racial and ethnic differences may substantially impact the process of ACP. In North America, research has demonstrated that Blacks, Hispanics, and Whites all appear to agree with the purpose of ACP.[110] However, most studies have found that Blacks and Hispanics are less likely than Whites to engage in ACP or to complete ADs.[111–114] Communication of values and goals of care may be particularly difficult for those of whom English is a second language. The designation of a healthcare surrogate was the most common form of AD in Blacks and Hispanics.[110] It has been shown that non-White racial groups are less knowledgeable about ADs[110,112] and more frequently learn about ADs from the media rather than from their physicians. Hispanics are more likely to prefer family-centred decision-making than other racial groups[112] and are more likely to defer decisions to their families.[110] Blacks are more likely to feel that they would receive less care if they had an AD than Hispanics and Whites.[110]

Cultural variations in the concept of autonomy, decision-making, and the meaning of illness clearly have implications for ACP. Given the high prevalence of ESRD in many ethnic minority groups, the ACP process must be sensitive to these cultural contexts.

4.9 Interventions to increase the use and effectiveness of advance care planning

There is a paucity of data on how to increase the use and value of ACP. The literature has focussed primarily on efforts to increase the completion of ADs – a fundamentally flawed endeavour given that the completion of an AD does not guarantee that the critical components of ACP have been addressed.[96] Efforts to increase AD completion have primarily been educational interventions. These were more likely to elicit patient preferences for EoL care when severely ill patients were targeted (i.e. there was clear clinical relevance) and when multi-component approaches were used in the context of ongoing discussions (i.e. ACP).[27,115,116] A retrospective audit of a community-wide education programme integrating ACP found AD completion increased from 15% to 85% during the intervention; the median time between AD documentation and death was 1.2 years. Almost all ADs requested that treatment be forgone as death neared, and treatment followed these instructions in 98% of cases.[117] Educational interventions in isolation have been mostly unsuccessful in altering either attitudes to or completion of ADs.[115] Providing dialysis patients with written material on ADs does not alter attitudes to ADs and only transiently improves perceived understanding of EoL-care issues.[118] A randomized, controlled trial of 203 dialysis patients found that peer mentoring increased completion of ADs, increased comfort discussing ADs, and improved subjective well-being and anxiety among the Black participants. These benefits of peer mentoring were not observed among the White patients.[45] It remains unclear how best to increase the prevalence of effective facilitated ACP in patients with ESRD.

Increasing the use and effectiveness of ACP will require substantial behavioural change. Health information technology, social marketing, and legal intervention/policy change are three mechanisms proposed to induce such behavioural change.[119] Health information technology may facilitate completion and implementation of ADs by providing automated reminders, sharing information across providers with a uniform instrument, and promoting adherence to guideline-based care.[120] Automated physician reminders of ADs resulted in an almost eightfold increase in the odds of having an AD discussion with 45% of these discussions resulting in the completion of an AD.[121] Another study evaluated a multifaceted automated intervention that not only prompted physicians to have ACP discussions but also sent out educational material on ADs to patients prior to their appointment with their physician.[122] This resulted in more ACP discussions (64% vs. 38%, $p < 0.001$) and more documentation of these discussions (47% vs. 24%, $p < 0.001$).

Social marketing is the planning and implementation of programmes designed to bring about voluntary social/behavioural change and has proven successful in achieving behavioural change with respect to other health issues. The "Respecting Choices" campaign in the United States is an example of social marketing that was successful in positively influencing both patient and care-provider thinking around ACP and ADs.[117,123] Legislative changes and the development of policy are typically required to encourage and guide these processes. However, it has yet to be determined how health information technology, social marketing, and policy changes in the context of ACP in ESRD will influence actual EoL care.

4.10 Role of legislation and policy in advance care planning

4.10.1 Legal aspects and policy of advance care planning in North America

In the US, the Patient Self-Determination Act of 1990 failed to increase the completion of ADs; so the utility of legislative actions to mandate ACP remains questionable. Many factors have contributed to the general failure of ADs, including the inconsistent honouring of ADs and the failure of ADs to accompany patients across sites of care. In an effort to ensure that patients' wishes for life-sustaining care and interventions are honoured, the POLST (Physicians Orders for Life Sustaining Treatment) programme was developed in Oregon and the form was released in 1995.[124] These documents were designed to convert patients' treatment preferences into medical orders that are transferable throughout the healthcare system. POLST is now used by all hospices in Oregon and by 95% of nursing homes. Seven states and a few municipalities use some form of POLST, and in 18 states POLST is under development (www.polst.org).[125] Local regulations and statutes dictate the form of the document. Most of the POLST documents are composed of four sections addressing resuscitation status, medical interventions (comfort care only, limited, or aggressive interventions), antibiotics, and artificial hydration and nutrition. The final section of the one-page document notes the decision-makers for the documented goals of care and assigns some reason for the choices (patient's request or known preference, patient's best interests, medical futility, etc.). Signatures of the physician (or physician assistant or nurse practitioner) and patient or patient surrogate complete the document.

Every province and territory in Canada (with the exception of Nunavut) has legislation giving legal recognition to the appointment of a healthcare agent or proxy.[126] ADs are also widely accepted not only as a way to identify preferences for EoL care but also as a general framework for decision-making near the end of life. Even in the absence of legislation, it is now fairly clear that at common law a patient's previously stated wishes with respect to EoL decisions, expressed at a time when the patient was competent, have legal force and must be respected.[126]

4.10.2 Legal aspects and policy of advance care planning in the United Kingdom

The UK has seen a movement in the last 50 years from clinicians emphasizing 'best interests' decision-making to promoting patients' autonomy and involvement at all stages of their care and treatment. The roots of this transformation relate to societal and attitudinal shifts which have changed the balance of power between medicine and the public. The highly publicized framework of the 'good death' produced by the prominent charity 'Age Concern'[127] is a prime example of the way in which pressure groups contributed to this shift. 'Age Concern' subsequently reported the case of a woman with cancer who found that a do-not-resuscitate order had been written in her notes without her knowledge.[128] This incident was followed by a public and media storm that was remarkable for its longevity. Subsequently, professional bodies published guidance that made it clear that patients and their family care-givers should be involved in care decisions.[129] There has also been a plethora of policy statements and new legislation in which 'choice' and 'control' during EoL care feature prominently.

The Mental Capacity Act[15] has, for the first time in England and Wales, created provisions for antecedent control[130] through the device of an ADRT (colloquially known as a 'living will') or an LPA. There is a great deal of work ongoing in the UK to bring these possibilities to wider awareness amongst user groups and the general public. These and wider elements of ACP, such as the development of models of communication practice and exchange in which ACP discussions are afforded a key role, have been emphasized in the first End of Life Care Strategy for England,[131] building on early work completed by a nationwide practice-development initiative – the National End of Life Care Programme.[132] Widespread practice and uptake of ACP remains to be seen although national guidelines on ACP have recently been published.[133]

4.11 Outcomes of advance care planning in end-stage renal disease

On the whole, there is little evidence of positive outcomes associated with ADs *unless* there is also supplemental work to change attitudes, influence the quality of communication between patients and their care-givers, or embed processes whereby the directive/statement is flagged in the healthcare system.

To our knowledge, there are no published clinical trials of a multidimensional ACP intervention in ESRD or of the impact of ACP on important clinical outcomes. However, there are qualitative data that strongly support the value of ACP in ESRD in that ACP allows patients to prepare for death, strengthen relationships with loved ones, achieve a sense of control, and relieve burdens placed on others.[13,16,134] There are also data that show that facilitated ACP through the provision of timely, appropriate information can positively enhance, rather than diminish, ESRD patients' hope.[16] It is recognized that hope can make a positive difference in patients' experiences with illness, facilitate the coping process, and enhance health-related quality of life. [135–138] ACP discussions may also strengthen patient–physician relationships and provide a closeness that both patients and physicians find rewarding.[16,43] In a study of 182 patients, ADs were more prevalent among chronic haemodialysis (HD) patients who withdrew from dialysis in a reconciled fashion than amongst patients who died suddenly and unexpectedly or who died without a reconciled decision to forego life-sustaining treatment.[139] Patients who had ADs were more likely to have made their own medical decisions rather than relying on relatives or other agents and tended to be those with a spouse or in a relationship.

Knowledge of the impact of ACP on EoL care for other groups of patients is also limited. A randomized, control trial executing the California Durable Power of Attorney for Health Care and having a summary placed in the patient's medical record had no effect on the well-being, health status, or medical treatments of 204 patients with life-threatening illnesses (defined by a 5-year life expectancy of no better than 50% as judged by the physician).[140]

ACP intervention using the 'Respecting Choices' programme achieved higher congruence between surrogates and patients in their understanding of patients' EoL preferences (76% vs. 55%); greater patient knowledge about ACP, less willingness to undergo life-sustaining treatments for a new serious medical problem, and less willingness to tolerate poor health states at 2 months follow-up.[141]

Prospective cohort studies indicate that ACP has positive outcomes on the limited aspects of EoL care that have been explored. Implementation of the CHOICES ACP and palliative care programme demonstrated increased hospice length of stay, less time spent in hospital, and more deaths occurring at home.[142] The systematic, community-wide Respecting Choices ACP programme showed significantly increased congruence in decision-making between patients and care-givers, and greater satisfaction with, and less conflict about, these EoL decisions.[95,123] This study included elderly patients with ESRD. POLST orders with regard to CPR were universally accepted in a study of 180 nursing-home residents. These patients received remarkably high levels of comfort care and low rates (15%) of transfer for aggressive life-extending treatments.[143] In an observational study of advanced cancer patients, EoL discussions were not associated with higher rates of major depression or worry and were associated with lower rates of ventilation, resuscitation, ICU admission, as well as earlier hospice enrollment.[144] Although this was not an interventional study and patient self-selection bias impact data, results are encouraging.

4.12 Conclusion

Traditional views of ACP centred on the completion of written ADs and presumed that discussions leading to ADs occurred within the patient–physician relationship. Contemporary investigation into ACP has taught us that such discussions occur within the patient–family relationship and that patients and families have a much broader view of the goals of ACP. Because ADs cannot anticipate all contingencies, are not always followed, often do not accompany patients throughout healthcare systems, and are completed by only a third of ESRD patients, they are no longer an appropriate goal of ACP. Physicians and dialysis-care providers need to continue to facilitate ACP among their patients and families in part because patients and families expect healthcare professionals to introduce the subject. Facilitated ACP can be an important avenue to communication amongst families, patients, and healthcare providers and can offer opportunities to foster quality care, particularly EoL care. The typical illness trajectory of ESRD often provides multiple opportunities to introduce ACP in the dialysis unit. Our patients deserve the highest quality of care we can provide: ACP is integral to providing high-quality ESRD care.

References

1 Canadian Institute for Health Information. Canadian Organ Replacement Registry: Dialysis and Renal Transplantation. Ottawa, ON; 2002.

2 U.S. Renal Data System, National Institutes of Health, National Institute of Diabetes and Digestive and Kidney Diseases (2007). USRDS 2007 Annual Data Report: Atlas of Chronic Kidney Disease and End-Stage Renal Disease in the United States. Bethesda, MD.

3 Davison SN (2002). Quality end-of-life care in dialysis units. *Semin Dial*, Jan, **15**(1), 41–4.

4 Davison SN, Jhangri GS, Johnson JA (2006). Cross-sectional validity of a modified Edmonton symptom assessment system in dialysis patients: a simple assessment of symptom burden. *Kidney Int*, May, **69**(9),1621–5.

5 Davison SN, Jhangri GS, Johnson JA (2006). Longitudinal validation of a modified Edmonton symptom assessment system (ESAS) in haemodialysis patients. *Nephrol Dial Transplant*, Nov, **21**(11), 3189–95.

6 Fainsinger R, Davison SN, Brenneis C (2003). A supportive care model for dialysis patients. *Palliat Med J*,**17**(1), 81–2.

7 Chater S, Davison SN, Germain MJ, et al. (2006). Withdrawal from dialysis: a palliative care perspective. *Clin Nephrol*, **66**(5), 364–72.

8 Cohen LM, Germain MJ, Poppel DM, et al. (2000). Dying Well after discontinuing the life support treatment of dialysis. *Arch Intern Med*, **160**(16), 2513–18.

9 Cohen LM, Germain M, Poppel DM, et al. (2000). Dialysis discontinuation and palliative care. *Am J Kidney Dis*, **36**, 140–4.

10 Moss AH (2002). ESRD Peer Workgroup: Recommendations to the Field, Final Report.

11 Germain MJ, Cohen LM, Davison SN (2007). Withholding and withdrawal from dialysis: what we know about how our patients die. *Semin Dial*, May, **20**(3),195–9.

12 Emanuel EJ, Emanuel LL (1990). Living wills: Past, present, and future. *J Clin Ethics*, **1**(1), 9–19.

13 Singer PA, Martin DK, Lavery JV, et al. (1998). Reconceptualizing advanced care planning from the patient's perspective. *Arch Intern Med*, **158**, 879–84.

14 Levine DZ (1999). "Springing back" advance care planning in dialysis. *Am J Kidney Dis*, May, **33**(5), 980–91.

15 Office of Public Sector Information (2005). Mental Capacity Act 2005.

16 Davison SN (2006). Facilitating advance care planning for patients with end-stage renal disease: the patient perspective. *Clin J Am Soc Nephrol*, Sep, **1**(5), 1023–8.

17 Davison SN, Simpson C (2006). Hope and advance care planning in patients with end stage renal disease: qualitative interview study. *Brit Med J*, Oct 28, **333**(7574), 886.

18 Emanuel LL, Alpert HR, Baldwin DC, et al. (2000). What terminally ill patients care about: toward a validated construct of patients' perspectives. *J Palliat Med*, **3**(4), 419–31.

19 Etchells E, Sharpe G, Walsh P, et al. (1996). Bioethics for clinicians: 1. Consent. *CMAJ*, Jul 15, **155**(2), 177–80.

20 Lazar NM, Greiner GG, Robertson G, et al. (1996). Bioethics for clinicians: 5. Substitute decision-making. *CMAJ*, Nov 15, **155**(10), 1435–7.

21 Singer PA, Robertson G, Roy DJ (1996). Bioethics for clinicians: 6. Advance care planning. *CMAJ*, Dec 15, **155**(12), 1689–92.

22 Fagerlin A, Schneider CE (2004). The failure of the living will. *Hastings Center Report* Mar, **34**(2), 30–42.

23 Reilly RB, Teasdale TA, McCullough LB (1994). Projecting patients' preferences from living wills: an invalid strategy for management of dementia with life-threatening illness. *J Am Geriatr Soc*, Sep, **42**(9), 997–1003.

24 Hines SC, Glover JJ, Babrow AS, et al. (2001). Improving advance care planning by accommodating family preferences. *J Palliat Med*, **4**(4), 481–9.

25 A controlled trial to improve care for seriously ill hospitalized patients (1995). The study to understand prognoses and preferences for outcomes and risks of treatments (SUPPORT). The SUPPORT Principal Investigators. *JAMA*, Nov 22, **274**(20), 1591–8.

26 Virmani J, Schneiderman LJ, Kaplan RM (1994). Relationship of advance directives to physician–patient communication. *Arch Intern Med*, Apr 25, **154**, 909–13.

27 Hanson LC, Tulsky JA, Danis M (1997). Can clinical interventions change care at the end of life? *Ann Intern Med*, Mar 1, **126**(5), 381–8.

28 Gillick MR (1995). A broader role for advance medical planning. *Ann Intern Med*, **123**, 621–4.

29 Holley JL, Stackiewicz L, Dacko C, et al. (1997). Factors influencing dialysis patients' completion of advanced directives. *Am J Kidney Dis*, **3**, 356–60.

30 Holley JL, Nespor S, Rault R (1993). Chronic in-center hemodialysis patients' attitudes knowledge and behavior towards advanced directives. *J Am Soc Nephrol*, **3**, 1405–8.

31 Cohen LM, McCue JD, Germain M, et al. (1997). Denying the dying. Advance directives and dialysis discontinuation. *Psychosomatics*, **38**(1),27–34.

32 Cohen LM, Germain M, Woods A, et al. (1993). Patient attitudes and psychological considerations in dialysis discontinuation. *Psychosomatics*, **34**, 395–401.

33 Holley JL, Hines SC, Glover JJ, et al. (1999). Failure of advance care planning to elicit patients' preferences for withdrawal from dialysis. *Am J Kidney Dis*, Apr 1, **33**(4), 688–93.

34 Sekkarie MA, Moss AH (1998). Withholding and withdrawing dialysis: the role of physician speciality and education and patient functional status. *Am J Kidney Dis*, **31**, 464–72.

35 Moss AH, Holley JL, Upton MB (1992). Outcomes of cardiopulmonary resuscitation in dialysis patients. *J Am Soc Nephrol*, **3**(6), 1238–43.

36 Lai M, Hung K, Huang J, et al. (1999). Clinical findings and outcomes of intra-hemodialysis cardiopulmonary resuscitation. *Am J Nephrol*, **19**(4), 468–73.

37 Lafrance JP, Nolin L, Senecal L, et al. (2006). Predictors and outcome of cardiopulmonary resuscitation (CPR) calls in a large haemodialysis unit over a seven-year period. *Nephrol Dial Transplant*, Apr, **21**(4), 1006–12.

38 Moss AH, Hozayen O, King K, et al. (2001). Attitudes of patients toward cardiopulmonary resuscitation in the dialysis unit. *Am J Kidney Dis*, Oct 1, **38**(4), 847–52.

39 Ostermann ME, Nelson SR (2003). Haemodialysis patients' views on their resuscitation status. *Nephrol Dial Transplant*, Aug, **18**(8), 1644–7.

40 Perry E, Buck C, Newsome J, et al. (1995). Dialysis staff influence patients in formulating their advance directives. *Am J Kidney Dis*, Feb 1, **25**(2), 262–8.

41 Cohen LM, Dobscha SK, Hails KC, et al. (2002). Depression and suicidal ideation in patients who discontinue the life-support treatment of dialysis. *Psychosom Med*, Nov 1, **64**(6), 889–96.

42 Rutecki GW, Rodriguez L, Cugino A, et al. (1994). End of life issues in ESRD. A study of three decision variables that affect patient attitude. *ASAIO J*, **40**, M798–M802.

43 Hines SC, Glover JJ, Babrow AS, et al. (2001). Improving advance care planning by accommodating family preferences. *J Palliat Med*, **4**(4), 481–9.

44 Fried TR, Bradley EH, Towle VR (2003). Valuing the outcomes of treatment. *Arch Intern Med*, Sep 22, **163**, 2073–8.

45 Perry E, Swartz J, Brown S, et al. (2005). Peer mentoring: a culturally sensitive approach to end-of-life planning for long-term dialysis patients. *Am J Kidney Dis*, Jul, **46**(1), 111-19.

46 Pruchno RA, Lemay EP, Jr., Feild L, et al. (2006). Predictors of patient treatment preferences and spouse substituted judgments: the case of dialysis continuation. *Med Decis Making*, Mar, **26**(2), 112–21.

47 Miura Y, Asai A, Matsushima M, et al. (2006). Families' and physicians' predictions of dialysis patients' preferences regarding life-sustaining treatments in Japan. *Am J Kidney Dis*, Jan, **47**(1), 122–30.

48 Miles SH, Koepp R, Weber EP (1996). Advance end-of-life treatment planning. *Arch Intern Med*, May 27, **156**, 1062–8.

49 Tulsky JA, Fischer GS, Rose MR, et al. (1998). Opening the black box: How do physicians communicate about advance directives? *Ann Intern Med*, **129**(6), 441–9.

50 Tulsky JA, Chesney MA, Lo B (1995). How do medical residents discuss resuscitation with patients? *J Gen Intern Med*, Aug 1, **10**, 436–42.

51 Miles SH, Bannick-Mohrland S, Lurie N (1990). Advance-Treatment planning discussions with Nursing Home Residents: Pilot experience with simulated interviews. *J Clin Ethics*, **1**, 108–12.

52 Curtis JR, Engelberg RA, Nielsen EL, et al. (2004). Patient–physician communication about end-of-life care for patients with severe COPD. *Eur Respir J*, Aug, **24**(2), 200–5.

53 DeNour AK (1982). Psychosocial adjustment to illness scale (PAIS): A study of chronic hemodialysis patients. *J Psychosom Res*, **26**(1), 11–22.

54 Oldenburg B, MacDonald GJ, Perkins RJ (1988). Prediction of quality of life in a cohort of end-stage renal disease patients. *J Clin Epidemiol*, **41**(6), 555–64.

55 Derogatis LR, Fleming MP (1996). Psychological Adjustment to Illness Scale: PAIS and PAIS-SR. In Spilker B (ed.) *Quality of life and pharmacoeconomics in clinical trials* 2nd ed. pp. 287–99. Philadelphia: Lippincott-Raven.

56 Zabalegui A (1999). Coping strategies and psychological distress in patients with advanced cancer. *Oncol Nurs Forum*, **26**(9), 1511–18.

57 Singer PA, Martin DK, Kelner M (1999). Quality end-of-life care. Patients' perspectives. *JAMA*, Jan 13, **281**(2), 163–8.

58 Parkerson GRJr, Gutman RA (1997). Perceived mental health and disablement of primary care and end-stage renal disease patients. *Int J Psychiatr Med*, **27**(1), 33–45.

59 Fricchione GL, Howanitz E, Jandorf L, et al. (1992). Psychological adjustment to end-stage renal disease and the implications of denial. *Psychosomatics*, **33**(1), 85–91.

60 Levy NB (1981). Psychological reactions to machine dependency: Hemodialysis. *Psychiatr Clin North Am*, **4**(2), 351–63.

61 Seamark DA, Seamark CJ, Halpin DM (2007). Palliative care in chronic obstructive pulmonary disease: a review for clinicians. *J R Soc Med*, May, 100(5), 225–33.

62 Coppola KM, Ditto PH, Danks JH, et al. (2001). Accuracy of primary care and hospital-based physicians' predictions of elderly outpatients' treatment preferences with and without advance directives. *Arch Intern Med*, **161**(3), 431–40.

63 Rosenfeld KE, Wenger NS, Phillips RS, et al. (1996). Factors associated with change in resuscitation preference of seriously ill patients. The SUPPORT Investigators. Study to Understand Prognoses and Preferences for Outcomes and Risks of Treatments. *Arch Intern Med*, Jul 22, **156**(14), 1558–64.

64 Alpert HR, Hoijtink H, Fischer GS, et al.(1996). Psychometric analysis of an advance directive. *Med Care*, Oct, **34**(10), 1057–65.

65 McParland E, Likourezos A, Chichin E, et al. (2003). Stability of preferences regarding life-sustaining treatment: a two-year prospective study of nursing home residents. *Mt Sinai J Med*, Mar, **70**(2), 85–92.

66 Weissman JS, Haas JS, Fowler FJ, Jr., et al. (1999). The stability of preferences for life-sustaining care among persons with AIDS in the Boston Health Study. *Med Decis Making*, Jan, **19**(1), 16–26.

67 Murphy DJ, Burrows D, Santilli S, et al (1994). The influence of the probability of survival on patients' preferences regarding cardiopulmonary resuscitation. *N Engl J Med*, Feb 24, **330**(8), 545–9.

68 Swartz R, Perry E (1998). Advance directives in end-stage renal disease inherently involve family and staff. *Adv Ren Replace Ther*, Apr 1, **5**(2), 109–19.

69 Butow PN, Maclean M, Dunn SM, et al. (1997). The dynamics of change: cancer patients' preferences for information, involvement and support. *Ann Oncol*, Sep, **8**(9), 857–63.

70 Prendergast TJ, Puntillo KA (2002). Withdrawal of life support: intensive caring at the end of life. *JAMA*, Dec 4, **288**(21), 2732–40.

71 Detmar SB, Muller MJ, Schornagel JH, et al. (2002). Role of health-related quality of life in palliative chemotherapy treatment decisions. *J Clin Oncol*, Feb 15, **20**(4), 1056–62.

72 Lockhart LK, Bookwala J, Fagerlin A, et al. (2001). Older adults' attitudes toward death: links to perceptions of health and concerns about end-of-life issues. *Omega* (Westport), **43**(4), 331–47.

73 Teno JM, Weitzen S, Fennell ML, et al. (2001). Dying trajectory in the last year of life: does cancer trajectory fit other diseases? *J Palliat Med*, **4**(4), 457–64.

74 Danis M, Garrett J, Harris R, et al. (1994). Stability of choices about life-sustaining treatments. *Ann Intern Med*, Apr 1, **120**(7), 567–73.

75 Davison SN, Torgunrud C (2007). The creation of an advance care planning process for patients with ESRD. *Am J Kidney Dis*, Jan, **49**(1), 27–36.

76 Lunney JR, Lynn J, Foley DJ, et al. (2003). Patterns of functional decline at the end of life. *JAMA*, May 14, **289**(18),2387–92.

77 Murray SA, Kendall M, Boyd K, et al. (2005). Illness trajectories and palliative care. *Brit Med J*, Apr 30, **330**(7498), 1007–11.

78 Moss AH, Ganjoo J, Sharma S, et al. (2008). Utility of the "surprise" question to identify dialysis patients with high mortality. *Clin J Am Soc Nephrol*, Sep, **3**(5), 1379–84.

79 Moss AH, Holley JL, Davison SN, et al. (2004). Palliative care. *Am J Kidney Dis*, Jan, **43**(1), 172–3.

80 Pfeifer MP, Sidorov JE, Smith AC, et al. (1994). The discussion of end-of-life medical care by primary care patients and physicians: a multicenter study using structured qualitative interviews. The EOL Study Group. *J Gen Intern Med*, **9**(2), 82–8.

81 Sehgal A, Galbraith A, Chesney M, et al. (1992). How strictly do dialysis patients want their advance directives followed? *JAMA*, **267**(1), 59–63.

82 Fine A, Fontaine B, Kraushar MM, et al. (2005). Nephrologists should voluntarily divulge survival data to potential dialysis patients: a questionnaire study. *Perit Dial Int*, May, **25**(3), 269–73.

83 Apatira L, Boyd EA, Malvar G, et al. (2008). Hope, truth, and preparing for death: perspectives of surrogate decision makers. *Ann Intern Med*, Dec 16, **149**(12), 861–8.

84 Johnston SC, Pfeifer MP, McNutt R, (for the End-of-Life Study Group) (1995). The discussion about advance directives. Patient and physician opinions regarding when and how it should be conducted. *Arch Intern Med*, May 22, **155**, 1025–30.

85 Hofmann JC, Wenger NS, Davis RB, et al. (1997). Patient preferences for communication with physicians about end-of-life decisions. SUPPORT Investigators. Study to understand prognoses and preference for outcomes and risks of treatment. *Ann Intern Med*, **127**(1), 1–12.

86 Finucane TE, Shumway JM, Powers RL, et al. (1988). Planning with elderly outpatients for contingencies of severe illness: a survey and clinical trial. *J Gen Intern Med*, Jul, **3**(4), 322–5.

87 Smucker WD, Ditto PH, Moore KA, et al. (1993). Elderly outpatients respond favorably to a physician-initiated advance directive discussion. *J Am Board Fam Prac*, **6**, 473–82.

88 Tilden VP, Tolle SW, Garland MJ, et al. (1995). Decisions about life-sustaining treatment. *Arch Intern Med*, Mar 27, **155**, 633–8.

89 Hines SC, Glover JJ, Holley JL, et al. (1999). Dialysis patients' preferences for family-based advance care planning. *Ann Intern Med*, May 18, **130**(10), 825–8.

90 Hawkins NA, Ditto PH, Danks JH, et al. (2005). Micromanaging death: process preferences, values, and goals in end-of-life medical decision making. *Gerontologist*, Feb, **45**(1), 107–17.

91 Singer PA, Thiel EC, Naylor DC, et al. (1995). Life-sustaining treatment preferences of hemodialysis patients: Implications for advanced directives. *J Am Soc Nephrol*, **6**, 1410–17.

92 Volandes AE, Abbo ED (2007). Flipping the default: a novel approach to cardiopulmonary resuscitation in end-stage dementia. *J Clin Ethics*, **18**(2), 122–39.

93 Sachs GA, Shega JW, Cox-Hayley D (2004). Barriers to excellent end-of-life care for patients with dementia. *J Gen Intern Med*, **19**(10), 1057–63.

94 Briggs L (2003). Shifting the focus of advance care planning: Using an in-depth interview to build and strengthen relationships. *Innov End-of-Life Care*, Mar, **5**(2), 1–16.

95 Lynn J, Goldstein NE (2003). Advance care planning for fatal chronic illness: avoiding commonplace errors and unwarranted suffering. *Ann Intern Med*, May 20, **138**(10), 812–18.

96 Weiner JS, Cole SA (2004). ACare: a communication training program for shared decision making along a life-limiting illness. *Palliat Support Care*, Sep, **2**(3), 231–41.

97 Welch G, Rose G, Ernst D (2006). Motivational Interviewing and Diabetes: What Is It, How Is It Used, and Does It Work? *Diabetes Spectr*, Jan 1, **19**(1), 5–11.

98 Back AL, Arnold RM, Baile WF, et al. (2007). Efficacy of communication skills training for giving bad news and discussing transitions to palliative care. *Arch Intern Med*, Mar 12, **167**(5), 453–60.

99 Tulsky JA, Alexander SC, Olsen MK, et al. (2008). Can oncologists be taught to respond to patients negative emotions? Results of the SCOPE trial. American Academy on Communication in HealthCare Conference.Madison, WI.

100 Weijer C, Singer PA, Dickens BM, et al. (1998). Bioethics for clinicians: 16. Dealing with demands for inappropriate treatment. *CMAJ*, Oct 6, **159**(7), 817–21.

101 Blackhall LJ, Frank G, Murphy ST, et al. (1999). Ethnicity and attitudes towards life sustaining technology. *Soc Sci Med*, Jun, **48**(12), 1779–89.

102 Davison SN, Holley JL (2008). Ethical issues in the care of vulnerable chronic kidney disease patients: the elderly, cognitively impaired, and those from different cultural backgrounds. *Adv Chronic Kidney Dis*, Apr, **15**(2), 177–85.

103 Fox S, Swazey JP (1984). Medical morality is not bioethics – medical ethics in China and the United States. *Perspect in Biol Med*, **27**(3), 336–60.

104 Coward H, Sidhu T (2000). Bioethics for clinicians: 19. Hinduism and Sikhism. *CMAJ*, Oct 31, **163**(9), 1167–70.

105 Kelly L, Minty A (2007). End-of-life issues for aboriginal patients: a literature review. *Can Fam Physician*, Sep, **53**(9), 1459–65.

106 Brant CC (1990). Native ethics and rules of behaviour. *Can J Psychiatry*, Aug, **35**(6), 534–9.

107 Newbold KB (1999). Disability and use of support services within the Canadian aboriginal population. *Health Soc Care Community*, Jul, **7**(4), 291–300.

108 Witherspoon G (1977). *Language and art in the Navajo universe*. University of Michigan Press.

109 Caralis PV, Davis B, Wright K, et al. (1993). The influence of ethnicity and race on attitudes toward advance directives, life-prolonging treatments, and euthanasia. *J Clin Ethics*, **4**(2), 155–65.

110 Hanson LC, Rodgman E (1996). The use of living wills at the end of life. A national study. *Arch Intern Med*, May 13, **156**(9), 1018–22.

111 Kwak J, Haley WE (2005). Current research findings on end-of-life decision making among racially or ethnically diverse groups. *Gerontologist*, Oct, **45**(5), 634–41.

112 Perkins HS, Geppert CM, Gonzales A, et al. (2002). Cross-cultural similarities and differences in attitudes about advance care planning. *J Gen Intern Med*, Jan, **17**(1), 48–57.

113 Winzelberg GS, Hanson LC, Tulsky JA (2005). Beyond autonomy: diversifying end-of-life decision-making approaches to serve patients and families. *J Am Geriatr Soc*, Jun, **53**(6), 1046–50.

114 Guo B, Harstall C (2004). Advance Directives for End-of-Life Care in the Elderly: Effectiveness of Delivery Models. Alberta Heritage Foundation for Medical Research; 2004. Report No.: Information Paper 20.

115 Hanson LC, Danis M, Garrett J (1997). What is wrong with end-of-life care? Opinions of bereaved family members. *J Am Geriatric Soc*, 45, 1339–44.

116 Hammes BJ, Rooney BL (1998). Death and end-of-life planning in one midwestern community. *Arch Intern Med*, **158**, 383–90.

117 Holley JL, Nespor S, Rault R (1993). The effects of providing chronic hemodialysis patients with material on advance directives. *Am J Kidney Dis*, Sep 1, **22**(3), 413–18.

118 Wilkinson A, Wenger N, Shugarman LR (2007). Literature Review on Advance Directives.

119 Chaudhry B, Wang J, Wu S, et al. (2006). Systematic review: impact of health information technology on quality, efficiency, and costs of medical care. *Ann Intern Med*, May 16, **144**(10), 742–52.

120 Dexter PR, Wolinsky FD, Gramelspacher GP, et al. (1998). Effectiveness of computer-generated reminders for increasing discussions about advance directives and completion of advance directive forms. A randomized, controlled trial. *Ann Intern Med*, Jan 15, **128**(2), 102–10.

121 Pearlman RA, Starks H, Cain KC, et al. (2005). Improvements in advance care planning in the Veterans Affairs System: results of a multifaceted intervention. *Arch Intern Med*, Mar 28, **165**(6), 667–74.

122 Briggs LA, Kirchhoff KT, Hammes BJ, et al. (2004). Patient-centered advance care planning in special patient populations: a pilot study. *J Prof Nurs*, Jan, **20**(1), 47–58.

123 Hickman SE, Tolle SW, Brummel-Smith K, et al. (2004). Use of the Physician Orders for Life-Sustaining Treatment program in Oregon nursing facilities: beyond resuscitation status. *J Am Geriatr Soc*, Sep, **52**(9), 1424–9.

124 Lee MA, Brummel-Smith K, Meyer J, et al. (2000). Physician orders for life-sustaining treatment (POLST): outcomes in a PACE program. Program of All-Inclusive Care for the Elderly. *J Am Geriatr Soc*, Oct, **48**(10), 1219–25.

125 Picard EL, Robertson GR (2007). *Legal liability of doctors and hospitals in Canada.* 4th ed. Toronto: Carswell.

126 Age Concern (1999). *The future of health and care of older people: the best is yet to come.* The Millennium Papers. London.

127 Bates L (2000). Cancer patient's fury at doctor who 'wrote her off on hospital's death ward'. The Guardian, Apr 13.

128 British Medical Association (2007). Withholding and withdrawing life-prolonging medical treatment: guidance for decision making. Manchester: Hammicks BMA. Report No.: 3.

129 Dworkin R (1993). *Life's dominion. An argument about abortion and euthanasia.* London: Harper Collins.

130 Department of Health (2008). End of Life Care Strategy – promoting high quality care for all adults at the end of life. Department of Health; Jul 16.

131 UK Department of Health. The National End of Life Care Programme. Internet 2008 [cited 2008 Dec 5]; Available from: URL: http://www.endoflifecareforadults.nhs.uk/eolc/

132 Royal College of General Practitioners, British Geriatric Society, Royal College of Physicians, et al. (2009). Advance Care Planning: National Guideline. Royal College of Physicians.

133 Martin DK, Thiel EC, Singer PA (1999). A new model of advance care planning: Observations from people with HIV. *Arch Intern Med*, **159**, 86–92.

134 Herth KA (1989). The relationship between level of hope and level of coping response and other variables in patients with cancer. *Oncol Nurs Forum*, **16**(1), 67–72.

135 Elliott TR, Witty TE, Herrick S, et al. (1991). Negotiating reality after physical loss: hope, depression, and disability. *J Pers Soc Psychol*, **61**(4), 608–13.

136 Staats S (1991). Quality of life and affect in older persons: hope, time frames, and training effects. *Curr Psychol: Res Rev*, **10**(1,2), 21–30.

137 Bruhn JG (1984). Therapeutic value of hope. *South Med J*, **77**(2), 215–19.

138 Swartz RD, Perry E (1993). Advanced directives are associated with "Good Deaths" in chronic dialysis patients. *J Am Soc Nephrol*, **3**, 1623–30.

139 Schneiderman LJ, Kronick R, Kaplan RM, et al. (1992). Effects of offering advance directives on medical treatments and costs. *Ann Intern Med*, **117**(7), 599–606.

140 Schwartz CE, Wheeler HB, Hammes B, et al. (2002). Early intervention in planning end-of-life care with ambulatory geriatric patients: results of a pilot trial. *Arch Intern Med*, **162**(14), 1611–18.

141 Stuart B, D'Onofrio CN, Boatman S, et al. (2003). CHOICES: promoting early access to end-of-life care through home-based transition management. *J Palliat Med*, Aug, **6**(4), 671–83.

142 Tolle SW, Tilden VP, Nelson CA, et al. (1998). A prospective study of the efficacy of the physician order form for life-sustaining treatment. *J Am Geriatr Soc*, Sep, **46**(9), 1097–102.

143 Wright AA, Zhang B, Ray A, et al. (2008). Associations between end-of-life discussions, patient mental health, medical care near death, and caregiver bereavement adjustment. *JAMA*, Oct 8, **300**(14), 1665–73.

144 Ditto PH, Jacobson JA, Smucker WD, et al. (2006). Context changes choices: a prospective study of the effects of hospitalization on life-sustaining treatment preferences. *Med Decis Making*, Jul, **26**(4), 313–22.

145 Puchalski CM, Zhong Z, Jacobs MM, et al. (2000). Patients who want their family and physician to make resuscitation decisions for them: Observations from SUPPORT and HELP. *JAGS*, **48**, S84–S90.

146 Ditto PH, Danks JH, Smucker WD, et al. (2001). Advance directives as acts of communication: A randomized controlled trial. *Arch Intern Med*, **161**(3), 421–30.

147 Asch A (2005). Recognizing death while affirming life: can end of life reform uphold a disabled person's interest in continued life? *Hastings Cent Rep*, Nov, Spec No, S31–S36.

148 Christakis NA, Asch DA (1995). Medical specialists prefer to withdraw familiar technologies when discontinuing life support. *J Gen Intern Med*, Sep, **10**(9), 491–4.

149 Rocker GM, Curtis JR (2003). Caring for the dying in the intensive care unit: in search of clarity. *JAMA*, Aug, **290**(6), 820–2.

150 Morrison RS, Morrison EW, Glickman DF (1994). Physician reluctance to discuss advance directives. An empiric investigation of potential barriers. *Arch Intern Med*, Oct, **154**(20), 2311–18.

151 Davison SN, Jhangri GS, Holley JL, et al. (2006). Nephrologists' reported preparedness for end-of-life decision-making. *Clin J Am Soc Nephrol*, Nov, **1**(6), 1256–62.

152 Feeg VD, Elebiary H (2005). Exploratory study on end-of-life issues: barriers to palliative care and advance directives. *Am J Hosp Palliat Care*, Mar, **22**(2), 119–24.

Chapter 5

What determines a good outcome? The selection of patients for renal replacement therapy

Terry Feest

5.1 A good outcome

A "good" outcome in renal replacement therapy (RRT) is most commonly measured in terms of the survival of the patient after starting treatment. This is easily measured, can be reported by large national registries, and is relatively simple to study in local audits. It is a measure which is easily understood by the general public and, perhaps more importantly, by politicians. Unfortunately this simple concept of a good outcome may lead to inappropriate practice of medicine, especially for a treatment such as RRT which is of high cost and often practised within the context of limited resources.

5.1.1 Limited resources

As RRT is very expensive, in a resource-limited health service it would appear reasonable to argue that it is appropriate to offer treatment to those who would most benefit. In practice health services are cash limited, even in developed countries. This is manifest by the limited availability of some expensive treatments in socialized healthcare systems such as the United Kingdom (UK), Australasia, and – to a lesser extent – Canada, and by the unequal access to healthcare in less regulated systems as in the USA. If it is accepted that those who would benefit most are simply those who would live longest this would bar most elderly people from starting RRT because, in statistical terms, increasing age confers a shorter life expectancy. People with other significant co-morbid conditions such as diabetes or malignancy or severe heart disease – which might otherwise shorten life – would also be excluded from treatment.

Case histories

The following case histories illustrate the limitations of defining a good outcome simply in terms of survival.

Case 1 – Mrs AA at age 78 presented with a 3-day history of increasing shortness of breath due to pulmonary oedema. She was found to be in oliguric renal failure, with serum creatinine 1500. Renal ultrasound showed normal size kidneys. Chest X-ray revealed a very large right hilar shadow suggestive of carcinoma of the lung. She received haemodialysis pending urgent chest investigations. Investigations showed squamous cell carcinoma of the right lung, and she was referred for radiotherapy.

With dialysis, her dyspnoea completely regressed and she felt well. There were no symptoms from the carcinoma. As she was feeling well she requested to continue dialysis so that she could visit her extended family and tidy her affairs. She said she would wish to stop dialysis once she developed symptoms from the carcinoma of the lung. After 7 weeks of dialysis she began to develop dyspnoea and pain related to her carcinoma, and withdrew from treatment with full supportive palliative care.

Case 2 – Mr. BB aged 66 had a history of mitral regurgitation, atrial fibrillation, and left ventricular failure. He had stenosis of the left anterior descending coronary artery and needed mitral valve replacement. He also had an 80% stenosis of his left renal artery and diffuse disease in the right renal artery. He rapidly became severely unwell with marked deterioration in renal function.

Left renal angioplasty was not successful in improving renal function. He then developed bacterial endocarditis, and thrombocytopaenia due to bone marrow suppression. The unanimous view of the cardiac physicians and surgeons was that he was not suitable for cardiac surgery and had a very poor prognosis. He was hypotensive, could rarely stand or tolerate a full dialysis session due to low blood pressure and poor cardiac output. It was the opinion of the attending renal physicians that RRT was not appropriate. Despite extensive and detailed counselling with the patient, his wife, and family, the patient was determined to undertake regular haemodialysis, and his wife fully supported this. As a series of problems arose, the patient and his wife were adamant that he wished to continue dialysis, and he refused to discuss the issue. Because of this, they would not accept palliative care or counselling. The patient continued on RRT for 5 months until he died, during which time he did not leave hospital. The entire prolonged hospital admission caused considerable distress to the patient, and the relatives were unable to come to terms with the death and the circumstances surrounding it for nearly 2 years.

The first case had a short prognosis and would not have been offered dialysis according to many of the guidelines which have been published, but this history must be considered a good outcome. Despite the fact that the patient lived for a predictably short period of time, and had malignancy at the start of dialysis, the use of technology to give the patient a few weeks of extra life was of great benefit to both the patient and to the family. This case demonstrates that a "good outcome" must be defined beyond simple length of survival.

The second patient lived considerably longer than first, but was unhappy throughout. There was great distress for the family, and this continued long after the death of the patient. The caring team were unable to reconcile the fears and wishes of the patient and his family with his inevitable death. It was not possible to apply either appropriate care or selection. This longer survival must be considered a poor outcome.

5.1.2 Summary

In assessing a good outcome of RRT, it is essential to consider both the quality of life offered, and the length of life. Tools for assessing quality of life in RRT will be discussed in subsequent chapters. When a patient first presents for dialysis it is a very hard task to predict either likely length of life or the quality of life which might be achieved. This will be discussed later in this chapter.

Perhaps a good outcome would be achievement of the aim of Quality Requirement 4 of the English National Service Framework for Renal Services:

> To support people with established renal failure to live life as fully as possible and enable then to die with dignity in a setting of their choice.[1]

5.2 Patient autonomy, rationing, and selection

5.2.1 Patient autonomy

In a healthcare system with unlimited resource, it is possible to offer true patient autonomy, allowing patients to make an informed choice about whether or not they wish to start RRT. Not everyone with established renal failure will elect to undertake RRT. Many patients will have such severe co-morbid conditions that RRT will simply prolong a difficult and painful life for a few weeks. Patients with impaired mental ability may be unable to comprehend the treatment offered them, and simply see it as a torture which is inflicted upon them 3 times a week. Many patients may wish, therefore, to select themselves not to receive RRT, but nevertheless their remaining life could be improved by appropriate supportive care, e.g. anaemia management, management of pruritus, nausea, pain relief.

In practice, healthcare systems rarely, if ever, have unlimited resource.

5.2.2 Rationing

Rationing is the implicit or explicit denial of beneficial or marginally beneficial medical treatment as a result of insufficient resources to provide treatment for all.

Renal replacement therapy is an expensive process which consumes a huge resource for a small number of patients. In the UK nearly 3% of the NHS budget is spent on RRT for less than 0.06% of the population, and the expenditure is rising. Even in the developed world, healthcare resources are limited and in most countries there is not enough resource for all patients with established renal failure to receive RRT. In these circumstances it is inevitable that a degree of patient autonomy is lost, as treatment may not be available for all those who might elect to receive it. Selection for treatment then becomes partly a rationing process: this may be overt with clear guidelines and rules or covert with physicians being subconsciously influenced by the knowledge of lack of resource. It is important to understand when selection starts to become involved with rationing.

There is general agreement that rationing should not be according to social worth, age, or ability to pay, but if necessary, could be justified according to potential medical benefit. [2] Even in the USA, there is evidence that physicians may still be responsible for selected aspects of terminal care independent of patient choice,[3] and with the advent of managed care there is concern that dialysis will be rationed.[2] In a climate in which some form of rationing may be inevitable, it is essential that the criteria for judgement are explicit and that transactions are transparent. This needs practice guidelines.[2,4,5] One such set of guidelines was produced by the Renal Physicians Association of the USA[6] and will be considered later in this chapter.

5.2.3 The concept of selection

The concept of selection of patients for treatment does not fit comfortably with modern practice of medicine, which places the patients at the centre of any decision-making process about their care. Nephrologists have moved towards a general consensus that there should be a process of shared decision-making and informed consent for initiation of RRT.[6–9]

The term "selection" implies the patient is a passive bystander whilst someone – usually the doctor – decides whether or not to offer this potentially life-saving treatment. Many believe that this paternalistic concept should not be applied to patients, who must be able to choose whether or not they want dialysis therapy.[9] Nevertheless, paternalism may still persist. In a 1-year prospective study in the UK reported in 2000,[10] of 88 patients referred for consideration of dialysis 11 were not started on RRT, six of these patients were older than 80, and only one had been seen earlier in a renal clinic. Of these 11 not treated, four were considered incapable of making a decision: only one of the other seven was offered a choice.

The Renal Physicians Association (of the USA) states: "A patient physician relationship that promotes shared decision making is recommended for all patients. Participants in shared decision making should involve at a minimum the patient and the physician. If a patient lacks decision-making capacity, the decisions should involve the legal agent. With the patients consent shared decision making may include family members or friends and other members of the renal care team".[6]

5.2.4 **Selection practices**

5.2.4.1 History

In 1982,[11] Berlyne famously observed that few people over the age of 50 could obtain RRT in the UK, and the UK National Health Service became notable, amongst others, for limiting resources available for RRT, causing the necessity for rationing of renal care. It was recognized that age was commonly used as a selection criteria for access to therapy.[12] The criteria for allocating the scarce resources were not in the public domain, if indeed they were explicit in the minds of nephrologists. Decisions seemed to be dominated by clinicians, but were considered often to be imperfect, and ultimately political.[13]

In the last three decades the situation has changed markedly, and in the UK and many other countries there has been a dramatic increase in the number of patients accepted for RRT, but with little change for younger people who were relatively readily accepted for treatment in the early days of RRT.[14–17] The most marked change is in the acceptance rate of the elderly, which shows a sixfold increase across some 20 years. Fig. 1.3, Chapter 1, illustrates clearly how age was widely used as a criterion for limiting access to care in the early 1980s. It also shows the impact of the recommendation issued by the UK government in 1993 that age was not an acceptable criterion for limiting access to therapy.[18] Acceptance rates for diabetics have also dramatically increased.

5.2.4.2 Factors influencing decision-making

There have been many studies, usually by means of vignette case history questionnaires, which have compared the attitude of referring physicians and nephrologists to selection for dialysis. [3–5,19–26] Overall it was expectation of medical benefit, and not social considerations, which was the main driver in decision-making.[5,24,26] The major factors influencing decisions to recommend non-commencement of dialysis were severe heart disease and severely impaired neurological function. Theory and practice also differ. It is interesting that in 1984 when the age specific acceptance rate for the over-65s in the UK was very low, the physicians were theoretically willing to accept some of the older patients in this study, suggesting practice differed from principle.[19]

A Canadian study in 1994[21] demonstrated that age, as well as co-existing disease, influenced the likelihood of referral. It also concluded that, in Canada, rationing decisions were being made which prevented access to treatment by patients who might have benefited from it. Even in the USA where acceptance policies were much more liberal, 94% of unit directors reported that they were prepared to make decisions to withhold dialysis. There was marked variation in attitudes and the criteria used for selection,[5] highlighting again the need for explicit guidelines to assist in more open and uniform decision-making.

A survey of dialysis decision-making in Canada, the UK, and the USA in 1998[4] showed that US nephrologists were more likely to offer dialysis than Canadian or British nephrologists, and ranked patient/family wishes and fear of lawsuit higher in decision-making than Canadian or British nephrologists. The Americans less frequently used their perceptions of the patient's likely quality of life to make decisions. Two percent of American nephrologists and 12% of Canadian and British nephrologists had had to refuse dialysis to possibly suitable patients in the last year due to lack of resources. The variation in nephrologists' reported attitudes in the three countries was not great enough to account for the wide variation in acceptance rates among the countries. It was concluded that this variation was partly influenced by financial constraints, and other factors such as differences in rates of referral to the specialist centres.

In the USA, it was clear that nephrologists were more comfortable withdrawing dialysis than withholding it.[5,24]

5.2.4.3 The role of referring physicians

Research early in the development of RRT showed that the low acceptance rate in the UK was largely due to under-referral of patients to dialysis and transplant units rather than to refusal by consultant renal physicians to treat patients.[19] Attitudes have liberalized significantly since this was published in 1984, but a study in 1996[27] demonstrated that there was still a reluctance of generalists to refer to renal physicians, whose attitudes towards acceptance of treatment were much more liberal.

In 2000, another study of attitudes in the USA, Canada, and the UK showed that 35% of Canadian and US physicians would operate an age restriction for referral to a specialist, compared with 51% in the UK.[25] Family physicians were still acting as gatekeepers to the system, taking into account the patient's life circumstances, often in concert with the patients and their family. In the USA and Canada, there was still evidence that patients who might benefit from dialysis were not always offered it,[4,20,22], and that non-referral by primary care physicians was still an important, although diminishing, factor in 2001. The reported attitudes of Canadian and US nephrologists were very similar, despite the differing treatment rates in the two countries – again suggesting that attitudes towards acceptance may differ from real practice.

That the attitude of referring physicians may still be an important factor in 2009 is illustrated by referrals to the Bristol Renal Unit, which are all sent to the same team of 10 nephrologists. Annual acceptance rates for RRT rates in one health authority served by the unit are 114 per million, and in another are consistently low although slowly rising, currently at around 76 per million.[17] Given that the populations served are relatively similar and that all are served by the same nephrologists, the major difference in acceptance rate is likely to be due to under-referral by general practitioners and/or general physicians in some areas.

5.2.4.4 Inappropriate application of care

From the 1980s the situation changed: dialysis is more freely available and there is a perception that patients who are too sick to benefit may be receiving treatment. By the mid-1990s many nephrologists and renal nurses believed that at least 15% of patients on dialysis had such a poor quality of life they should not be receiving the treatment.[28–30] This raises issues about the appropriateness of counselling and information offered to patients approaching established renal failure. A study in Virginia in 1998 suggested only 7% of patients were counselled not to accept treatment.[23]

Inappropriate application of care may also be avoided if dialysis is not always offered as a choice. There are those who believe that deciding not to offer dialysis is a fundamental responsibility of the nephrologist,[30] and that failure to make these decisions will harm patients, their families, other patients, and staff. Advocates of this approach accept that saying "no" will demand both careful assessment of the patient and the medical literature on the outcomes of dialysis for someone in the patient's condition. The nephrologist is then obliged to fully explain to the patient why dialysis treatment is not offered. Implementing this advice would be difficult, as there is severe doubt whether the medical literature is adequate to enable nephrologists to predict which patients will experience more harm than benefit on dialysis, and so make such decisions.

5.2.4.5 Current national and regional variations

The current differences between countries (as discussed in Chapter 1) need to be interpreted with caution; it should not be assumed that those with lower acceptance rates for dialysis are turning away suitable patients. A study was undertaken to explore the difference between the crude annual acceptance rates in 2005 between the UK (105 per million population) and Germany (194 per million population).[31] Much of the difference in RRT incidence between Germany and England and Wales is explained by a greater prevalence of diabetes, hypertension, and vascular disease in the German general population, particularly those older than 65 years, and lower competing mortality risk. In addition, there was no funding for renal supportive care in Germany with the result that this was rarely offered to patients. If the number of patients receiving supportive care were added to the UK acceptance rate, then all but 15% of the difference in acceptance rates between the two countries would be explained without the need to invoke rationing within the UK.

5.2.5 Summary

In the development of dialysis programmes in the last 30 years, it is clear that selection for treatment has been significantly influenced by the need for economic rationing. When the first dialysis programme was established in Seattle a citizens committee was set up to allocate places. Analysis showed that perceptions of social worth were influential in decisions.[32] In a fair society, access to treatment should be free and not amenable to manipulation by the more able or socially privileged as happened in the UK in the 1980s.[33] As more facilities have been made available, acceptance has become more liberal: concurrently beliefs about who might benefit have also changed, indicating that such apparently clinical decisions are influenced, often subconsciously, by resource and budget constraints.

In the last decade, limited resource has become less of an issue in many countries, although it is still present. Nevertheless, attitudes to selection have been variable and often not reflected in real practice, which has tended to be more restrictive than the quoted underlying principle. Levinsky reminds us[34] that physicians have not been appointed to resolve economic issues, and that recommendations regarding dialysis must be based on clinical criteria, and not on subconscious (or even overt) prejudices or perceptions of social worth.

Practice has moved away from selection towards patient autonomy – the patient making an informed choice, with appropriate counselling from the nephrologist and others. There will be cases where, as in case 2 above, the patient or family may not be able to accept that advice, but it is hoped this is rare.

Even if the nephrologist restricts his/her role to that of informing the autonomous patient, what criteria are to be used to inform a patient, and possibly to advise against accepting treatment? This chapter shows that such criteria have historically been covert and variable, and susceptible to economic and political influences. Even if it is accepted that the major criterion should be an expectation of an acceptable quality of life for a given length of time, is it possible to define and predict this in an individual case?

5.3 Is it possible to predict individual outcomes?

Without good predictive tools it is very difficult to offer appropriate information to the more frail patients who present to nephrologists with progressive or established renal failure.

Several factors have been shown to have value in predicting outcome of patients starting RRT.

5.3.1 Age

Whilst age was widely used to exclude people in the early development of dialysis, there is now a majority view amongst nephrologists[4] and governments[18] that age alone is not an acceptable

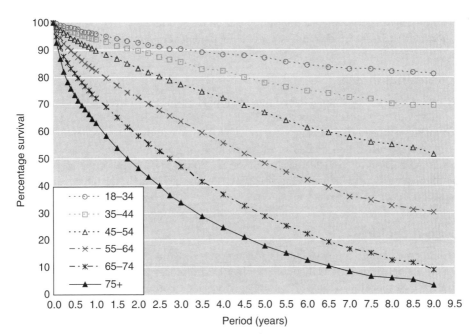

Fig. 5.1 Kaplan–Meier 9-year survival of incident UK renal replacement therapy patients 1997–2005 combined cohort (from day 0).
Source: From the UK Renal Registry 10th Annual Report 2007[16].

criterion for selection. The concept of fitness rather than chronological age should be applied. Whilst older patients starting dialysis have a shorter prognosis than younger patients (Fig. 5.1),[16] their relative risk of death compared with the general population of the same age is much less than that of younger patients (Fig. 5.2).[35] In addition, some older patients live a long time on treatment. Whilst some older patients are fit, there are many with other significant

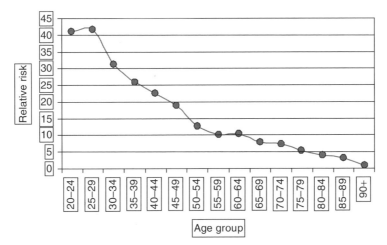

Fig. 5.2 Relative risk of death in Established Renal Failure Patients compared with the general population in England and Wales.
Source: From the UK Renal Registry[36].

co-morbidity factors giving them a poor prognosis on the stratification techniques. It is the sum of co-morbidity present which renders many older patients of poor prognosis, rather than age itself.

5.3.2 Terminal illness

Many patients present with established renal failure at a time when they have other terminal illness leading to very short life expectancy. Case 1 in this chapter is an example. A few weeks of additional life may be of considerable value to such patients. A study of such patients[36] showed that 62% treated rated their quality of life as good or improved, but only 27% were alive at 5 months. An analysis of cost effectiveness, however, showed that except for the best prognostic group the cost per quality-adjusted life year (QALY) gained was well over the commonly used threshold acceptability of $50 000.

5.3.3 Co-morbidity

A hospital-based cohort study of factors affecting survival and morbidity in patients starting dialysis in a single unit in the UK published in 1999 identified factors significantly affecting survival,[37] which included a poor Karnofsky performance score at presentation, and myeloma. Unplanned presentation for dialysis was also a risk factor. Using several factors, a high-risk group of 26 patients was defined, which had a 19.2% 1-year survival. This paper appropriately gave important impetus to the supportive or palliative renal care movement in the UK. However, it should be noted that five of these 26 high-risk patients did have good long-term survival with apparent good quality of life. Thus excluding this group of 26 patients from dialysis would have excluded a significant number who had a good outcome.

Several risk-stratification systems have been developed to try to predict survival in different groups of patients, to identify those with good or bad prognosis, and to allow correction for case mix in comparison of survival between centres.[38–40] Whilst they do identify groups of patients at high risk, they were not designed for the purpose of selecting individual patients suitable for receiving treatment. A systematic literature review identified several individual factors as predictors of early death – in particular, low serum albumin, poor functional status, and acute myocardial infarct.[6] Patients with an above-knee amputation may have a 73% 1-year mortality. However, interpretation of even an objective measure such as the serum albumin must now be done with caution, given the considerable variation in dialysis patients between the two most commonly used methods of measuring the serum albumin.[41]

The "surprise" question has also been advocated as a means of assessing prognosis.[42] A study investigated whether the "surprise" question, "Would I be surprised if this patient died in the next year?" identifies patients who are at high risk for early mortality. The 1-year mortality of the "yes" group was 11% compared with 29% of the "no" group. It was concluded that the "surprise" question is effective in identifying sicker dialysis patients who have a high risk for early mortality and should receive priority for palliative care interventions. However, the prediction was too imprecise to be reliable in an individual, and is dependent on the skill of the respondent, and the threshold for "surprise". Is one surprised at an event one considers to be a 20%, 40%, or 60% probability?

Another study, in an attempt to identify patients at risk of 6-month mortality from starting dialysis, used three prognostic indicators – the serum albumin, the Charlson Comorbidity Index, and a modified surprise question.[43] This approach did separate a high-risk group from a low-risk group, but even in the high-risk group chosen for a probability of death within 6 months the 6-month survival was around 80%. This again shows that, in statistical terms, it is possible to identify high- and low-risk groups, but that the precision is not sufficient to be able to say with certainty to any one individual that they will live a very short time.

Case histories

The difficulties of predicting individual patient outcomes are illustrated by the following two case histories.

Case 3 – A 60-year-old man with no previous history suffered a severe myocardial infarct. He developed a major ventricular septal defect and profound hypotension, and was transferred to the Regional Cardiothoracic Surgery Unit. Two attempts at closure of the septal defect were not entirely successful and he was left with a small defect and persistent hypotension. He remained in cardiac intensive and high-density care units for 3 months. During his profound hypotension, he developed anuria, there was cortical necrosis of his kidneys, and his renal function did not recover. He was considered to have a dreadful cardiac prognosis.

The patient expressed the wish to try dialysis. Multiple central lines had already been used in the intensive care unit (ICU) and he was profoundly hypotensive, so he opted for peritoneal dialysis. This was started and within 3 weeks he had a mild episode of peritonitis which was successfully treated. He was then discharged from hospital and despite persisting hypotension, remained reasonably well and was not admitted to hospital for a further year. There was then one admission with low-grade peritonitis which recovered rapidly. Eighteen months after starting dialysis he developed myelodysplasia which is now transforming to acute myeloid leukaemia. For those 18 months he has remained ambulant, at home, and independent.

This apparently hopeless case was at home on peritoneal dialysis for 18 months, during which time he did not need hospital admission, and was very grateful to have been given this extension of reasonable life. He then had an acute illness and died.

Case 4 – An 86-year-old woman presented with established renal failure of unknown cause. She initially started peritoneal dialysis but had several episodes of peritonitis over the subsequent year and was transferred to haemo-dialysis. Following the death of her husband she moved to live nearer her son and continued therapy at another renal unit. She was on dialysis for 9 years and died of a short illness at age 95. She was mobile, independent, and thoroughly enjoyed life for that time, particularly participating in the care of her grandchildren. In the course of her 9 years of haemodialysis, she twice needed revision of her vascular access. She was not admitted to hospital for over 4 years prior to her terminal illness.

This elderly lady may have been refused RRT by many centres, especially 12 years ago when her treatment started. Her excellent response to treatment would not have been predicted by any of the systems used for predicting outcomes.

5.3.4 **Quality of life**

Predicting the quality of life which may be attained for patients starting dialysis is notoriously difficult. Furthermore, it has been widely shown that physicians and healthcare professionals' perceptions of a patient's quality of life are usually lower than those of the patients themselves. It is regrettable that many renal units do not perform any formal assessment of quality of life or function in their patients, either before or after starting RRT, especially as a relatively simple measure such as the Karnofsky score has been shown to be of useful predictive value in terms of outcome.[37] There is growing awareness of the desirability of such measurements, as is indicated by the recommendation for their use in the Standards for Renal Replacement Therapy issued by the UK Renal Association in 2003.[44]

5.3.4.1 The role of the patient

The patients themselves are the ones who are best placed to determine whether the quality of life they achieve is sufficient to wish to continue therapy. It is important that patients feel no coercion to accept treatment. If a supportive relationship is maintained between the renal team and the patient which respects the patient's autonomy, then the patient will decide whether or not they wish to continue attending for treatment. In that circumstance it is both presumptuous and unnecessary for the renal team to attempt to make decisions for the patient as to whether their quality of life is worthwhile.

Case 5 – *A 75-year-old woman had a long history of thoracic surgery and respiratory problems. She needed to use continuous positive airway pressure (CPAP) ventilatory support at night, but led an active and independent life. She then developed a severe chest infection and was admitted to an ICU. Associated with the infection, she developed acute renal failure on the background of moderate chronic renal impairment. A nephrologist had suggested haemofiltration to support this, but the intensive care team was uneasy about starting further interventional therapy. A second nephrologist was asked for a further opinion. He stated that he would give this after reading the notes and talking with the patient. On his way to visit the patient he met the patient's elder sister. She asked, "What are they going to do to my sister?" The nephrologist responded by saying that he did not know, he was first going to ask the patient what she wanted. At this point the sister burst into tears, saying "Nobody ever asks us old people what we want". After discussion with the patient it was agreed that she would undergo haemofiltration or dialysis for a short period to see if she obtained renal recovery. She agreed that if her kidneys did not recover that long-term RRT would not be appropriate. The patient received RRT for 5 days. Her kidneys recovered, and she is now once more at home and independent.*

This case illustrates the widespread anticipation that things will be done to patients by doctors and therapeutic systems, without recognition that the central figure in such decisions and who must be consulted is the patient. It was consultation with the patient that resolved the situation and enabled a wise decision to be made.

5.4 Guidelines

Guidelines for decision-making on initiation of dialysis may be issued for a variety of reasons. They may be for political purposes, for cost containment and appropriate use of scarce resources, or for good professional practice in the interest of patients.

5.4.1 Political guidelines

Governments may issue political statements, which are effectively guidelines. For example, in 1993, the Department of Health in the UK stated that age was not an acceptable criterion for judging the suitability for dialysis.[18]

The Wiltshire Health Authority in the UK, faced with considerable cost constraints, issued guidelines for initiation of treatment[45] with the aim "To prioritise entry onto the programme for those patients who have the most likelihood of health gain from treatment, based on potential life years to be gained from treatment". The three criteria published were:

1 Anticipated survival of at least 12 months

2 Absence of significant co-morbidity

3 The capability of independent living

This was very little different from the approach of the local renal units, although referring physicians appeared to be much more restrictive at the time. One effect of this guideline was not to limit care, but to emphasize which patients should expect care.

5.4.2 Professional guidelines

There have been few professional consensus guidelines issued. Lowance, in 1993,[46] believed that doctors with high technology were guilty of having "tunnel vision in dealings with patients" and that physicians often did things to patients simply because they were able to do them, rather than because they were necessarily correct. It was suggested when counselling patients with impending established renal failure that they should be advised against accepting dialysis if:

1 The patient is physiologically or chronologically old with an estimated life expectancy of less than 2 years.

2 The patient is demented or has impending dementia with no expectations of gaining cognitive function

3 The patient's life expectancy is less than 2 years because of the existence of co-existing disease, such as advanced diabetes, vascular disease, heart disease, acquiredimmune deficiency syndrome (AIDS), cancer, or other systemic illnesses.

4 The patient has a co-existing illness that will produce intractable pain or suffering should artificial support prolong life long enough to allow this to occur even though the life expectancy with support may be beyond 2 years.

It was intended to apply these guidelines in a "sensible" manner. These recommendations were the personal view of one experienced nephrologist, not a consensus statement.

In 1994, Hirsch et al.[20] published their experience of advising when dialysis was not considered appropriate. In this prospective study in one unit in Canada, in 1992, one-quarter of patients referred to a dialysis unit were not accepted to the programme. Patients not accepted were predominantly female, with very poor functional capacity as judged by the Karnofsky scale, had a mean age of 74 years, and suffered from a combination of cardiovascular and renovascular disease. Very few of those not accepted survived more than 6 months. Based on their experience, the authors suggested the following guidelines for advising against dialysis:

1 Non-uraemic dementia

2 Metastatic or non-resectable solid malignancy or refractory haematologic malignancy

3 End-stage irreversible liver, heart, or lung disease – patient confined to bed or chair needing assistance for activities of daily living

4 Irreversible neurological disease significantly restricting mobility and activities of daily living – e.g. major stroke

5 Multisystem failure making survival extremely unlikely

6 Need to sedate or restrain on each dialysis to maintain functioning access.

These two sets of guidelines, and the Wiltshire guidelines, would have excluded cases 1, 3, and 4 in this chapter who had good outcomes from their treatment.

Somewhat more recently, following a detailed literature review and consultation, the Renal Physicians Association (RPA; of the USA) and the American Society of Nephrology (ASN) issued a clinical practice guideline on shared decision-making in the appropriate initiation or withdrawal from dialysis.[6] The recommendations are laid out in the introduction to ethical case analysis Page xvi. They summarize the converging approaches discussed earlier in this chapter. Recommendations 5, 8, and 9 are of particular interest. Advance directives, whilst relatively common in the USA, are infrequently written in the UK.

5.4.2.1 Standard from the Renal Association of the UK

Similar recommendations are embodied in the current guidelines from the Renal Association.[47]

> Non-dialytic treatment of patients with established renal failure should be regarded as a specific management option and not as "no treatment". This implies that patients should continue to receive

regular follow-up and have a clear treatment plan. Management goals should include prolonging survival where possible and optimising quality of life. The treatment plan should also include timely arrangements for palliative and end of life care. Such arrangements should be made in close consultation with patients and their families."

This standard stresses the concept that the "no-dialysis" option is not a withdrawal of care, but the decision for an active alternative route of care. This approach is also incorporated in the National Service Framework for Renal Services for England.[1]

5.5 The "no dialysis" option

One of the improvements in renal care in the last decade has been the growing interest in the "no dialysis option" – often called renal palliative or supportive care and now to be termed conservative kidney care in the UK. This is discussed further in Chapter 13.

5.6 Counselling to facilitate informed patient choice

The most difficult part of the "no dialysis option" is to provide appropriate and unbiased counselling for the patient. This is discussed in Chapter 12.

5.7 Conclusion

Patients, the renal team, politicians, and health service managers may not entirely agree on what constitutes a "good "outcome" in RRT. A "good" outcome cannot simply be judged on length of life obtained; quality of life, even if short, is equally important. The case histories demonstrate that provision of short periods of dialysis life even in patients with severe co-morbidities can be very rewarding for patients and families: this is often not reflected in the practices of healthcare systems.

In 2009, it is no longer acceptable to the general public or to many governments for nephrologists to make unilateral decisions whether or not to offer patients treatment. The nephrologist must respect the patient's autonomy, and be willing to present carefully considered information concerning likely outcomes sensitively, such that the patient, together with the family, can make a supported and informed decision whether or not to accept RRT. With both intensive medical and psychological support to maximize the quality of remaining life for the patient and the family, a good outcome should be achieved in the large majority of patients, whether or not dialysis is accepted.

Ethical case analysis

The challenge in trying to establish a framework for selecting patients for RRT is that major ethical principles conflict. In some cases such as that of Mr BB (Case 2 in this chapter), the principle of respect for patient autonomy conflicts with non-maleficence, justice, and professional integrity. Despite extensive counselling, Mr BB undertook a course of dialysis therapy that the renal physicians thought likely to cause more harm than good. In the terms of the RPA/ASN guidelines, dialysis was not medically indicated for Mr BB because the expected benefits did not justify the risks. Mr BB experienced considerable distress during his course of dialysis, and he never improved enough to be discharged from the hospital. In terms of quality of life and quantity of life, Mr BB did not benefit from dialysis. The judgement of his nephrologists that dialysis was not appropriate for him was vindicated. Use of the process for conflict resolution in the RPA/ASN guideline (recommendation 5) might have helped in dialysis decision-making with this patient and his family. Unresolved psychosocial and spiritual issues were probably present.

With regard to the case of Mrs AA (Case 1 in this chapter), recommendation 7 of the RPA/ASN guideline is applicable. The RPA/ASN Guideline Working Group resisted using a diagnosis of a terminal illness from a non-renal cause as a reason to preclude dialysis in all cases. The guideline working group anticipated cases just like Mrs AA. She used the 7 weeks of extended life with dialysis to accomplish the tasks of life closure. Dialysis provided her with the opportunity to strengthen her personal relationships and leave a legacy of good memories for her family. Mrs AA clearly benefitted from her dialysis. The extension of life that dialysis afforded for Mr BB did not have such a positive effect. In all likelihood, intensive counselling based on exploring the issues raised in a 'patient as person' would have benefitted him more than dialysis.

It is likely that increased attention to psychosocial and spiritual issues in Mr. BB's prolonged hospital dying would have been the most helpful to his family who had unreconciled grieving months later. In the USA there is a growing trend to use hospital ethics committee consultation to resolve conflicts over what the healthcare team considers family requests for medically ineffective treatment. Research has shown that hospital ethics committee intervention in these circumstances can be successful.[48]

References

1 National Service Framework for Renal Services – Part Two: Chronic kidney disease acute renal failure and end of life care. 2007 http://www.dh.gov.uk/en/Publicationsandstatistics/Publications/PublicationsPolicyAndGuidance/Browsable/DH_4102941.

2 Glover JJ, Moss AH (1998). Rationing dialysis in the United States: possible implications of capitated systems. *Adv Ren Replace Ther*, **5**(4), 341–9.

3 Rutecki GW, et al. (1997). Nephrologists' subjective attitudes towards end-of-life issues and the conduct of terminal care. *Clin Nephrol*, **48**(3), 173–80.

4 McKenzie JK, et al. (1998). Dialysis decision making in Canada, the United Kingdom, and the United States. *Am J Kidney Dis*, **31**(1), 12–18.

5 Moss AH, et al. (1993). Variation in the attitudes of dialysis unit medical directors toward decisions to withhold and withdraw dialysis. *J Am Soc Nephrol*, **4**(2), 229–34.

6 Renal Physicians Association and American Society of Nephrology (2000). Clinical Practice Guideline on Shared Decision-Making in the Appropriate Initiation of and Withdrawal from Dialysis. Washington DC: Renal Physicians Association and American Society of Nephrology.

7 Kee F, et al. (2000). Stewardship or clinical freedom? variations in dialysis decision making. *Nephrol Dial Transplant*, **15**(10), 1647–57.

8 Lelie A (2000). Decision-making in nephrology: shared decision making? *Patient Educ Couns*, **39**(1), 81–9.

9 Lowance DC (2002). Withholding and withdrawal of dialysis in the elderly. *Semin Dial*, **15**(2), 88–90.

10 Main J (2000). Deciding not to start dialysis – a one year prospective study in Teesside. *J Nephrol*, **13**(2), 137–41.

11 Berlyne G (1982). *Nephron*, **31**, 189–190.

12 Baker R (1994). BNHS (British National Health Service) age rationing: a riposte to Bates. *Health Care Anal*, **2**(1), 39–41.

13 Halper T (1985). Life and death in a welfare state: end-stage renal disease in the United Kingdom. *Milbank Mem Fund Q Health Soc*, **63**(1), 52–93.

14 Ansell D, et al. (2005). The Eight Annual Report of the UK Renal Registry. www.renalreg.com.

15 Ansell D, et al. (2006). The Ninth Annual Report of the UK Renal Registry. www.renalreg.com.

16 Ansell D, et al. (2007). The Tenth Annual Report of the UK Renal Registry. www.renalreg.com.

17 Ansell D, Tomson C (2008). The Eleventh Annual Report of the UK Renal Registry. www.renalreg.com.

18 Department of Health (1994). Report of the Health Care Strategy Unit Review of Renal Services. Part I. Department of Health: London.

19 Challah S, et al. (1984). Negative selection of patients for dialysis and transplantation in the United Kingdom. *BMJ*, **288**(6424), 119–22.

20 Hirsch DJ, et al. (1994). Experience with not offering dialysis to patients with a poor prognosis. *Am J Kidney Dis*, **23**(3), 463–6.

21 Mendelssohn DC, Kua BT, Singer PA (1995). Referral for dialysis in Ontario. *Arch Intern Med*, **155**(22), 2473–8.

22 Sekkarie M, Cosma M, Mendelssohn D (2001). Nonreferral and nonacceptance to dialysis by primary care physicians and nephrologists in Canada and the United States. *Am J Kidney Dis*, **38**(1), 36–41.

23 Sekkarie MA, Moss AH (1998). Withholding and withdrawing dialysis: the role of physician specialty and education and patient functional status. *Am J Kidney Dis*, **31**(3), 464–72.

24 Singer PA (1992). Nephrologists' experience with and attitudes towards decisions to forego dialysis. The End-Stage Renal Disease Network of New England. *J Am Soc Nephrol*, **2**(7), 1235–40.

25 Wilson R, et al. (2001). End-stage renal disease: factors affecting referral decisions by family physicians in Canada, the United States, and Britain. *Am J Kidney Dis*, **38**(1), 42–8.

26 Holley JL, Foulks CJ, Moss AH (1991). Nephrologists' reported attitudes about factors influencing recommendations to initiate or withdraw dialysis. *J Am Soc Nephrol*, **1**(12), 1284–8.

27 Parry RG, et al. (1996). Referral of elderly patients with severe renal failure: questionnaire survey of physicians. *BMJ*, **313**(7055), 466.

28 Badzek L, et al. (2000). Inappropriate use of dialysis for some elderly patients: Nephrology nurses' perceptions and concerns. *Nephrol Nursing J*, **27**, 462–70.

29 Friedman E (1993). We treat too many dialysis patients but ESRD Program is still a success. *Nephrol News Issues*, **7**, 41–2.

30 Moss A, (2003). Too many patients who are too sick to benefit start chronic dialysis nephrologists need to learn to "just say no". *Am J Kidney Dis*, **41**(4), 723–7.

31 Caskey FJ et al. (2006). Exploring the differences in epidemiology of treated ESRD between Germany and England and Wales. *Am J Kidney Dis*, **47**(3), 445–54.

32 Sanders D, Dukeminier JJ (1968). Medical advance and legal lag: Hemodialysis and kidney transplantation. *UCLA Law Rev*, **15**, 357–413.

33 Aaron HJ, S.W., (1984). *The painful prescription: rationing hospital care*. Brookings Institution. Washington, DC.

34 Levinsky NG (2003). Too many patients who are too sick to benefit start chronic dialysis nephrologists need to learn to "just say no". *Am J Kidney Dis*, **41**(4), 728–32.

35 Ansell D, Feest T, Byrne C (2003). The Sixth Annual Report of the UK Renal Registry., Bristol: The UK Renal Registry.

36 Hamel MB, et al. (1997). Outcomes and cost-effectiveness of initiating dialysis and continuing aggressive care in seriously ill hospitalized adults. SUPPORT Investigators. Study to Understand Prognoses and Preferences for Outcomes and Risks of Treatments. *Ann Intern Med*, **127**(3), 195–202.

37 Chandna SM, et al. (1999). Is there a rationale for rationing chronic dialysis? A hospital based cohort study of factors affecting survival and morbidity. *Brit Med J*, **318**(7178), 217–23.

38 Beddhu S, et al. (2000). A simple comorbidity scale predicts clinical outcomes and costs in dialysis patients. *Am J Med*, **108**(8), 609–13.

39 Fried L, Bernardini J, Piraino B (2001). Charlson comorbidity index as a predictor of outcomes in incident peritoneal dialysis patients. *Am J Kidney Dis*, **37**(2), 337–42.

40 Khan IH, et al. (1998). Comparing outcomes in renal replacement therapy: how should we correct for case mix? [published erratum appears in *Am J Kidney Dis*, May, **31**(5), 900]. *Am J Kidney Dis*, **31**(3), 473–8.

41 Ansell D, Feest T, Byrne C (2002). The Fifth Annual Report of the UK Renal Registry. Bristol: The UK Renal Registry.

42 Moss AH, et al. (2008). Utility of the "surprise" question to identify dialysis patients with high mortality. *Clin J Am Soc Nephrol*, **3**(5), 1379–84.

43 Germain MJ, et al. (2008). Predicting 6 Month Mortality in Hemodialysis (HD) Patients: Identifying Patients Eligible for Hospice Services. Renal Week abstracts 2008. http://www.abstracts2view.com/asn/view.php?nu=ASN08L1_4081a.

44 Renal Association (2003). Treatment of patients with renal failure: recommended standards and audit measures. Renal Association and Royal College of Physicians, London.

45 Farmery E, Milner P (1997). *Renal replacement therapy: purchasing review and recommendations.* Devizes: Wiltshire Health Authority.

46 Lowance DC (1993). Factors and guidelines to be considered in offering treatment to patients with end-stage renal disease: a personal opinion. *Am J Kidney Dis*, **21**(6), 679–83.

47 Renal Association (2008). Renal Assocaition Guidelines – Chronic Kidney Disease. Renal Association Guidelines.http://www.renal.org/pages/pages/guidelines/current/ckd.php#SUMMARY_3.

48 Fine RL, Mayo TW (2003). Resolution of futility by due process: early experience with the Texas Advance Directives Act. *Ann Intern Med*, **138**, 743–6.

Chapter 6

Health-related quality of life and the patient with chronic kidney disease

Fredric O Finkelstein and Susan H Finkelstein

6.1 Introduction

The health-related quality of life (HRQOL) of the patient with chronic kidney disease (CKD) has been attracting increasing interest in recent years. This relates to a variety of factors. There has been an increasing standardization of instruments used to assess the HRQOL of patients with chronic illnesses and there has been a better understanding on the part of clinicians of the interpretation of these instruments. It is now clearly recognized that there is a strong association amongst various HRQOL measures and patient outcomes as well as the cost of providing care for patients with medical illnesses. In addition, there is recognition of the importance of these measures for the patients themselves, the effectiveness of the care provided to patients, and the patients' perceptions of the care provided for them.

Quality of life has been defined by the World Health Organization as an individual's perception of their position in life in the context of the culture and value systems in which they live and in relation to their goals, expectations, standards, and concerns; it refers to a state of physical, psychological, and social well-being and not merely the absence of disease or infirmity. HRQOL can be defined as the extent to which one's usual or expected physical, social, or emotional well-being (quality of life) is affected by a medical condition or its treatment. The assessment of HRQOL depends to a large extent on patient-reported outcomes (PROs); these can be defined as measurements of any aspect of a patient's health status that comes directly from the patient (i.e. without the interpretation of the response by a physician or anyone else).

HRQOL needs to be viewed as a multidimensional concept, involving four overlapping components (Fig. 6.1). The physical component refers to the level of physical activity, sense of physical well-being, overall health, and energy/vitality level of the patients. The psychological component refers to the cognitive and emotional functioning (e.g. depression, anxiety, interpersonal relationships) of the individual. The social component refers to performance of societal functions, activities of daily living, and responsibilities within and without the home. In addition, the treatment-related component refers to the impact of a specific therapy on a patient's life and the patient's satisfaction with the care he or she is receiving. All of these components need to be viewed in the context of the individual's social, emotional, and cultural environment.

6.2 Health-related quality of life and outcomes

The importance of HRQOL measurements in terms of their association with the outcomes of patients with end-stage renal disease (ESRD) is now well documented. The Dialysis Outcomes and Practice Patterns Study (DOPPS) have clearly shown a strong relationship amongst the mental component score (MCS) and physical component score (PCS) of the Short Form-36 (SF-36)

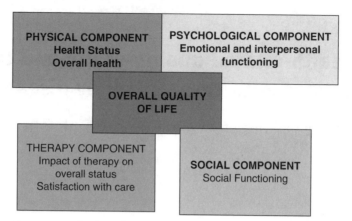

Fig. 6.1 Schematic conceptualization of HRQOL.

questionnaire and mortality and hospitalizations of ESRD patients.[1] Thus, haemodialysis (HD) patients with PCS of 25 or less have a 1.9- and 1.6-fold greater chance of dying or being hospitalized than patients with scores over 46. Similarly, HD patients with MCS of 34 or less have a 1.5- and 1.2-fold greater chance of dying or being hospitalized than patients with scores over 50.

A single global question asking about general health ("How would you say your health is in general?") has been noted to strongly correlate with outcomes in the de Nederlandse Coöperatieve Studie naar de Adequaatheid van Dialyse (NECOSAD) database. Patients replying 'poor' had a 3.6-fold greater risk of death compared to patients replying 'excellent' or 'very good', after correcting for a wide number of variables, including co-morbidities, age, serum albumin level, and primary kidney disease.[2]

Depressive symptoms have also been associated with mortality and hospitalization in ESRD patients. The DOPPS, using the Center for Epidemiological Studies Depression Screening Index (CES-D) questionnaire to assess for the presence of depressive symptoms has shown that HD patients with scores of 15–30 have a 1.8 higher mortality rate that patients with scores of 0–4.[3] These findings confirmed prior studies using the Beck Depression Inventory (BDI) and a time-dependent analysis in a cohort of HD patients.[4]

These questionnaires screen just for the presence of depressive symptoms and not for the presence of clinical depression. Thus, the recent paper by Hedayati et al. is of particular importance.[5] These investigators studied 98 prevalent HD patients with a structured interview and used the Diagnostic Statistical Manual of Mental Disorders IV (DSM-1V) criteria to diagnosis clinical depression. The patients were followed for up to a year; 27% patients were diagnosed with clinical depression. After adjustments for age, co-morbidity, gender, dialysis duration, and race, patients with depression were 2.07 (confidence interval: 1.1–3.9) times more likely to reach the composite outcome of death or first hospitalization.

The reasons for the association of depression and poorer outcomes are likely multifactorial. Firstly, there is greater likelihood of withdrawal from dialysis. In the DOPPS, patients with CES-D scores between 15 and 30 had a more than twofold greater chance of withdrawing from dialysis than those with scores between 0 and 4.[3] Secondly, there is greater likelihood of reduced compliance with a pre-specified medical regimen. This has been well documented for patients with cardiac disease.[6] Peritonitis rates are substantially higher in chronic peritoneal dialysis (PD) patients with high BDI scores, perhaps reflecting reduced compliance with their dialysis regimen in patients with higher scores.[7] Thus, PD patients with BDI scores greater than or equal to 11 had a 2.7-fold greater chance of developing peritonitis than PD patients with lower BDI scores, after correcting for a variety of co-morbidities.

Thirdly, there is a well-established association between depression and inflammatory markers. For example, recent studies have demonstrated a strong association between major depression and elevated C-reactive protein (CRP) levels and between CRP and mortality in the general population (8). In dialysis patients in our facilities, elevated CRP levels have been noted in patients with elevated BDI scores (unpublished data). The relationship between elevated CRP levels and cardiovascular disease is well established. In addition, depression itself – independent of other risk factors – has been correlated with vascular calcifications.[9]

6.3 Health-related quality of life as an outcome measure in clinical trials

There has been a recent interest in exploring newer dialysis modalities, such as more frequent HD and nocturnal HD – both being done in-centre as well as at home. Clinical trials have been organized to study these therapies and investigators have realized that HRQOL measures need to be viewed as important primary outcome measures. Thus, the Frequent Hemodialysis Network study, sponsored by the National Institutes of Health, is a randomized trial exploring differences between conventional HD and both 6 times/week in-centre HD and 5 or 6 nights/week home nocturnal HD.[10] One of the two primary outcome measures involves the physical health composite score (PHC) of the SF-36 and three of the nine secondary outcome measures utilize HRQOL measures (BDI, PHC, and a trail-making test of cognitive function).

The Alberta Trial of Nocturnal HD[11] used a variety of HRQOL domains as secondary end-points in their randomized trial of home nocturnal HD. Their end-points included an overall quality of life and global health perception from the EuroQOL-5D questionnaire and four selected domains from the Kidney Disease Quality of Life questionnaire (KDQOL; effects of kidney disease, burden of kidney disease, sleep, and kidney disease-related symptoms/problems).

The Following Rehabilitation, Economics, and Everyday Dialysis Outcome Measurements (FREEDOM) study is looking at a variety of HRQOL domains in a large, cohort based study of 500 patients being treated with 6 times/week home HD with the NxStage HD machine.[12] Various HRQOL domains are being monitored including the BDI, SF-36, global quality-of-life assessment, time to resume normal activities after each dialysis session, sleep, and restless-leg syndrome.

There is also an increasing interest in in-centre, 3 times/week nocturnal HD, since this treatment has been associated with reduced rates of ultrafiltration, improved blood pressure, and phosphate control, and possibly improved, selected quality-of-life measures.[13] For example, the time to resume usual activities after a dialysis session appears to be shorter for patients on in-centre nocturnal HD than on conventional HD, perhaps reflecting the more gradual ultrafiltration and solute removal with this therapy (*ibid*).

6.4 Health-related-quality-of-life measurements

When deciding which instruments to use to assess HRQOL of CKD patients, it is important to keep in mind the following points. First, it is essential to remind oneself "What it is you are trying to measure?" and "What are the goals of measuring HRQOL?" It is also important to remember that there is a difference in using objective versus subjective measurements. Objective measures are more scientifically valid but may not capture a patient's experience. Subjective measures, such as PROs are of special interest, but their interpretation is difficult and currently is being reevaluated by a committee designated by the Food and Drug Administration in the US. It is also important to distinguish between patient and physician/nurse perceptions, again emphasizing the value of PROs. As an example, the inability of healthcare providers to properly assess the symptoms and complaints of patients has recently been emphasized.[14]

The validity of the instrument to be used also needs to be considered. What is the reported experience with instrument? What is its documented reliability? What is the 'face value' of the instrument"? Does it appear to ask questions concerning the areas you are interested in studying? What is the responsiveness (sensitivity, discriminatory ability, etc.) of the instrument to answer the questions being asked? There is often a lack of a 'gold standard' for many HRQOL measures and thus one needs to accept the answers at their face value. What is most important is to consider carefully the question one is asking and then match the instrument that best addresses that question.

The use of generic instruments and their performance compared to disease or treatment specific ones also needs to be considered. Generic instruments have been developed for use in the general population with a variety of diseases (e.g. SF-36, Health Utility Index) and cover a wide variety of domains. The problem with generic instruments is that they may not focus enough attention on areas of difficulty presented by the specific problems of CKD patients or the treatment modalities for these patients. Disease-specific questionnaires, such as the KDQOL, focus on symptoms that are more specifically related to patients with CKD and/or their treatment. For example, several specific questions used in the CHOICE study (the CHEQ questionnaire), were included after a series of focus groups with ESRD patients identified specific domains of concern for these patients.[15]

Symptom-specific questionnaires focus on particular symptoms associated specifically with CKD or its treatment. A good example involves depression. Clinical depression has been observed in between 25% and 30% of patients with ESRD.[5,16] Thus, using depression-specific questionnaires to examine the HRQOL of patients with CKD is indeed reasonable. In order to assess the presence of depressive symptoms, the BDI, CES-D, and patient health questionnaires (PHQ9) have all been utilized in studies of CKD patients. A remarkably high incidence of depressive symptoms has been noted in these patients, although with the caveat that certain somatic symptoms such as fatigue and poor sleep can be reported even by well-dialysed patients. In one large study, e.g. the mean ± BDI scores for 370 dialysis patients was 12 ± 3.2.[16] Another good example of a specific question is one discussed by Lindsay concerning the time it takes patients to resume their usual activities after conclusion of a dialysis session.[17] The mean time for patients maintained on conventional 3 times/week HD is over 6 h. This question has been particularly useful in assessing some of the newer HD therapies, since the time to recovery after a dialysis session is markedly shorter in patients undergoing more frequent HD.[17]

6.4.1 Generic health-related-quality-of-life measurement

The most widely used generic HRQOL instrument is the SF-36. The domains measured by the SF-36 include four physical domains (physical functioning, role limitations due to physical health (role–physical), general health perceptions, and pain) and four mental domains (energy/fatigue (vitality), social functioning, emotional well-being (mental health), and role limitations due to emotional problems). The physical and mental domains from the SF-36 questions are summarized in physical- and mental-component summary scores, which are standardized to the general US population (mean ± SD score of 50 ± 10).[18] This instrument is of particular value since there are numerous publications documenting the values in ESRD and CKD patients from around the world; it has proved a source of excellent data documenting the relationship of SF-36 scores to a variety of outcomes as well as data documenting the impact of various treatment programmes on scores.

It is now well documented from many studies that dialysis patients have significantly lower or worse scores than the general population on the SF-36 questionnaire, indicating a significant impairment in HRQOL. This is particularly so for the physical domains of this instrument. For example, mean scores in the DOPPS study for HD patients on the physical component score of SF-36 was 33.1 compared to a score of 50 for the general population.[19] Of the four physical components of the SF-36, physical function scores were 41, physical role scores 32, physical pain scores 59, and general health scores 40, compared to scores of 100 for the general population. Mental health scores of the SF-36 were not as strikingly reduced. For example, the mental-health component score of HD patients was 46.6 compared to a score of 50 for normal individuals.[19] The most reduced score of the four mental component scores was the score of 43 for vitality while the mental health score was 67 compared to scores of 100 for the control population.

Other instruments that have been used include the Health Utilities Index (HUI) and global assessment of health or quality of life. The HUI is a 21-item questionnaire that is composed of eight attributes felt to be important by the general population (vision, hearing, ambulation, dexterity, emotion, cognition, pain, and speech). Responses are then converted into an overall utility score. This score can be compared across disease states. For example, a recent study suggests that that HUI scores for the general population is 0.93, for patients with coronary heart disease it is 0.87, for patients with glomerular filtration rates (GFRs) of 30–60 it is 0.67, for patients with GFR of <30 it is 0.54, for patients with a stroke it is 0.54, and for patients with Alzheimer's disease it is 0.22.[20]

Global assessments of quality of life by patients have been thought to be particularly useful in that they capture the patients' global perspective of their quality of life and they may be sensitive to changes in treatment regimens.[21,22] Global assessments of health may also be useful and have been shown to strongly correlate with patient outcomes, as noted above.[2]

6.4.2 Disease-specific and symptom-specific health-related quality of life measurements

Disease-specific instruments require that we identify specific domains that are of concern for the patient with kidney disease. One approach is to develop a questionnaire with many questions that addresses a variety of targeted domains. For example, the KDQOL-Short Form targets domains specifically for patients with kidney disease (based on the 43 kidney-disease-specific questions). These domains include work status, quality of social interactions, burden of kidney disease, social support, cognitive function, sexual function, sleep, effects of kidney disease (overall health), and symptoms/problem list. The scores are aggregated and transformed linearly to a 0–100 possible range, with higher scores indicating better status. Another approach is to target specific domains that have been identified as being problem areas for patients with CKD. One example would be depression, which is a problem for between 25% and 30% of ESRD patients. In this regard, it is important to remember that questionnaires inform us about the presence of clinical symptoms (pessimism, anhedonia, sadness; complaints of feeling helpless and hopeless; changes in sleep, concentrating ability, appetite, activity level, and libido; and problems with marital and family relationships). The actual diagnosis of clinical depression requires a structured interview, such as the Structured Clinical Interview for Depression (SCID) or Hamilton. Questionnaires, though, can be a useful way to screen for depression. For example, BDI scores greater than or equal to 16 and PHQ-9 scores greater than or equal to 10 have a nearly 90% sensitivity and specificity for diagnosing clinical depression in ESRD patients.[23]

Other domains that are particularly relevant for the patient with kidney disease include

♦ fatigue and vitality, physical functioning, sleep, cognitive functioning, and sexual functioning,

♦ length of time to resume normal functioning after dialysis treatment, and

♦ restless legs.

These domains have all been well documented to be problem areas for patients with CKD and may well be important ingredients in the patients' perception of their quality of life. Particular mention needs to be made of cognitive difficulties, since problems with cognitive function are now recognized as being a major problem area for CKD patients. Furthermore, cognitive difficulties may interfere with the assessment of various quality-of-life domains that depend on the patients reporting symptoms. More attention needs to be paid to cognitive dysfunction and its impact on how care and support is provided to CKD patients. Providing support for patients to maximize their HRQOL requires that providers understand the impact of cognitive deficits on patients and how these deficits, in turn, impact on the care provided by the nephrology community and the patients' care-givers.

6.4.3 Health-related quality of life and dialysis modality

It is now recognized that the HRQOL problems of ESRD patients are related in part to the treatments the patients receive. This may be because of the inadequate solute removal rates of the dialysis therapy, the impact and effect of the treatment itself, or the associated co-morbidities associated with CKD. This area has attracted considerably more attention recently as researchers have been investigating the impact of different dialysis regimens on individual patient's HRQOL measures.[24]

The HRQOL of patients maintained on conventional, 3 times/week HD have been compared in several studies to patients maintained on PD. The results of these studies have been variable, but in large part have suggested that standard HRQOL measures – when corrected for co-morbidities – do not appear to different for PD patients compared to HD patients, at least for the initial year or so of therapy. Results beyond this time period get difficult to interpret because there is a moderate transfer rate from PD to HD and a very small transfer rate from HD to PD. Of all the patients started on PD, only 50% are still receiving therapy at 24 months, because of death, transplantation, or transfer to HD.[25] Thus, patients remaining on PD may be 'selected' in a sense, since those not doing well may be those transferring to HD.

Nevertheless, there appears to be agreement that patients are more satisfied with PD than HD and that PD has less of a negative impact on patients' lives than HD.[26,27] This satisfaction applies to both the patients' satisfaction with the dialysis facility and staff and care they receive, and to their satisfaction with the overall treatment regimen itself.

There has been an increased interest in modifying conventional 3 times/week HD therapy to improve the outcome of patients by using more frequent regimens at home or in-centre and/or using longer dialysis treatments at night 3 or more times per week. Newer dialysis machines are being used to facilitate home HD.[12] Part of the stimulus for these therapies relates to the concern of the nephrology community over the poor HRQOL of patients maintained on conventional HD. There is an increasing interest in exploring whether measured HRQOL can be improved by modifying the HD regimen.

Home HD has certain clear advantages. The treatment is done in the patients' home and the patient has control of his treatment. There is often an increased frequency of therapy and a reduced rate of ultrafiltration. The latter is particularly important since recent studies from London, Ontario, have focussed attention on the notion of time to recovery after a dialysis treatment (i.e. the time to resume usual activities after an HD treatment).[17] These studies noted that patients treated with 3 times/week conventional HD take on average 6 h to resume their usual activities after completing an HD session. In contrast, patients treated with short daily HD or 5 or 6 times/week nocturnal HD take less than 1 h to recover after an individual dialysis session. This reduction is strongly correlated with selected, other HRQOL measures, such as fatigue and vitality.

There are certain obvious negative aspects of more frequent HD. These include an increased burden of therapy in terms of frequency or home treatment, a negative impact on the partner, a negative impact of the treatment on a patients' life-style, and a potential for increased risk of complications of therapy, such as bleeding, access issues, etc. The impact of home HD on the care-giver has received surprising little attention, but may well have an important impact on the overall quality of life of both the care-giver and the patient.[28] This is an area that deserves further investigation, particularly as the use of home therapies expands in the coming years.

6.5 Interventions to improve health-related quality of life

Although poor HRQOL measures have been associated with poor outcomes in dialysis patients, it is surprising that few studies employing treatments specifically directed at improving HRQOL have been reported. Furthermore, the impact of these newer treatment plans on patient outcomes has not as yet been reported. This in part reflects the difficulties in organizing well-planned studies aimed specifically to document the impact of treatment of impaired HRQOL of patients with complex medical illnesses.

Certain specific treatment programmes have been discussed in the literature, including treatment of depression, anaemia, and physical functioning, and modifications in the dialysis treatment regimen itself. In the present review, we will focus on three selected interventional programmes to improve the HRQOL of patients with CKD – depression, anaemia, and more frequent HD.

6.5.1 Depression

Management of depression is discussed in Chapter 11.

6.5.2 Anaemia

The use of erythropoesis-stimulating agents (ESAs) in patients with CKD has recently been called into question. Recent studies in patients with CKD have prompted the Food and Drug Administration (FDA) in the US to suggest that the benefits of these drugs have not been well documented and that increases in haemoglobin levels to values over 12 gm/dl may be associated with increased morbidity and mortality (FDA Advisory warning, 11/8/07). Furthermore, the FDA has indicated that the studies that have suggested that HRQOL improves with treatment for anaemia have not been satisfactorily conducted and have consequently discounted these studies in providing guidelines for the use of ESAs in CKD patients. Some studies, moreover, have in fact suggested the HRQOL may not improve with increases in haemoglobin levels,[29] e.g. the recent Correction of Hemoglobin and Outcomes in Renal Insufficiency (CHOIR) study examining various HRQOL measures in CKD patients randomized to target haemoglobin levels of 11.3 and 13.5 demonstrated no difference in quality of life between the higher and lower target groups.[29]

Two recent studies have readdressed this issue. One study was a cross-sectional study examining over 1100 CKD patients and correlated various HRQOL domains with haemoglobin levels.[30] The findings indicated that in Stage 3–5 CKD patients not on dialysis, there is a significant improvement in various quality-of-life domains as haemoglobin levels increase from less than 11 to 11–12 and higher, and these improvements persist in selected domains after correction for variety of factors including the use of ESAs, and other co-morbidities. The authors felt that the findings supported other studies suggesting that there is a relationship between haemoglobin levels and various quality-of-life domains; and that the greatest improvement in quality of life occurs with the increase in haemoglobin level to the 11–12 gm% range.[31]

The second study was a review article concerning HRQOL and anaemia treatment in CKD patients.[32] These authors underscore the difficulty in interpreting the data concerning anaemia treatment and HRQOL and emphasize the lack of uniformity in the findings. This relates in turn to a variety of demographic and methodological differences in the various studies, including differences in baseline health status, instruments used to assess HRQOL, and haemoglobin targets. Nevertheless, certain patterns exist in the various studies that have been published suggesting that the HRQOL domains that are most improved with ESAs relate to physical symptoms, vitality, energy, and physical activity. There is some improvement in domains of social functioning and mental health, but little improvement in emotional functioning and pain. Other more specific domains that have been reported to improve with ESA therapy include sleep, cognitive functioning, and sexual functioning. Interestingly, the maximal increase in HRQOL per incremental increase in haemoglobin appears to occur in the range of 10–12 g/dl.[32] Normalization of haemoglobin levels to 12–14 g/dl provided some additional, but blunted improvements, supporting the findings in the study cited above.

6.5.3 More frequent haemodialysis

The impact of more frequent HD on HRQOL of ESRD patients has been the subject of much interest and discussion.[33] It appears likely that there are changes that occur in various quality-of-life domains with a change in the HD frequency from 3 times/week to 6 times/week. The studies that have been reported thus far have involved small numbers of patients. Different quality-of-life instruments have been used in the different studies and the findings have not been consistent. Perhaps the most striking finding is the reduction in the time to recovery of function (time to resume usual activities after the end of a HD treatment).[17] Other HRQOL domains that have been effected by more frequent HD include depressive symptoms, selected dimensions on the KDQOL (such as patient satisfaction, physical health, and general health perception), and patient's global assessment of their quality of life. Some investigators have emphasized that it is important to talk to patients and listen to what they report to be the impact that a change in therapy is having on their lives, since patients appear to report improvements that may not be captured in standardized HRQOL instruments.[22,34]

Two recent important studies deserve special mention. In the Alberta Trial, 52 ESRD patients were randomized to conventional HD or frequent nocturnal HD done without home monitoring, 5–6 times/week for a minimum of 6 h for each treatment.[11,35] Predetermined HRQOL measures were assessed, including the EuroQOL-5D Index Score (a measure of overall quality of life), the Euro5D visual analogue scale (global health perception), and four domains from the KDQOL questionnaire (effects of kidney disease, burden of kidney disease, sleep, and kidney-disease-related symptoms/problems). Following 6 months of therapy, the results indicated no significant change in EuroQOL index question or in the EuroQOL visual analogue scale but an improvement in effects of kidney disease (8.6 point difference) and burden of kidney disease (9.8 point increase). There were non-significant improvements in all domains on the SF-36, including the physical component and mental component scores.

The second study is the preliminary analysis of the FREEDOM study.[12] As noted above, this is a cohort study which plans to examine 500 patients treated with short, daily HD with the NxStage dialysis machine. A 4-month interim analysis of various quality-of-life measures was planned and this analysis showed a significant reduction in BDI scores, an improvement in global perception of quality of life, improvement in PCS and MCS scores from the SF-36, and a dramatic decrease in the time to recovery after a dialysis session from over 6 h to about 1 h.

Thus, the impact of more frequent HD on HRQOL measures is somewhat uncertain, but the data suggests that there is clearly an improvement in selected domains. It is, therefore, important to make sure that future studies documenting the outcomes of more frequent HD focus attention on appropriate HRQOL domains to critically examine the impact on the change in therapy on medical outcomes as well as HRQOL.

6.6 Conclusion

HRQOL of patients with CKD is an arena that is now receiving much more attention. The HRQOL problems of patients with CKD are now well documented and can be assessed using a variety of quality-of-life instruments. Recent studies have begun to explore ways to improve the HRQOL of patients with CKD. While several therapeutic approaches have been suggested, it remains uncertain if these approaches can be applied to a large number of CKD patients and whether these interventions will result in an improvement in medical outcomes. Of particular interest are the newer dialysis treatments that are being utilized; the impact of these therapies on HRQOL of ESRD patients needs to be carefully studied.

References

1 Mapes D, Lopes AA, Satayathum S, et al. (2003). Health-related quality of life as a predictor of mortality and hospitalization: the Dialysis Outcomes and Practice Patterns Study (DOPPS). *Kidney Int*, **64**, 339–49.

2 Thong MS, Kaptein AA, Benyamini Y, et al. (2008). Netherlands Cooperative Study on the Adequacy of Dialysis (NECOSAD) Study Group Association between a self-rated health question and mortality in young and old dialysis patients: a cohort study. *Am J Kidney Dis*, **52**, 111.

3 Lopes AA, Albert JM, Young EW, et al. (2004). Screening for depression in hemodialysis patients: associations with diagnosis, treatment, and outcomes in the DOPPS. *Kidney Int*, **66**, 2047–53.

4 Kimmel P, Peterson RA, Weihs KL, et al. (2000). Multiple measurements of depression predict mortality in a longitudinal study of chronic hemodialysis outpatients. *Kidney Int*, **57**, 2093–8.

5 Hedayati SS, Bosworth H, Briley L, et al. (2008). Death or hospitalization of patients on chronic hemodialysis is associated with a physician-based diagnosis of depression. *Kidney Int*, **74**, 930–6.

6 Gehi A, Haas D, Pipken S, et al. (2005). Depression and medication adherence in outpatients with coronary heart disease: findings from the Heart and Soul Study. *Arch Intern Med*, **165**, 2508–13.

7 Troidle L, Watnick S, Wuerth DB, et al. (2003). Depression and its association with peritonitis in long-term peritoneal dialysis patients. *Am J Kidney Dis*, **42**, 350–4.

8 Ford DE, Erlinger TP (2004). Depression and C-reactive protein in US adults: data from the third national health and nutrition examination survey. *Arch Intern Med*, **164**, 1010–14.

9 Agatisa PK, Matthews KA, Bromberger JT, et al. (2005). Coronary and aortic calcification in women with a history of major depression *Arch Intern Med*, **165**, 1229–36.

10 Suri RS, Garg AX, Chertow GM, et al. (2007). Frequent Hemodialysis Network Trial Group. Frequent Hemodialysis Network (FHN) randomized trials: study design. *Kidney Int*, **71**, 349–59.

11 Cullerton B, Walsh M, Klarenbach SW, et al. (2007). Effect of frequent nocturnal hemodialysis vs. conventional hemodialysis on left ventricular mass and quality of life: a randomized controlled trial. *JAMA,* **298**, 1291–9.

12 Jaber BL, Finkelstein FO, Glickman JD, et al. for the FREEDOM Study Group (2009). Scope and Design of the Following Rehabilitation, Economics and Everyday-Dialysis Outcome Measurements (FREEDOM) Study. *Am J Kidney Dis,* **53**, 310–20.

13 Troidle L, Hotchkiss M, Finkelstein FO (2007). A thrice weekly in-center nocturnal hemodialysis program. *Adv Chronic Kidney Dis,* **14**, 244–8.

14 Weisbord, Fried SD, Linda F, et al. (2007). Renal Provider Recognition of Symptoms in Patients on Maintenance Hemodialysis. *Clin J Am Soc Nephrol,* **2**, 960–7.

15 Wu AW, Fink NE, Cagney KA, et al. (2001). Developing a health-related quality-of-life measure for end-stage renal disease: The CHOICE Health Experience Questionnaire. *Am J Kidney Dis,* **37**, 11–21.

16 Wuerth D, Finkelstein SH, Finkelstein FO (2003). Chronic Peritoneal Dialysis Patients Diagnosed with Clinical Depression: Results of Pharmacological Therapy. *Semin Dial,* **16**, 424–7.

17 Lindsay RM, Heidenheim PA, Nesrallah H, et al. (2006). Minutes to recovery after a hemodialysis session: a simple health-related quality of life question that is reliable, valid and sensitive to change. *Clin J Am Soc Nephrol,* **1**, 952–9.

18 Ware J, Kosinski M, Keller S (1994). *SF36 Physical and Mental Health summary scales. A User's Manual,* 2nd Ed. Moston, MA: The Health Institute, New England Medical Center.

19 Perlman R, Finkelstein FO, Liu L et al. (2005). Quality of life in chronic kidney disease: a cross-sectional analysis of the Renal Research Institute CKD study. *Am J Kidney Dis,* **45**, 658–66.

20 Gorodetskaya I, Zenios Z, McCulloch CE, et al. (2006). Health-related quality of life and estimates of utility in chronic kidney disease. *Kidney Int,* **68**, 2801–8.

21 Concato J, Feinstein AR (1997). Asking patients what they like: overlooked attributes of patient satisfaction with primary care. *Am J Med,* **102**, 399–406.

22 Reynolds J, Homel P, Cantey L, et al. (2004). A One Year Trial of In-Center Daily Hemodialysis with an Emphasis on Quality of Life. *Blood Purif,* **22**, 320–8.

23 Watnick S, Wang PL, Demadura T, et al. (2005). Validation of two depression screening tools in dialysis patients. *Am J Kidney Dis,* **46**, 919–24.

24 Finkelstein FO, Wuerth D, Finkelstein SH (2007). Quality of life assessments in hemodialysis and peritoneal dialysis patients: an important dimension of patient choice. *Semin Dial,* **20**, 211–13.

25 Brown EA, Davies SJ, Rutherford P, et al. for the EAPOS Group (2003). Survival of functionally anuric patients on automated peritoneal dialysis: the European APD Outcome Study. *J Am Soc Nephrol,* **14**, 2948–57.

26 Rubin HR, Fink NE, Plantinga LC, et al. (2004). Patient ratings of dialysis care with peritoneal dialysis vs. hemodialysis. *JAMA,* **291**, 697–703.

27 Juergensen E, Wuerth D, Finkelstein SH, et al. (2006). Hemodialysis and peritoneal dialysis: patients' assessment of their satisfaction with therapy and the impact of the therapy on their lives. *Clin J Am Soc Nephrol,* **1**, 1191–6.

28 Gayomali C, Sutherland S, Finkelstein FO (2008). The challenge for the caregiver of the patient with chronic kidney disease. *Nephrol Dial Transplant,* **23**, 3749–51.

29 Singh AK, Szczech L, Tang KL, et al. (2006). Correction of anemia with epoetin alfa in chronic kidney disease. *N Engl J Med,* **355**, 2085–98.

30 Finkelstein FO, Story K, Firanek C, et al. (2009). Health-related quality of life and hemoglobin levels in chronic kidney disease patients. *Clin J Am Soc Nephrol,* **4**, 33–8.

31 Lefebvre P, Vekeman F, Sarokham B, et al. (2006). Relationship between hemoglobin level and quality of life in anemic patients with chronic kidney disease receiving epoetin alfa. *Curr Med Res Opin.* **22**, 1929–37.

32 Leaf DE, Goldfarb DS (2008). Interpretation and review of health-related quality of life data in CKD patients receiving treatment for anemia. *Kidney Int*, **75**, 15–24.

33 Finkelstein FO, Finkelstein SH, Wuerth D, et al. (2007). Effects of Home Hemodialysis on Health-Related Quality of Life Measures. *Semin Dial*, **20**, 265–8.

34 Kutner NG (2004). Quality of life and daily hemodialysis. *Semin Dial*, **17**: 92-8.

35 Manns BJ, Walsh MW, Cullerton BF, et al. (2009). Nocturnal hemodialysis does not improve overall measures of quality of life compared to conventional hemodialysis. *Kidney Int*, in press.

Chapter 7

Symptoms in renal disease; their epidemiology, assessment, and management

Fliss Murtagh and Steven D Weisbord

7.1 Introduction

Patients with chronic kidney disease (CKD), particularly those with end-stage renal disease (ESRD) are among the most symptomatic of any chronic disease group.[1] Identifying and controlling symptoms is a high priority for patients and families,[2] and notably improves their quality of life.[3] For those with ESRD, excellent symptom management becomes an increasingly high priority as the duration of time they remain dependent on chronic renal replacement therapy (RRT) increases.[2,4] It is also important to recognize that, while RRT provides major benefit, including symptom relief, it will not always ameliorate or abolish symptoms and may sometimes contribute to them.

7.2 Causes for symptoms in end-stage renal disease

Symptoms arise in advanced renal disease for a number of reasons; they may be a direct consequence of the renal disease, a consequence of dialysis, or due to co-morbid conditions. Co-morbidity is increasingly important as the ESRD population becomes older and is more likely to have multiple and often chronic medical conditions.

7.2.1 Symptoms directly related to renal disease

Prior to dialysis (or if dialysis is subsequently withheld or withdrawn), uraemia can affect all organ systems, leading to symptoms such as pruritus, fatigue, gastrointestinal symptoms, sexual dysfunction,[5] uropathy, and arthropathy.[6] Experience with daily or nocturnal dialysis has demonstrated a significant reduction in uraemic symptoms, although distressing symptoms may remain or develop.[7]

Few symptoms can be easily attributable to one cause alone, however. For example, itch or pruritus is commonly attributed to uraemia (although 'CKD-associated pruritus' may be a more accurate term[8] because the pathogenesis remains uncertain and it is not clearly a direct consequence of uraemia). There is evidence, however, that about a third of patients with pruritus report intensification of the symptom during or immediately following dialysis.[9] Similarly, symptoms arising directly from the renal disease may interact with a co-morbid condition to give rise to a worsening and more complex symptom picture. Examples are fluid overload because of renal failure exacerbated by cardiac failure, or uraemic neuropathy complicated by co-existing diabetic neuropathy.

7.2.2 Symptoms related to dialysis

Intradialytic symptoms are those relating directly to the dialysis procedure. Approximately 40% of haemodialysis sessions are associated with symptomatic hypotension, cramps, nausea and vomiting, and pruritus. In addition, post-dialysis hypotension and a 'washed-out' feeling lasting up to 24 h are common. Other symptoms, such as headache, may be very common (affecting up to 70% of haemodialysis patients), but are often difficult to classify and attribute to specific causes.[10]

Those symptoms occurring early in the dialysis are commonly related to a lack of appropriate vasoconstriction, whilst those occurring later may be related to or caused by the target dry weight being too low. Many of these symptoms are reduced or eliminated by peritoneal dialysis, or by frequent, slow haemodialysis – such as nocturnal or daily. Shorter dialysis treatments, high-flux dialysis, elderly patients, and high co-morbid burden correlate with increased symptoms on dialysis. Recent studies have supported the value of changes in the dialysis prescription in decreasing intradialytic symptoms. Monitoring blood volume, decreasing the dialysis temperature, and modelling of dialysate sodium and ultrafiltration rates are effective and inexpensive.[11,12]

Some specific symptoms may occur in relation to dialysis. Symptomatic hypotension can occur early in dialysis, often in association with rapid or large intravascular volume changes. Loss of autonomic nervous system control can sometimes play a part. Hypotensive symptoms later in dialysis are more usually related to the target dry weight being too low. Pruritus may worsen during or just after dialysis, and has been associated with inadequate dialysis. Anorexia is also common in dialysis patients, and it may indicate uraemia and inadequate dialysis, although it is more often multi-factorial, with other factors (such as anaemia, depression, taste disturbance, dry mouth, gastrointestinal symptoms, or gastroparesis) likely to play a part. Constipation is common for dialysis patients, and immobility, fluid restriction, dietary restrictions, and/or medication (such as aluminium and calcium phosphate binders, iron supplements, and opioids) may all contribute.

7.2.3 Symptoms due to co-morbid conditions

Because of limited symptom research, it is not always clear whether uraemia, dialysis, or co-morbid conditions are the most dominant cause of each symptom, and for many patients a combination of causes and triggers does, in reality, together contribute to their overall symptom burden. Co-morbid conditions do, however, play a major part in causing symptoms, particularly for the older patient, who may have vascular disease, cardiac problems, diabetes mellitus, or other co-morbidities. Some of the commoner co-morbid conditions which contribute to symptom burden include diabetic gastroparesis, other diabetic neuropathies, other diabetic complications, cardiovascular disease, and peripheral vascular disease.

Diabetic patients with ESRD have often had their diabetes for many years, and may have other complications in addition to their renal impairment. Diabetic gastroparesis due to autonomic nerve damage is common in long-standing diabetes, and is characterized by anorexia, early satiety (feeling full), nausea, and sometimes vomiting. Advanced uraemia itself also leads to delayed gastric emptying, which can contribute to this problem. Delayed gastric emptying may itself go on to cause gastric reflux and dyspepsia. Diabetic patients also suffer from other neuropathies. Autonomic neuropathy can also affect the mid- and lower gut, leading to an enteropathy characterized by alternating diarrhoea and constipation, and sometimes faecal incontinence. Non-autonomic diabetic neuropathies that affect the peripheral nerves may take a number of different forms, including polyneuropathies, radiculopathies, or mononeuropathies. Paraesthesia – with sensory disturbance or loss, and sometimes associated pain – is a typical presentation of these non-autonomic neurological complications, whilst motor impairment occurs late in the course of the condition. The neuropathic pain associated with diabetic neuropathies can be severe, persistent, and difficult to control. Skin and soft-tissue problems are also common in the diabetic patient; decubitus ulcers or diabetic foot may occur and amputation may sometimes be required. The severity of these skin and soft-tissue problems may be such that these pains too are difficult to control.

Cardiovascular disease encompasses a wide range of clinical problems, including coronary artery disease, cerebrovascular disease, peripheral vascular disease, congestive heart failure, and left ventricular hypertrophy. All forms of cardiovascular disease are notably more common in those with CKD, and the risk of cardiac events in patients with ESRD is estimated to be about 3–5 times higher than in the general population.[13] Cardiovascular causes account for about 45% of deaths in those on dialysis, and the proportion is similar or even higher for those managed conservatively, without dialysis. The main symptoms associated with cardiovascular disease are pain, breathlessness, and hypotension, although this depends very much on the particular presentation and problems of the individual patient. Peripheral vascular disease, if present, is a particular challenge because it is often far advanced before symptoms develop. Pain (ranging from intermittent claudication to rest pain), ischaemic ulceration, and gangrene are easier to prevent rather than relieve. Smoking cessation and regular exercise are important even in advanced peripheral vascular disease, and preventative foot care is of paramount importance (as for the diabetic patient).

Calciphylaxis is a problem seen most often either in dialysis patients or immediately following transplantation. It is infrequent but when it does occur, it can be extremely painful. Small vessels are calcified and become occluded, with ischaemic necrosis of the surrounding tissue. Skin changes occur, with livedo reticularis and palpable tender subcutaneous nodules, which most often affect the lower trunk and lower extremities.[14] (See also Chapter 8.)

Hypotension from a variety of causes may be a common contributory factor in falls, especially for older patients. Hypotension occurs most often in relation to dialysis, but may also occur in diabetes (the postural hypotension caused by diabetic autonomic neuropathy), and be precipitated by medications such as beta-blockers, calcium-channel blockers, and nitrates.

7.3 Symptom prevalence

How common symptoms are depends to some extent on which CKD population is being considered. Although little comparative study has been made of symptoms across the different stages of CKD, those with more advanced disease are likely to be most symptomatic. Fig. 7.1 illustrates the prevalence of common symptoms in three populations with advanced CKD: those on dialysis,[15] those with Stage 5 CKD managed conservatively (without dialysis),[16] and those withdrawing from dialysis in the last 24 h of life.[17]

7.3.1 Prevalence of anxiety and depression

Although anxiety and depression (particularly depression) have been widely studied in ESRD, their exact prevalence remains contentious, and this is reflected in the wide range of reported prevalence for these conditions.

Most evidence comes from dialysis populations. Anxiety is reported as occurring in 12–52%[3,18–24] and depression in 5–71%[3,20–39] of dialysis patients. Much of this variation reflects differences in the populations assessed, the definitions of anxiety and depression used, and the instruments used to detect them. For instance, studies using formal diagnostic criteria (as defined in the Diagnostic and Statistical Manual of Mental Disorders 4th edition (DSM-IV))

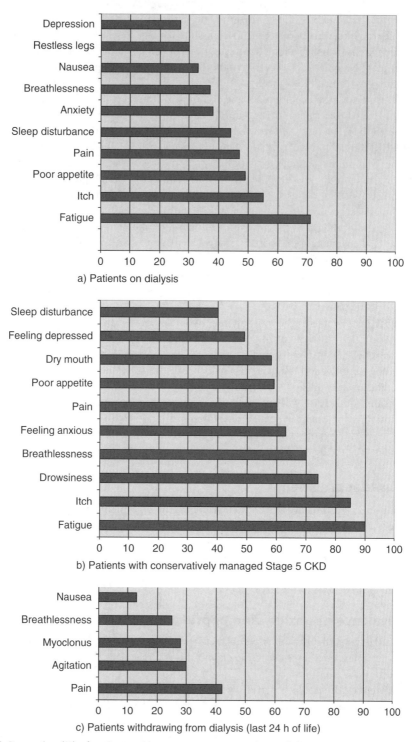

Fig. 7.1 Proportion (%) of patients with common symptoms in renal disease.

suggest that 27–46% of haemodialysis patients have an anxiety disorder,[18,19] and 26–30% have a depressive disorder.[39] Screening tools, such as the Beck Depression Inventory, tend to identify a somewhat higher proportion (45–50%) of potential depression than diagnostic tools, depending on the level of cut-off used in the screening tool.[26,38] It is important to distinguish between the formal diagnosis of anxiety or depressive disorder (less common), and more non-specific symptoms of feeling anxious or depressed (which are inevitably more common). Both need to be determined; the former because formal anxiety or depressive disorders need defined interventions, proactive management, and detailed, skilled follow-up, the latter because it is important to know from the patients themselves what is troubling to them. While feelings of anxiety and sadness may not necessarily reflect full-blown anxiety or depression, these symptoms will still need to be addressed, such as through information, communication, and preparation, or through psychological and social support. However for clinical and research purposes, they should be carefully distinguished.

Patients managed without dialysis probably have similar levels of anxiety and depression, although evidence remains limited, and the prevalence of anxiety and depression likely increases over time.[15] They have a high prevalence of the symptoms of feeling anxious or sad (63% and 50%, respectively), and 45% have depressive scores above the standard cut-off on the Geriatric Depression Scale.[15]

7.3.2 Prevalence of pain

In the past, data on pain prevalence has sometimes been collected within studies of quality of life, where pain is just one of the many domains influencing quality of life. However, pain prevalence is more accurately determined with a specific, validated pain- or symptom-assessment measure. When used both in dialysis populations and the general population, quality of life measures do, however, indicate that (after adjustment for age and gender) dialysis patients experience notably more pain than their counterparts in the general population.[40–42]

Now that specific validated pain measures are beginning to be more widely adopted, it is becoming clear that pain is a common problem for patients with advanced renal disease. Studies from Canada,[43] Italy,[44] and the US[45] have reported 48–50% of all haemodialysis patients reporting pain using, respectively, the McGill Pain Questionnaire, a numerical pain score, and the Dialysis Symptom Index; each convincingly demonstrate that pain is more common in dialysis patients than previously recognized. Pain prevalence has also been identified in this more rigorous way in patients with Stage 5 CKD managed without dialysis, revealing a similar baseline pain prevalence of 53%,[46] although pain prevalence was demonstrated to increase markedly over time, increasing to affect 73% of all conservatively managed Stage 5 CKD patients by the month before death, with over half of these reporting severe pain.[15] Studies of patients withdrawing from dialysis suggest pain affects about 50% of patients,[47,48] allowing for the reduced accuracy of proxy measures.[49]

It is important to understand, not only the overall prevalence, but also the nature and patterns of pain experienced by patients. Pain which is recurrent or persistent is more likely to be intrusive and will impair quality of life of patients more substantially.[50] For this reason, longitudinal study of pain (as well as other symptoms) is particularly important. The majority of studies to date is cross-sectional, and provides only a 'snapshot' of pain at any one time point. The few longitudinal studies of pain indicate that worsening or fluctuating pain over time contributes substantially to deterioration in both physical and mental components of quality of life.[15,45] This is discussed more fully in Chapter 8.

7.3.3 Prevalence of pruritus

Numerous cross-sectional studies provide evidence on the prevalence of itch.[3,9,23,52–68] Together, these studies (most of which are small, mostly involving <300 participants) suggest that pruritus affects between 28% and 60% of patients on haemodialysis, and between 50% and 68% of those on peritoneal dialysis. Four studies report higher prevalence (between 70% and 74%) among haemodialysis patients,[24,69–71] but this may reflect the longer periods of prevalence used in these studies. Pruritus prevalence in those with Stage 5 CKD managed without dialysis was also shown to be high (74%) in a study using a shorter period of prevalence (pruritus occurring in the previous week), suggesting it is more prevalent in this population.[46]

There has also been some suggestion that the prevalence of pruritus has been decreasing over time, parallel with advances in techniques and efficiency of dialysis. A recent epidemiological study of >18 000 patients refutes this, however, indicating that between 36% and 50% of all haemodialysis patients report moderate to extreme pruritus, despite the continuing advances in dialysis techniques.[72] Given the size of this study, it provides the most reliable evidence as to pruritus prevalence in haemodialysis patients, and confirms that the mid-range from the smaller studies provides the most accurate prevalence data. More importantly, it demonstrates that pruritus is associated with worse physical and mental quality of life domains, and a 17% higher mortality risk, mediated in part through disturbances in sleep quality.[72] This finding is supported elsewhere, with clear indication that severe pruritus is associated with worse prognosis. [73] Pruritus is, therefore, not only a common symptom, often distressing to patients, but it has implications beyond impairment of quality of life, of worse prognosis and survival.[74]

7.3.4 Prevalence of restless legs

The reported prevalence of the symptom of restless legs among dialysis patients varies considerably, from 12% to 58%.[24,58,59,65,75–83] This compares with prevalence of at least 10–15% in the general population.[84] For this symptom, perhaps more than any other, reported prevalence depends heavily on the definition used. Earlier studies have tended to use less well-defined criteria, while more recent studies have used the specific criteria developed by the International Restless Legs Syndrome Study Group (IRLSSG) to define restless legs syndrome (RLS).[85] These latter studies indicate a somewhat lower prevalence of the syndrome of restless legs amongst patients receiving dialysis, between 12% and 22%.[74] Amongst transplanted patients, the incidence of RLS is lower, at about 5%.[85] Of those with Stage 5 disease and not receiving dialysis, 48% report the symptom of restless legs,[46] although this reflects the less defined symptom as reported by patients, rather than formal IRLSSG criteria.

As with pruritus, there is some indication that RLS is associated with poorer prognosis which may again be mediated partly through impaired quality of sleep.[79]

7.3.5 Prevalence of sleep disturbance

Sleep disturbance is a common problem in patients with ESRD but it is hard to determine the exact prevalence of this problem because of the challenges of definition. Insomnia affects at least 10–15% of the general population,[86] but the prevalence of sleep disturbance in renal patients is notably higher. Several studies have described prevalence,[23,52,53,59,62,65,82,86–97] and findings range from 20% to 83% of dialysis patients affected by sleep problems. This wide range reflects variable periods of prevalence – from point prevalence (symptom currently present) up to sleep disturbance at some time in the preceding 3 months. Definitions range from simple patient report of a 'sleep problem' to more specific definitions such as 'at least one of the following: problems initiating or maintaining sleep, early or difficulty waking, tiredness on waking, daytime sleepiness'.

Whatever definition is used, however, it is clear that this is a symptom which troubles many dialysis patients. Given the concerns regarding the relationship between poor quality of sleep and worse prognosis,[73] it is important that sleep problems are assessed and addressed carefully, together with the other symptoms which tend to cluster with sleep disturbance (pruritus and RLS in particular). All probably interact to adversely impact quality of life for individual patients.

Those Stage-5 CKD patients who opt not to have dialysis and are managed conservatively also have a high prevalence of sleep disturbance, with 41% experiencing some difficulty with sleep, and 21% (of all conservatively managed patients) reporting severely distressing sleep disturbance. [46] Over time, the prevalence of sleep problems seems to remain constant in this conservatively managed population, with similar proportions affected in the month before death as earlier in Stage 5 disease.[15]

Poor sleep has been shown to be associated with depression in renal patients,[86] and polysomnographic studies suggest that obstructive sleep apnoea is disproportionately common in dialysis patients.[98] Other studies of selected ESRD populations show prevalence of sleep apnoea up to 50%,[99] and this may contribute to daytime fatigue and sleepiness, as well exacerbating the cardiovascular complications of ESRD. The reasons for this high prevalence of sleep apnoea are unclear – it may be directly linked to the renal disease, with both destabilization of central ventilatory control and a degree of upper airway occlusion. There is also some suggestion that sleep patterns change early in CKD, so that sleep disturbance is common in the early stages, as well as advanced CKD, although the reasons for this are poorly understood.[100]

7.3.6 Prevalence of tiredness or fatigue

Tiredness or fatigue is also a symptom which is difficult to define, and therefore to quantify. Despite this, there is evidence that it is one of the most common symptoms experienced by renal patients; in most studies, between 70% and 97% of dialysis patients are affected by fatigue. [13,22,101,102] A very high proportion of conservatively managed stage-5 CKD patients are also affected by fatigue, with 90% of patients affected by fatigue, and 35% of all patients severely distressed by this.[15] Qualitative studies also suggest it is one of the most difficult symptoms for patients to cope with.[15,102]

Renal professionals may often be unaware of the presence and severity of fatigue in their patients,[103] especially since it may be less apparent than other, more tangible, symptoms. However, careful identification and assessment is important because of the high prevalence of this symptom, its major impact, and because it may be potentially treatable.

7.3.7 The prevalence of other symptoms

There are a number of other key symptoms which have been shown to be important for patients with advanced renal disease. Because the majority of studies of symptom prevalence focus on one or two symptoms of interest, rather than the whole range of symptoms experienced by the patients, there is much less evidence on the epidemiology of these remaining symptoms. Some studies have evaluated the whole range of symptoms, and provide data on how common these other symptoms are.[3,13,24,46,53,62] These symptoms include nausea and vomiting, drowsiness, breathlessness, leg oedema, dry mouth, lack of appetite and altered taste, poor concentration, dry skin, and constipation. Sexual dysfunction is also common (more fully described in the first edition of this book). Some symptoms, e.g. breathlessness, are frequently linked to co-morbidity, such as co-existing cardiac or respiratory disease, and their prevalence very much reflects the demographics of the population, with older populations and those conservatively managed (without dialysis) displaying a notably higher prevalence of these symptoms.[15]

7.4 **Assessment of symptoms**

There is growing evidence that symptoms in renal disease are under-recognized. A recently published study indicates that renal professionals substantially underestimate both the presence and the severity of the symptoms that their patients experience.[104] Appropriate, clinically relevant and valid instruments are essential to measure symptoms, both in clinical practice and the research setting.

7.4.1 **Symptom measurement tools**

A variety of tools have been used to evaluate symptoms in renal disease. Over two decades ago, Parfrey and colleagues developed a tool to capture the overall health status of patients with ESRD, including symptoms.[52–54,105] This questionnaire assessed the presence and severity of key symptoms, and also included emotional and psychological dimensions, the patient's life satisfaction, and a simple 0–100 visual quality-of-life scale.[54] However, it did not include certain symptoms important in renal disease (such as restless legs or poor appetite), and it used terms which were rather medical for a patient-completed measure, such as 'dyspnoea' and 'angina'. Perhaps for these reasons, it was not widely adopted, and other, more patient-centred instruments have been used instead. These include instruments which have been widely used in other advanced diseases, such as the Edmonton Symptom Assessment System[51,54,106] and the Memorial Symptom Assessment Scale short form.[3,46]

Other measures have been adapted and validated specifically for use in those with renal disease. These include the Dialysis Symptom Index, developed from the Memorial Symptom Assessment Scale by Weisbord,[107] and the renal version of the Patient Outcome Scale (symptom module), derived from the generic version of the Patient (or Palliative) Outcome Scale which is used across a wide number of conditions and countries.[108] Both are patient-completed tools, and each of these symptom measures validated in renal populations will be briefly discussed here (see Appendix for both tools).

7.4.1.1 The Edmonton Symptom Assessment System

The Edmonton Symptom Assessment System (ESAS) measures nine physical and emotional symptoms (pain, tiredness, nausea, depression, anxiety, drowsiness, appetite, well-being, and shortness of breath).[109] Each symptom is scored on a visual analogue scale from 0 (absence of the symptom) to 10 (worse possible level of the symptom). It was originally developed and validated for cancer patients, but has been modified and validated for renal patients by Davison and colleagues.[106] The modification includes the addition of a 10th item, itching (scored in the same way), and their original work also included a further unlabelled item for the patient to define themselves, to ensure key symptoms were not being missed.

This tool has the advantage of brevity and simplicity, although some patients (depending on the population) may find visual analogue scales less easy to use.[110] It has been validated in the dialysis population, and the wide use of this tool in other populations facilitates comparison across different conditions.

7.4.1.2 The Memorial Symptom Assessment Scale and the Dialysis Symptom Index

The Memorial Symptom Assessment Scale was also originally developed for cancer patients, and measures the frequency, severity, and distress of 32 common physical and psychological symptoms. [111] Chang et al. developed a short form (MSAS-SF), with the same number of items but focussing predominantly on severity and distress of symptoms, rather than frequency.[112] Weisbord and colleagues undertook a detailed development process to modify the MSAS-SF for use in the dialysis population. This revised instrument is called the Dialysis Symptom Index (DSI).[107] The DSI is a 30-item index that assesses the presence and severity of 30 individual physical and emotional symptoms. It provides an estimate of the prevalence and severity of these individual symptoms as well as an overall symptom burden and symptom severity score. The DSI has been shown to be a reliable and valid tool to assess symptoms in the haemodialysis population.

Both MSAS-SF and DSI are longer than the ESAS, although each individual item within them is perhaps simpler to complete than a visual analogue scale (it requires the patient simply to indicate (by tick or check) the presence of a symptom, and if present the amount of distress the symptom caused in the last week; either 'no' distress, 'a little bit', 'somewhat', 'quite a bit', or 'very much' distress. The MSAS-SF offers considerable scope for comparison with other populations, since it is used widely across other advanced diseases.

7.4.1.3 The Patient Outcome Scale

The Patient Outcome Scale (POS) was developed as a brief measure for use in those with far advanced disease, for whom completion of questionnaires may be most burdensome and difficult. The original instrument extends beyond physical and psychological symptoms, to include information needs, family communication, and practical matters.[113] More recently, a symptom module (Patient Outcome Scale symptom (POSs)) has been developed [114] which scores 10 symptoms (pain, shortness of breath, weakness or lack of energy, nausea, vomiting, poor appetite, constipation, mouth problems, drowsiness, and immobility) as having 'no' effect, 'slight', 'moderate', 'severe', or 'overwhelming' effect. Patients can also specify additional symptoms if needed, and indicate what symptom is affecting them the most and which has improved the most. This provides additional useful information, especially in the clinical setting where a brief tool is needed, and scarce clinical time addressing symptoms may need to be prioritized to quickly focus on the most severe symptoms. POSs has been validated across a number of conditions, including renal disease.[15] The renal version includes seven additional symptoms; itch, difficulty sleeping, restless legs, feeling anxious, feeling depressed, skin changes, and diarrhoea.[108]

POSs is intermediate in length between ESAS and DSI, and is effective as a brief symptom assessment tool, even in an elderly renal population.[108] It also enables the most severe symptom to be highlighted and responded to rapidly.

7.4.1.4 Symptom-specific measures

Although there is considerable need for the whole range of symptoms which patients experience to be captured, there is a wider range of instruments which have been used to assess individual symptoms, such as pain, pruritus, or depression. It is important to recognize that these may provide a more detailed and accurate picture of each symptom, especially for research purposes. A range of measures are available for measurement of pain,[115,116] depression,[20,22,117] pruritus,[118] or RLS.[119] The Cambridge–Hopkins restless legs questionnaire is patient-completed and is based on the IRLSSG criteria, but also distinguishes RLS from other conditions, with good sensitivity and specificity.[119] A range of other measures for individual symptoms exist, and are useful for research purposes, but fairly brief validated measures which capture the whole range of symptoms may be most useful in the clinical setting.

7.5 **The management of symptoms**

Once symptoms have been identified and carefully assessed, they need to be actively managed. Evidence shows that management of symptoms is less than optimal for renal patients.[120,121]

Symptom assessment and management is an area which has received only limited clinical or research attention in the past, although this is changing, and research evidence, plus related symptom guidelines are now beginning to emerge for pain and end-of-life care.[122–124] There is some evidence on management derived from the renal population, while other evidence can be extrapolated (to a limited extent) from other populations with chronic disease. However, the renal impairment itself places a major constraint on use of medication, since many medicines are renally excreted, and may therefore accumulate substantially in renal impairment. Careful consideration needs to be given to the effect of dialysis on clearance for those on dialysis.

This section addresses the management of some of the more common symptoms which occur in patients with CKD. Management of pain is addressed in Chapter 8, that of anxiety and depression in Chapter 9, and symptom management in the last days of life – including controlling agitation and myoclonus – are discussed in Chapter 15.

7.5.1 Management of anorexia and dry mouth

Anorexia (loss of appetite) is a distressing symptom for patient and family. The pathogenesis of anorexia is complex and poorly understood,[125] but it is thought that uraemic toxins, altered amino acid patterns, leptin, ghrelin, and neuropeptide Y are involved.[126] There is some debate about the significance of anorexia as a prognostic factor: some evidence indicates that anorexia in dialysis patients is associated with increased risk of death,[127] but a large study of >1800 haemodialysis patients (the HEMO study) suggests this association is lost when co-morbidity is also considered.[128]

In practice, many factors can contribute, and good management requires a thorough and detailed assessment to identify reversible causes. Contributing (and potentially reversible) factors can include nausea or vomiting, constipation, uncontrolled pain, oesophagitis, dyspepsia, dry mouth, and oral candidiasis (common in far advanced disease). In older patients, poor condition or fit of dentures may also need addressing. Dry mouth needs to be actively managed; by ensuring the patient is not dehydrated, using an artificial saliva preparation 1–2 hourly, stopping medications which exacerbate dry mouth (such as cyclizine) whenever possible, and using ice chips to moisten the mouth (particularly useful if fluid restriction remains clinically important). If oral candidiasis is present, nystatin or fluconazole can be used to treat it, in accordance with local sensitivities to these drugs. Fluconazole should be given at a reduced dose of 50–100 mg daily (based on 50% of normal dose if glomerular filtration rate (GFR) is <10 or if the patient is on dialysis) short term (longer term is more likely to select out resistant strains and will cause more adverse effects). If there is taste disturbance, herbs or spices can help in seasoning. Plastic utensils may remove the unpleasant metallic taste sometimes experienced from metal cutlery. Psychological factors are also important, and anorexia may be a feature of underlying depression (which can be particularly difficult to diagnose in debilitated patients); this needs to be assessed fully.

Food is an integral part of social interaction and care. Family carers may need to understand that food intake will reduce as disease advances (especially near end-stage), and offering food too frequently or in the usual portion size can be counter productive. Smaller, attractively presented meals, offered more frequently, may be more palatable, with high-calorie foods in the small amounts that are managed (if diabetic control permits). Dietetic help is very useful in advising and supporting this approach, as well as providing the more usual renal dietary advice. Detailed dietetic assessment and support of CKD patients with anorexia has been shown to improve their biochemical outcomes.[129] Other advice includes trial of metoclopramide to improve gastric emptying, avoiding early satiety by not drinking with meals, and avoiding regular weighing, which can be demoralizing (unless it is important for fluid balance).

The next step to relieve anorexia is to ensure the patient is well-dialysed (a Kt/V of at least 1.2). An increase in the number of dialysis sessions to daily haemodialysis has also been shown to improve appetite and food intake.[130] There is some evidence, recently reviewed by Bossola et al.[126] that megestrol acetate (which improves appetite, and possibly nutritional status, in cancer patients) is effective in improving appetite in CKD patients, but the high rate of adverse effects in the renal population means it cannot be recommended for clinical use at present. Dietary supplementation, including with branched-chain amino acids, may offer future avenues for management.

7.5.2 Management of breathlessness

The most common causes of breathlessness or dyspnoea in the renal patient are anaemia, pulmonary oedema (related to fluid overload or to co-existing cardiovascular disease), or co-morbidity (cardiac or respiratory disease). Anaemia produces significant symptoms including dyspnoea, and although anaemia is likely to be due to renal failure in the CKD patient, other causes should be considered and excluded. It is important to identify the underlying cause of breathlessness, since treating the underlying cause is almost always the most appropriate and effective first line of management. If volume overload is identified as a cause or contributor, more frequent or longer dialysis, with ultrafiltration, can be helpful. If treatment of the underlying cause has been exhausted, then the situation may arise (particularly in far advanced disease or close to the end of life) where symptomatic measures to relieve breathlessness will be required. These include general and non-pharmacological measures, psychological support, and pharmacological measures.

General measures in advanced disease include sitting upright rather than lying (which maximizes vital capacity), using a fan or stream of cool air which can provide effective symptom relief,[131] inhaled oxygen if hypoxia is confirmed or suspected,[132] and a calm, settled environment. For the patient whose mobility is limited by breathlessness, physiotherapy and occupational therapy can help to maximize mobility and provide appropriate aids to improve function constrained by breathlessness. Since breathlessness is a profoundly unpleasant symptom, assessment and management of the underlying psychological state is important. Breathlessness is very commonly associated with anxiety, often in an escalating cycle (anxiety causing worsening dyspnoea, which triggers worsening anxiety, and so on). Information, education, and support of patient and family is therefore critical. Detailed explanation of how to cope with and respond to breathlessness should be integral to this. Regular use of relaxation techniques and complimentary therapies can be useful, according to patient preference.

As prognosis worsens, general and non-pharmacological measures will have less to offer, and pharmacological measures directed at the symptom of breathlessness itself may be more appropriate. This is usually only when treatment of the underlying cause of breathlessness has been exhausted. Note that untreated moderate or severe dyspnoea at the end of life is very distressing, and should be treated as actively as pain or any other distressing symptom. It is also important to remember that breathlessness is an increasingly important and dominant symptom in renal patients towards the end of life,[15] so it is important to plan with the patient who has had one or more episode of acute breathlessness (or steadily increasing breathlessness over time) how they would like to be treated if they become more symptomatic in the future. Not all patients will, for instance, choose to be admitted for maximal treatment with intravenous diuretics in the last days or weeks of life.

Pharmacological treatments directed specifically at breathlessness include opioids and benzodiazepines (especially if there is moderate or severe associated anxiety). Low-dose opioids are helpful in relieving breathlessness near the end of life in end-stage cardiac and respiratory disease,[133,134] and clinical experience suggests that this is true for renal patients too. However, there are considerable constraints on the use of opioids in renal patients; the guidance as for pain management should be followed (see Chapter 8), although dose of opioids for breathlessness is likely to be notably smaller (usually half or quarter the starting dose for pain) and titration upwards is undertaken to a lesser degree. If small doses are not at least partly effective, combining an opioid such as fentanyl with low-dose midazolam may bring relief where either alone is only partially effective. This is often a better strategy than increasing the dose, since adverse effects quickly increase as doses rise. These issues are discussed more fully in Chapter 15.

Benzodiazepines are useful when there is co-existing anxiety (as there often is), but again need to be used with care and in reduced doses. Shorter-acting benzodiazepines are recommended, such as lorazepam 0.5–1 mg orally or sublingually q.d.s. (if used sublingually, it has a quicker onset of action and may more readily restore a sense of control to the frightened and anxious patient). If the patient is in the last days of life, midazolam (at 25% of normal dose, if eGFR < 10) can be given subcutaneously and titrated according to effect. Midazolam can be given every 2–4 h, although CKD patients are sensitive to its effects and do not usually need frequent or large doses. A starting dose of 2.5 mg is common. If more than one or two doses are required, a subcutaneous infusion over 24 h is most practical.

7.5.3 Management of constipation

Constipation is common among CKD patients. The causes can be multi-factorial – fluid restriction, reduced mobility, medication (such as aluminium or calcium phosphate binders, iron supplements, and opioids), poor dietary intake, depression, and reduced muscle tone, through debility, can all contribute. The dietary restriction of high-potassium fruits and vegetables decreases the fibre content of food ingested. Management requires detailed assessment, treatment of reversible causes where appropriate/possible, acute management to overcome current constipation (including rectal measures), and then action to prevent further recurrence. Mobility and adequate dietary intake – including sufficient fibre and fluid (within the constraints of reduced fluid intake) – need to be encouraged. Table 7.1 shows which laxatives are useful. All are safe in dialysis, although other common laxatives which contain magnesium, citrate, or phosphate (not included in Table 7.1) should be avoided in ESRD. Often, a combination of softener or

Table 7.1 Laxatives for use in renal patients

Drug	Mode of action	Dose	Notes
Lactulose	Osmotic	10–20 ml bd	Ensure adequate oral intake for efficacy
Senna	Stimulant	1–2 tablets nocte or bd	Can cause colic
Bisacodyl	Stimulant	5–10 mg nocte or bd	Can cause colic
Docusate sodium	Softener	100–200 mg bd	
Polyethylene glycol	Osmotic	1–2 sachets	Short-term use only for resistant constipation or impaction (requires high fluid intake which may preclude use)

osmotic laxative with a stimulant is required. Polyethelene glycol (Movicol) is not ideal for renal patients because it requires high concurrent fluid intake, and also contains potassium. However, it may be useful in the short term for constipation which does not respond to other measures, or (in higher doses) for faecal impaction.

7.5.4 Management of fatigue

Fatigue is multi-dimensional,[135] with physical, cognitive, and emotional elements,[136] There is a complex relationship between fatigue, sleep disturbance, physical functioning, and depression in those with renal disease.[23,137] but it is poorly understood. It is not clear, for instance, whether the reduced physical functioning which occurs with renal disease itself causes fatigue, or whether in fact the symptom of fatigue is a consequence of poor function. Fatigue is an important symptom because it is very common, highly distressing to patients, and there are a number of causes which are potentially treatable. These causes can be classified as related to the renal disease, to dialysis itself, or related to co-morbid conditions. The renal disease may cause anaemia, hyperparathyroidism, and uraemia, all of which may directly contribute to fatigue. Secondary to these direct effects are dietary and fluid restrictions, impaired nutrition, and the side effects of medications, all of which may contribute to fatigue, even if they are not the predominant causes of it. For those on dialysis, dialysis inadequacy, post-dialysis fatigue, and the burden of dialysis itself may also play a part in instigating or perpetuating fatigue. Conditions unrelated to renal disease, such as hypothyroidism, should be considered and excluded. Non-pharmacological managements of fatigue – such as exercise, cognitive and psychological approaches, and complementary treatments – are important, especially as pharmacological interventions become increasingly limited.

A systematic review of the use of erythropoietin-stimulating agents demonstrates that, in renal patients, there is a consistent relationship between haematocrit and energy/fatigue domains in quality of life;[138] as haematocrit increases, so energy levels increase and fatigue reduces. When anaemia is due to CKD, which is likely if GFR < 30 ml/min/1.73 m^2 (<45 in diabetics) and no other cause, such as blood loss and folic acid or B12 deficiency, is identified, then active treatment with erythropoietin-stimulating agents is likely to improve fatigue. Haemoglobin should be maintained between 10.5 and 12.5 g/dl (per UK Renal Association guidelines). It is not clear, however, how long treatment should be maintained in those who are nearing end of life; most clinicians continue treatment while the patient still continues to gain symptomatic benefit.

7.5.5 Management of nausea and vomiting

Nausea and vomiting are extremely unpleasant symptoms. They may frequently be multi-factorial. Assessment requires a thorough history including establishing the history and pattern of both nausea and vomiting separately. The relationship between the two should also be established, as well as the frequency and volume of vomits, whether there is associated constipation, and a detailed medication history. Profound nausea and/or repeated vomiting will prevent absorption of any medications taken orally, and alternative routes (such as sublingual, rectal, or subcutaneous routes) need to be considered, at least until nausea and vomiting is controlled.

The first step is to identify the specific cause of nausea and vomiting where possible, since cause-directed treatment is most likely to succeed. If medication or toxins are causing nausea, then nausea is usually persistent and unremitting, and sometimes unaccompanied by vomiting. Uraemia, and a variety of drugs (including opioids, anti-convulsants, antibiotics, and anti-depressants) can cause this kind of persistent nausea. Gastroparesis or delayed gastric emptying (which may be caused by drugs such as opioids, as well as occurring secondary to diabetes mellitus,

Table 7.2 Anti-emetics used for CKD patients*

Suspected cause	Drug of choice	Oral dose	Notes
Gastroparesis, delayed gastric emptying	Metoclopramide	5–10 mg tds	Do not use in bowel obstruction with colic. Do not use with cyclizine. Increased risk of dystonia in CKD patients.
	Domperidone	20 mg tds	Domperidone can also be used rectally (30–60 mg bd or tds)
Uraemia	Haloperidol Levomepromazine	0.5–2 mg od or bd 6 mg od	Increased cerebral sensitivity in renal failure Sedative at higher doses
	5HT3 antagonists: Ondansetron Granisetron	8 mg bd 1 mg bd	Side effects of constipation and headaches may limit use
Drug induced	Haloperidol	0.5–3 mg od or bd	First step is to stop medication causing drug-induced nausea if possible.
	Cyclizine	25–50 mg tds (caution – adverse cardiac effects may need consideration given the high proportion of CKD patients with cardiac co-morbidity)	Note: opioid-induced nausea usually settles spontaneously after about 7–10 days on the opioid.
Gastritis (low threshold for treatment)	Omeprazole or other proton-pump inhibitor	20 mg od	

*Also see Chapters 8 and 15

for instance) usually presents with a history of post-prandial nausea or vomiting of undigested food which relieves nausea. Bloating, epigastric fullness, flatulence, hiccough, or heartburn may accompany this. Nausea related to gastritis is often associated with heartburn, dyspepsia, or epigastric pain. Constipation may exacerbate nausea and vomiting.

7.5.6 Management of pruritus

Although there are a number of studies into the pathogenesis and treatment of pruritus in CKD patients, its aetiology and pathogenesis remains unclear, and treatment options remain somewhat limited in their effectiveness.

Pruritus is thought to arise in C-fibres located in the skin and distinct from those which mediate pain; a subgroup of C-fibres has been identified which discharge in a pattern matching that induced by itch.[139] These C-fibres transmit via the contralateral spinothalamic tract to the brain (thalamus and hypothalamus) via the reticular formation.[140] Connections to distinct cortical areas (the anterior cingulate process, supplementary motor area, and inferior parietal lobe) then mediate – via motor areas – the powerful, almost involuntary, desire to scratch.

The difficulty is that pruritus could originate at any level within this convoluted pathway (in the skin at the level of the receptors, neuropathically in the afferent nerve pathway, neuropathically in central neural pathways, or centrally from psychogenic causes). In CKD-related itch, it appears that complex interacting factors operate at more than one place in the pathway,[140] so that it is extremely difficult to elucidate any one discrete cause for itch. Current hypotheses postulate abnormal inflammatory/immune processes, dysfunction in the opioid receptor system, and/or neuropathic processes within the nervous system itself.

Firstly, it is known that CKD leads to an immune system derangement, and it has been suggested that this results in a pro-inflammatory or inflammatory state that precipitates itch;[8] for this reason, immune modulators (such as ultraviolet (UV) B light, tacrolimus, and thalidomide) have been proposed to treat itch. These all act in various ways to decrease pro-inflammatory cytokines. This inflammatory hypothesis resonates with evidence that a high white blood cell count is predictive of itch in haemodialysis patients,[72] and dialysis patients on statins (which reduce serum pro-inflammatory cytokines) have lower levels of itch.[141] Others have shown that pro-inflammatory and inflammatory cytokines are associated with pruritus,[142] and that increasing levels of C-reactive protein correlate with severity of itch in dialysis patients.[55]

Secondly, a number of authors have proposed disturbance in the endogenous opioids system as a cause of itch.[8,143] It is well established that μ-opioids can induce itch, particularly spinally administered μ-opioid receptor agonists, and μ-opioid receptor antagonists can reduce itch.[144] In contrast, κ-opioid receptor agonists have been shown to have anti-pruritic effects in animals, and κ-opioid receptor antagonists enhance itch in animal studies.[144] It is for this reason that opioids such as butorphanol (which has μ-opioid antagonist and κ-opioid agonist action),[145] and opioids antagonists such as naloxone and naltrexone, have been proposed to treat itch. There is also some evidence that a new κ-opioid agonist (nalfurafine) may be useful.[146]

Thirdly, there is some evidence to support the link between itch and neuropathic processes. There are a number of features of itch which suggest a neuropathic process, and Akhyani and colleagues report association between clinical neuropathy and itch in haemodialysis patients.[9] Other studies have explored the use of neuropathic agents (lidocaine, gabapentin, and capsaicin) to treat itch, with some success. However, the neuropathic component could be a secondary, rather than primary, cause of CKD-related pruritus.

Lastly, the role of histamine in acute itch is long established. Acute histamine-induced itch is well described, and histamine receptors appear to sensitize at least some of the C-fibres which mediate itch. What is less clear is how this acute itch response relates to the chronic itch experienced by CKD-related pruritus. Nevertheless, anti-histamines are widely used in the management of CKD-related pruritus, with varying results.

A further important factor in CKD-related itch is xerosis, or dry skin. There is conflicting evidence about the relationship between xerosis and itch in CKD patients,[9,64,66] but it may be an important factor in older people with CKD.[147] In addition, although uraemia is the most likely cause of pruritus, other common causes of pruritus, such as skin disorders, skin infections such as scabies, and liver impairment, need to be considered if the symptom is not resolving.

Given the confusion and complexity in understanding the causes of pruritus in CKD, it is not surprising that it can be a difficult symptom to manage, with a variety of different treatments proposed, each of limited effectiveness. The first step in management is to optimize renal management; high phosphate may contribute to pruritus,[140] so attention to reducing phosphate levels may be important – consider dietary advice and the use of phosphate-binders. Hyperparathyroidism may also be a contributory factor and should be considered. Dry skin may both cause and contribute to pruritus, and so should be treated actively; liberal emollients should be used if dry skin is present. Older people living alone may find it hard to apply emollients easily; spray applications are often helpful in this instance. Preventive measures, such as nail care (keeping nails short), keeping cool (light clothing, and tepid baths or showers) are useful concurrent measures.

The evidence as to which medications are effective is limited, often conflicting, and no single preparation can be recommended above others. Choice of treatment for should be influenced by the stage of disease – for instance, UV light may be practical for those who remain relatively well, while anti-histamines may be more appropriate nearer end of life. Table 7.3 provides details of possible drug treatments and the evidence to support each. Whatever the evidence, individual patients do report significant benefit with some of these options. Time should be taken to discuss with the patient the need to persist with any one medication, and to explaining and minimizing side effects where possible. A clear plan of management, and persistence in following treatment through, goes a long way to helping patients cope with the distress that this symptoms can sometimes cause. The psychological and social dimensions of severe itch are considerable,[15] and psychological, family, and social support is an important component of management.

7.5.7 Management of restless legs

Restless legs syndrome is characterized by urge to move the legs, uncomfortable sensations in the legs, and worsening of symptoms at rest, especially during the night. The formal IRLSSG criteria are (1) urge to move the legs, usually with unpleasant sensations in the legs, (2) worse during periods of rest or inactivity like resting or sitting, (3) partial or total relief by physical activity, and (4) worse symptoms in the evening or night rather than the day.[84] The exact cause for restless legs is not understood as yet; it is widely accepted, however, that the dopaminergic system in the central nervous system is somehow disrupted.[74] There may also be a relationship between brain iron metabolism and RLS.[172] There is limited evidence in uraemic RLS that iron deficiency,[173] low parathyroid hormone,[76] hyperphosphataemia, and psychological factors[174] may all play a role. Treatment should involve correction of these factors, and reduction of potential exacerbating agents, such as caffeine, alcohol, nicotine, and certain drugs (sedative anti-histamines, metoclopramide, tricyclic antidepressants, selective serotonin uptake inhibitors, lithium and dopamine antagonists).[74] Calcium antagonists may also exacerbate RLS.[175]

There is very limited evidence about treatment of restless legs in CKD patients, and much of the evidence is extrapolated from patients with idiopathic restless legs.[176]

7.5.8 Management of sleep disturbance

A detailed history of any sleep disturbance is important, in order to identify sleep apnoea, RLS, and pruritus – which may be the underlying reason for the sleep disturbance; each of these need treating in their own right initially to resolve any sleep problems. General sleep-hygiene measures are important in addressing sleep disturbance; avoiding caffeine after lunch, reducing overall caffeine intake, avoiding alcohol (which is both depressant and stimulant), and avoiding day-time sleeping. If sleep apnoea is excluded, other exacerbating symptoms are treated optimally, and general measures are unsuccessful, then hypnotics may be necessary, ideally short term to attempt to re-establish sleep patterns. For those with a longer prognosis, hypnotics carry risk of dependence, and this needs consideration in management. The shorter acting hypnotics, such as zolpidem 5–10 mg, or temazepam 7.5–10 mg are preferable. These are generally safe in dialysis patients, although CKD patients may be more sensitive to benzodiazepines in general, and lower doses are often required than in the general population.

Table 7.3 Proposed treatments for pruritus in CKD patients

Drug	Dose	Evidence of effectiveness	Notes
Topical and external treatments			
Emollients (aqueous cream, Diprobase, Balneum, etc.)	Topical, applied liberally 2–4 times daily	In an uncontrolled study, 9 out of 21 dialysis patients with dry skin had marked reduction in itch following regular use of twice daily aqueous cream for 1 week[148] In a small controlled study, 10 haemodialysis patients with mild pruritus showed benefit from an aqueous gel applied twice daily for two weeks, compared with 10 control patients[149] In an uncontrolled study, 26 out of 30 dialysis patients had resolution of pruritus following baths using Balneum bath oil every 1–2 days for 4 weeks[150] In an uncontrolled study, eight out of 21 haemodialysis patients with dry skin and pruritus had resolution of pruritus following twice daily use of a lipid-based cream containing endocannabinoids for 3 weeks[151]	**RECOMMENDED FIRST LINE** especially if xerosis (dry skin) Use spray preparations for ease of application where appropriate (e.g. older patients living alone)
Capsaicin cream	0.025% cream applied qds	In a double-blind RCT with cross-over design, 19 haemodialysis patients with moderate-to-severe pruritus received 0.025% cream qds; 14 out of 17 showed marked improvement, although burning on application of the cream was problematic and caused two patients to drop out[152] Eight of nine haemodialysis patients in an uncontrolled study, and two out of 5 in a double-blind RCT reported complete resolution of pruritus following 0.025% cream qds[153]	**CONSIDER IF LOCALIZED RATHER THAN GENERALIZED ITCH** Capsaicin cream is best used when pruritus is localized, as it is not practical to apply it widely. It works by depleting Substance P, and some persistence is needed to continue use with local burning discomfort until it can take effect. Cost may be a limiting factor in its use.
Tacrolimus ointment	0.03% or 0.1% ointment bd	In a controlled study, three dialysis patients reported benefit following use of 0.03% ointment bd[154] In an uncontrolled study, 25 haemodialysis patients showed small reduction in pruritus scores following use of 0.1% then 0.03% ointment bd, although five out of 25 patients reported troublesome side effects (rash, tingling/burning)[155] In a double-blind RCT of 22 haemodialysis patients, the 0.1% ointment bd for 4 weeks showed no benefit over control[156]	**NOT RECOMMENDED** Little evidence to support use, and safety in longer term use is uncertain.

(Continued)

Table 7.3 (continued) Proposed treatments for pruritus in CKD patients

Drug	Dose	Evidence of effectiveness	Notes
UVB light		In an uncontrolled study, 32 out of 38 dialysis patients improved after UVB treatment twice weekly for 4 weeks[157,158] In an uncontrolled study, 17 dialysis patients given UVA or UVB light 3 times weekly for 2–3 min all had resolution of their pruritus[159]	**RECOMMENDED IF LOCALLY AVAILABLE** Some uncertainty regarding long-term effects.
Systemic therapy			
Anti-histamines, such as:		Evidence in respect of anti-histamines for pruritus is scanty, and much of the rationale for their use is extrapolated from other disease populations.	**IT IS CURRENT CLINCAL PRACTICE TO USE ANTI-HISTAMINES ALTHOUGH EVIDENCE DOES NOT SUPPORT THIS** May be useful mostly for their sedative effects, especially at night.
Cetirizine	10 mg od (5 mg if eGFR < 10)	In a double-blind RCT, cross-over design, 18 out of 27 patients showed remission of pruritus following treatment with terfenadine[160]	
Chlorpheniramine	4 mg qds (tds if eGFR < 10)	In an uncontrolled study, all five haemodialysis patients had reduction in pruritus following treatment with ketotifen over 6 weeks[161]	
Gabapentin	100–400 mg after dialysis sessions	In a double-blind RCT of 25 haemodialysis patients with itch, there was statistically significant reduction in itch scores in those treated with gabapentin thrice weekly following dialysis for 4 weeks[162] In a double-blind RCT of 34 haemodialysis patients with itch unresponsive to anti-histamines, there was statistically significant reduction in itch scores in those treated with gabapentin 400 mg twice weekly after dialysis for 4 weeks[163] Both studies reported no adverse effects	**RECOMMENDED FOR DIALYSIS PATIENTS** Needs substantial dose reduction in those on dialysis, and should be given only after dialysis. Accumulates rapidly in those not dialysed who have Stage 4 and 5 CKD; use with caution and in very low doses. In Stage 5 CKD without dialysis, it is preferable not to use it at all.

Drug	Dose	Evidence	Recommendation
5-HT3 receptor antagonists, such as:		In a double-blind RCT with cross-over design, 17 haemodialysis patients with pruritus of all levels of severity were given ondansetron 8 mg tds, and both placebo and treatment groups showed benefit with no statistically significant difference[164] In an uncontrolled study, 11 dialysis patients with moderate to severe pruritus were given ondansetron 4 mg bd and all responded within 2 weeks[63] In a double-blind RCT with cross-over design, 16 haemodialysis patients with persistent pruritus were given ondansetron 8 mg tds for 2 weeks, and pruritus scores did not change during treatment in either control or treatment groups[165] In an uncontrolled study of 14 haemodialysis patients with pruritus, granisteron 1 mg bd was given for 4 weeks, with significant reduction in itch from the first week of treatment[166]	**NOT RECOMMENDED** A few very small trials undertaken with conflicting results, and the RCTs in particular suggest no benefit. It could be considered in those with co-existing nausea since it is an effective anti-emetic. It is highly constipating (laxative should be co-prescribed).
Ondansetron	2–8 mg bd		
Granisetron	1 mg bd		
Naltrexone	50 mg daily	In a double-blind RCT with cross-over design, 15 haemodialysis patients with severe pruritus were given naltrexone 50 mg daily for 1 week. Pruritus improved following naltrexone, within the first 48 h of treatment[167] In a double-blind RCT with cross-over design, 23 dialysis pts with moderate to severe pruritus were given naltrexone 50 mg daily for 1 week. Pruritus reduced in both treatment and control phases with no statistically significant difference. The level of adverse effects was high, with gastrointestinal side effects occurring in 10 out of 23 patients[168] Naloxone has also been proposed, but only case study evidence exists[169]	**NOT RECOMMENDED** Evidence is conflicting and based on small studies, with concern about adverse effects. Opioid antagonists also cannot be given if opioids are to be used for pain management. Opioid receptor imbalance may become more relevant only in severe pruritus[170] and this may be one of the reasons for conflicting evidence.

(Continued)

Table 7.3 (continued) Proposed treatments for pruritus in CKD patients

Drug	Dose	Evidence of effectiveness	Notes
Thalidomide	100 mg at night	In a double-blind RCT with cross-over design, 29 haemodialysis patients received thalidomide daily for 1 week, and over half showed significant response in the thalidomide phase of the study[171]	**CONSIDER IF RESISTANT TO OTHER TREATMENTS** The evidence is very limited, and the risks and adverse effects of thalidomide should be considered carefully. Thalidomide has a risk of (reversible) peripheral neuropathy, and there is risk of teratogenic effects to those who are pregnant, even from handling tablets.
Nalfurafine	5 μg 3 times week-ly by infusion	In one double-blind placebo controlled RCT, 79 haemodialysis patients received nalfurafine thrice weekly after dialysis, over 4 weeks. In a second placebo controlled cross-over study, 34 haemodialysis patients received nalfurafine or placebo for 2 weeks before crossing over for a further 2 weeks.[146] In both studies, nalfurafine produced a statistically significant improvement in 'worst itching'	These findings are promising although nalfurafine is not widely available at the time of publication.

Table 7.4 Proposed treatments for restless legs in CKD patients

Drug	Starting dose	Evidence of effectiveness	Notes
Co-careldopa (levodopa with carbidopa)	12.5 mg/50 mg od	In a double-blind RCT cross-over study, 11 uraemic patients had improved sleep, quality of life, and reduced movements on levodopa 100–200 mg od with no adverse effects[177] In an RCT with just five haemodialysis patients, there were reduced movements and improved sleep on levodopa/carbidopa (25/100 mg)[178] In an uncontrolled study, eight haemodialysis patients on 25/100–25/250 mg of levodopa and carbidopa had reduced perception of RLS[179]	**RECOMMENDED** RLS may become, over time, worse in 80% of cases (augmentation). This correlates with greater accumulated dose of L-dopa, so treat with lowest dose for shortest duration.
Dopamine agonists: Pergolide Pramipexole Ropinirole	25 µg od 88 µ tds 250 µg tds	In an RCT, cross-over design, with 11 haemodialysis patients, ropinirole was better than levodopa in controlling the symptoms of RLS[180] In an uncontrolled study, the RLS symptoms of 10 haemodialysis patients improved with pramipexole[181] In a double-blind RCT, 16 haemodialysis patients with RLS had benefit from pergolide; nausea and nightmares were noted adverse effects[182]	**RECOMMENDED** Nausea common with pergolide, but in general augmentation is less likely to occur with the dopamine agonists than with levodopa, and the side effects may also be less. Long-term use may be precluded by restrictive cardiac valve disease and pulmonary fibrosis[74]
Clonazepam	250–500 µg od	In an uncontrolled study, 14 out of 15 patients with end-stage renal disease benefited from clonazepam 1–2 mg daily[183]	**CONSIDER IF OTHER TREATMENT INEFFECTIVE OR CONTRAINDICATED** Can cause day-time sleepiness and cognitive impairment
Gabapentin	100–400 mg (post dialysis)	In a controlled study comparing levodopa and gabapentin, with 15 haemodialysis patients, gabapentin was more effective[184] In a double-blind RCT with cross-over, comparing placebo and gabapentin, in 16 haemodialysis patients, gabapentin was more effective[185]	**RECOMMENDED IN DIALYSIS PATIENTS** Needs substantial dose reduction in those on dialysis, and should be given only following dialysis. Accumulates rapidly in those not dialysed who have Stage 4 and 5 CKD; use with caution and in very low doses. In Stage 5 CKD without dialysis, it is preferable not to use it at all.

7.6 **Conclusions**

For people with CKD, symptoms can arise directly from the renal disease itself, as a consequence of dialysis, or from co-morbid conditions (particularly in older patients). For any single individual, it is often a combination of causes which contributes to their overall symptom burden. Fatigue, itch, pain, and breathlessness are highly prevalent, and other physical symptoms (such as restless legs, muscle cramps, headaches, and dizziness) are particularly characteristic of renal disease. Mild psychological symptoms are also frequent in this population, and formal depressive illness – although seen less often – is notably more frequent than in the age-matched general population.

This chapter highlights the importance of regular and routine symptom assessment as an integral part of clinical practice. Symptom measures have been briefly reviewed, and the importance of assessing the whole range of symptoms underlined. Two symptom measures, the DSI and the renal version of the POSs module, are presented. Pharmacological management of symptoms is discussed in detail, since this is one of the most challenging aspects of the care of those on dialysis, withdrawing from dialysis, or managed conservatively, without dialysis. Although the emphasis has been on pharmacological management, it should be stressed that psychological, social, and spiritual aspects of management are also important, especially towards the end of life. It is for these reasons that care of renal patients is best managed with multi-professional teams, including counsellors and psychologists, occupational and physiotherapists, dieticians, and chaplains, and most importantly, professionals with both nephrology and palliative care skills.

References

1 Solano JP, Gomes B, Higginson IJ (2006). A comparison of symptom prevalence in far advanced cancer, AIDS, heart disease, chronic obstructive pulmonary disease and renal disease. *J Pain Symp Manag*, **31**(1), 58–69.

2 Steinhauser KE, Christakis NA, Clipp EC, et al. (2000). Factors considered important at the end of life by patients, family, physicians, and other care providers. *JAMA*, **284**(19), 2476–82.

3 Weisbord SD, Carmody SS, Bruns FJ, et al (2003). Symptom burden, quality of life, advance care planning and the potential value of palliative care in severely ill haemodialysis patients. *Nephrol Dialy Transplant*, **18** (7), 1345–52.

4 Singer PA, Martin DK, Kelner M (1999). Quality end-of-life care: patients' perspectives. *JAMA*, **281**(2), 163–8.

5 Palmer BF (1999). Sexual dysfunction in uremia. *J Am Soc Nephrol*, **10**(6), 1381–8.

6 Sarraf P, Kay J, Reginato AM (2008). Non-crystalline and crystalline rheumatic disorders in chronic kidney disease. *Curr Rheumatol Rep*, **10**(3), 235–48.

7 Kliger AS. (2009). New options to improve hemodialysis patient outcomes, *Clin.J Am.Soc Nephrol*, **4**(4), 694–5.

8 Patel TS, Freedman BI, Yosipovitch G (2007). An update on pruritus associated with CKD. *Am J Kidney Dis*, **50**(1), 11–20.

9 Akhyani M, Ganji MR, Samadi N, et al. (2005). Pruritus in hemodialysis patients. *BMC Dermatol*, **5**, 7.

10 Antoniazzi AL (2003). Headache and hemodialysis: a prospective study. *Headache*, **43**(2), 99–102.

11 Song JH, Park GH, Lee SY, et al. (2005). Effect of sodium balance and the combination of ultrafiltration profile during sodium profiling hemodialysis on the maintenance of the quality of dialysis and sodium and fluid balances. *J Am Soc Nephrol*, **16**(1), 237–46.

12 van der Sande FM, Wystrychowski G, Kooman JP, et al. (2009). Control of core temperature and blood pressure stability during hemodialysis. *Clin J Am Soc Nephrol*, **4**(1), 93–8.

13 Kundhal K, Lok CE (2005). Clinical epidemiology of cardiovascular disease in chronic kidney disease. Nephron Clin Pract, **101**(2), c47–52.

14 Nigwekar SU, Wolf M, Sterns RH, et al. (2008). Calciphylaxis from nonuremic causes: a systematic review. *Clin J Am Soc Nephrol*, **3**(4), 1139–43.

15 Murtagh FE, Addington-Hall J, Higginson IJ (2007). The prevalence of symptoms in end-stage renal disease: a systematic review. *Adv Chr Kidney Dis*, **14**(1), 82–99.

16 Murtagh FEM (2009). Understanding and improving quality of care for people with conservatively-managed Stage 5 Chronic Kidney Disease – the course of symptoms and other concerns over time. PhD thesis. King's College London.

17 Cohen LM, Germain M, Poppel DM, et al. (2000). Dialysis discontinuation and palliative care. *Am J Kidney Dis*, **36**(1), 140–4.

18 Cukor D, Coplan J, Brown C, et al (2008). Anxiety disorders in adults treated by hemodialysis: a single-center study. *Am J Kidney Dis*, **52**(1), 128–36.

19 Cukor D, Coplan J, Brown C, et al. (2007). Depression and anxiety in urban hemodialysis patients. *Clin J Am Soc Nephrol*, **2**(3), 484–90.

20 Martin CR, Thompson DR (2000). Prediction of quality of life in patients with end-stage renal disease. *Brit J Health Psychol*, **5**(1), 41–55.

21 Farmer CJ, Snowden SA, Parsons V (1980). The prevalence of psychiatric illness among patients on home haemodialysis. *Psychol Med*, **9**(3), 509–14.

22 Kutner NG, Fair PL, Kutner MH (1985). Assessing depression and anxiety in chronic dialysis patients. *J Psychosom Res*, **29**(1), 23–31.

23 McCann K, Boore JRP (2000). Fatigue in persons with renal failure who require maintenance haemodialysis. *J Adv Nurs*, **32**(5), 1132–42.

24 Curtin RB, Bultman DC, Thomas-Hawkins C, et al. (2002). Hemodialysis patients' symptom experiences: effects on physical and mental functioning. *Nephrol Nurs J: J Am Nephrol Nurses' Assoc*, **29**(6), 562.

25 Martin CR, Tweed AE, Metcalfe MS (2004). A psychometric evaluation of the Hospital Anxiety and Depression Scale in patients diagnosed with end-stage renal disease. *Brit J Clin Psychol*, **43**(1), 51–64.

26 Kimmel PL (2001). Psychosocial factors in dialysis patients. *Kidney Int*, **59**(4), 1599–613.

27 O'Donnell K, Chung JY (1997). The diagnosis of major depression in end-stage renal disease. *Psychother Psychosom*, **66**(1), 38–43.

28 Craven JL, Rodin GM, Littlefield C (1988). The Beck Depression Inventory as a screening device for major depression in renal dialysis patients. *Int J Psych Med*, **18**(4), 365–74.

29 Hong BA, Smith MD, Robson AM, et al. (1987). Depressive symptomatology and treatment in patients with end-stage renal disease. *Psychol Med*, **17**(1), 185–90.

30 Lopes AA, Bragg J, Young E, et al (2002). Depression as a predictor of mortality and hospitalization among hemodialysis patients in the United States and Europe. *Kidney Int*, **62**(1), 199–207.

31 Smith MD, Hong BA, Robson AM (1985). Diagnosis of depression in patients with end-stage renal disease. Comparative analysis. *Am J Med*, **79**(2), 160–6.

32 Watnick S, Kirwin P, Mahnensmith R, et al. (2003). The prevalence and treatment of depression among patients starting dialysis. *Am J Kidney Dis*, **41**(1), 105–10.

33 al Hihi E, Awad A, Hagedorn A (2003). Screening for depression in chronic hemodialysis patients. *Missouri Med*, **100**(3), 266–8.

34 Hinrichsen GA, Lieberman JA, Pollack S, et al. (1989). Depression in hemodialysis patients. *Psychosomatics: J Consult Liaison Psych*, **30**(3), 284–9.

35 Rodin G, Voshart K (1987). Depressive symptoms and functional impairment in the medically ill. *General Hospital Psych*, **9**(4), 251–8.

36 Walters BA, Hays RD, Spritzer KL, et al. (2002). Health-related quality of life, depressive symptoms, anemia, and malnutrition at hemodialysis initiation. *Am J Kidney Dis*, **40**(6), 1185–94.

37 Wuerth D, Finkelstein SH, Ciarcia J, et al. (2001). Identification and treatment of depression in a cohort of patients maintained on chronic peritoneal dialysis. *Am J Kidney Dis*, **37**(5), 1011–17.

38 Wuerth D, Finkelstein SH, Finkelstein FO (2005). The identification and treatment of depression in patients maintained on dialysis. *Semin Dial*, **18**(2), 142–6.

39 Chilcot J, Wellsted D, Da Silva-Gane M, et al. (2008). Depression on dialysis. *Nephron*, **108**(4), c256–64.

40 Merkus MP, Jager KJ, Dekker FW, et al. (1999). Quality of life over time in dialysis: the Netherlands Cooperative Study on the Adequacy of Dialysis. NECOSAD Study Group. *Kidney Int*, **56**(2), 720–8.

41 Diaz-Buxo JA, Lowrie EG, Lew NL, et al. (2000). Quality-of-life evaluation using Short Form 36: comparison in hemodialysis and peritoneal dialysis patients. *Am J Kidney Dis*, **35**(2), 293–300.

42 Meyer KB, Espindle DM, DeGiacomo JM, et al. (1994). Monitoring dialysis patients' health status. *Am J Kidney Dis*, **24**(2), 267–79.

43 Davison SN (2007). The prevalence and management of chronic pain in end-stage renal disease. *J Palliat Med*, **10**(6), 1277–87.

44 Mercadante S, Ferrantelli A, Tortorici C, et al. (2005). Incidence of chronic pain in patients with end-stage renal disease on dialysis. *J Pain Symp Manag*, **30**(4), 302–4.

45 Weisbord SD, Fried LF, Arnold RM, Fine MJ, Levenson DJ, Peterson RA, et al (2005). Prevalence, severity, and importance of physical and emotional symptoms in chronic hemodialysis patients. *J Am Soc Nephrol*, **16**(8), 2487–94.

46 Murtagh FE, Addington-Hall JM, Edmonds PM, Donohoe P, Carey I, Jenkins K, et al (2007). Symptoms in advanced renal disease: a cross-sectional survey of symptom prevalence in stage 5 chronic kidney disease managed without dialysis. *J Palliat Med*, **10**(6), 1266–76.

47 Cohen LM, Germain MJ, Poppel DM, et al. (2000). Dying well after discontinuing the life-support treatment of dialysis. *Arch Intern Med*, **160**(16), 2513–18.

48 Chater S, Davison SN, Germain MJ, et al. (2006). Withdrawal from dialysis: a palliative care perspective. *Clin Nephrol*, **66**(5), 364–72.

49 Klinkenberg M, Smit JH, Deeg DJ, et al. (2003). Proxy reporting in after-death interviews: the use of proxy respondents in retrospective assessment of chronic diseases and symptom burden in the terminal phase of life. *Palliat Med*, **17**(2), 191–201.

50 Devins GM, Armstrong SJ, Mandin H, et al. (1990). Recurrent pain, illness intrusiveness, and quality of life in end-stage renal disease. *Pain*, **42**(3), 279–85.

51 Davison SN, Jhangri GS, Johnson JA (2006). Longitudinal validation of a modified Edmonton symptom assessment system (ESAS) in haemodialysis patients. *Nephrol Dial Transplant*, **21**(11), 3189–95.

52 Parfrey PS, Vavasour H, Bullock M, et al. (1987). Symptoms in end-stage renal disease: dialysis v transplantation. *Transplant Proceed*, **19**(4), 3407–9.

53 Parfrey PS, Vavasour HM, Henry S, et al. (1988). Clinical features and severity of nonspecific symptoms in dialysis patients. *Nephron*, **50**(2), 121–8.

54 Parfrey PS, Vavasour H, Bullock M, et al. (1989). Development of a health questionnaire specific for end-stage renal disease. *Nephron*, **52**(1), 20–8.

55 Chiu YL, Chen HY, Chuang YF, et al. (2008). Association of uraemic pruritus with inflammation and hepatitis infection in haemodialysis patients. *Nephrol Dial Transplant*, **23**(11), 3685–9.

56 Razeghi E, Tavakolizadeh S, Ahmadi F (2008). Inflammation and pruritus in hemodialysis patients. *Saudi J Kidney Dis Transplant*, **19**(1), 62–6.

57 Frank A, Auslander GK, Weissgarten J (2003). Quality of Life of Patients with End-Stage Renal Disease at Various Stages of the Illness. *Soc Work Health Care*, **38**(2), 1–27.

58 Curtis BM, Barret BJ, Jindal K, et al. (2002). Canadian survey of clinical status at dialysis initiation 1998-1999: a multicenter prospective survey. *Clin Nephrol*, **58**(4), 282–8.

59 Virga G, Mastrosimone S, Amici G, et al. (1998). Symptoms in hemodialysis patients and their relationship with biochemical and demographic parameters. *Int J Artif Organs*, **21**(12), 788–93.

60 Balaskas EV, Chu M, Uldall RP, et al. (1993). Pruritus in continuous ambulatory peritoneal dialysis and hemodialysis patients. *Periton Dialy Int*, **13** (Suppl. 2), S527–32.

61 Masi CM, Cohen EP (1992). Dialysis efficacy and itching in renal failure. *Nephron*, **3**, 257–61.

62 Barrett BJ, Vavasour HM, Major A, et al. (1990). Clinical and psychological correlates of somatic symptoms in patients on dialysis. *Nephron*, **55** (1), 10–15.

63 Balaskas EV, Bamihas GI, Karamouzis M, et al. (1998). Histamine and serotonin in uremic pruritus: Effect of ondansetron in CAPD-pruritic patients. *Nephron*, **78**(4), 395–402.

64 Szepietowski JC, Sikora M, Kusztal M, et al. (2002). Uremic pruritus: a clinical study of maintenance hemodialysis patients. *J Dermatol*, **29**(10), 621–7.

65 Winkelman JW, Chertow GM, Lazarus JM (1996). Restless legs syndrome in end-stage renal disease. *Am J Kidney Dis*, **28**(3), 372–8.

66 Zucker I, Yosipovitch G, David M, et al. (2003). Prevalence and characterization of uremic pruritus in patients undergoing hemodialysis: uremic pruritus is still a major problem for patients with end-stage renal disease. *J Am Acad Dermatol*, **49**(5), 842–6.

67 Kosmadakis GC, Papakonstantinou S, Theodoros C, et al. (2008). Characteristics of uremic pruritus in hemodialysis patients: data from a single center. *Kidney Int*, **74**(7), 962.

68 Mistik S, Utas S, Ferahbas A, et al. (2006). An epidemiology study of patients with uremic pruritus. *Journal of the European Acad Dermat Venereol*, **20**(6), 672–8.

69 Dyachenko P, Shustak A, Rozenman D (2006). Hemodialysis-related pruritus and associated cutaneous manifestations. *Int J Dermat*, **45**(6), 664–7.

70 Merkus MP, Jager KJ, Dekker FW, et al. (1999). Physical symptoms and quality of life in patients on chronic dialysis: results of The Netherlands Cooperative Study on Adequacy of Dialysis (NECOSAD) *Nephrol Dialy Transplant*, **14**(5), 1163–70.

71 Subach RA, Marx MA (2002). Evaluation of uremic pruritus at an outpatient hemodialysis unit. *Ren Fail*, **24**(5), 609–14.

72 Pisoni RL, Wikstrom B, Elder SJ, et al. (2006). Pruritus in haemodialysis patients: International results from the Dialysis Outcomes and Practice Patterns Study (DOPPS). *Nephrol Dial Transplant*, **21**(12), 3495–505.

73 Narita I, Alchi B, Omori K, et al. (2006). Etiology and prognostic significance of severe uremic pruritus in chronic hemodialysis patients. *Kidney Int*, **69**(9), 1626–32.

74 Manenti L, Tansinda P, Vaglio A (2009). Uraemic pruritus: clinical characteristics, pathophysiology and treatment. *Drugs*, **69**(3), 251–63.

75 Molnar MZ, Novak M, Mucsi I (2006). Management of restless legs syndrome in patients on dialysis. *Drugs*, **66**(5), 607–24.

76 Rijsman RM, de Weerd AW, Stam CJ, et al. (2004). Periodic limb movement disorder and restless legs syndrome in dialysis patients. *Nephrology*, **9**(6), 353–61.

77 Collado-Seidel V, Kohnen R, Samtleben W, et al. (1998). Clinical and biochemical findings in uremic patients with and without restless legs syndrome. *Am J Kidney Dis*, **31**(2), 324–8.

78 Gigli GL, Adorati M, Dolso P, et al. (2004). Restless legs syndrome in end-stage renal disease. *Sleep Med*, **5**(3), 309–15.

79 Hui DS, Wong TY, Ko FW, et al. (2000). Prevalence of sleep disturbances in chinese patients with end-stage renal failure on continuous ambulatory peritoneal dialysis. *Am J Kidney Dis*, **36**(4), 783–8.

80 Cirignotta F, Mondini S, Santoro A, et al. (2002). Reliability of a questionnaire screening restless legs syndrome in patients on chronic dialysis. *Am J Kidney Dis*, **40**(2), 302–6.

81 Unruh ML, Levey AS, D'Ambrosio C, et al. (2004). Restless Legs Symptoms among Incident Dialysis Patients: Association with Lower Quality of Life and Shorter Survival. *Am J Kidney Dis*, **43**(5), 900–9.

82 Mucsi I, Molnar MZ, Rethelyi J, et al. (2004). Sleep disorders and illness intrusiveness in patients on chronic dialysis. *Nephrol Dialy Transplant*, **19**(7), 1815–22.

83 Siddiqui S, Kavanagh D, Traynor J, et al. (2004). Clinical Aspects of Restless Legs Syndrome in Patients on Chronic Haemodialysis. UK Renal Association conference proceedings, 2004 Annual Conference.

84 Medcalf P, Bhatia KP (2006). Restless legs syndrome. *BMJ*, **333**(7566), 457–8.

85 Allen RP, Picchietti D, Hening WA, et al. (2003). Restless legs syndrome: diagnostic criteria, special considerations, and epidemiology. A report from the restless legs syndrome diagnosis and epidemiology workshop at the National Institutes of Health. *Sleep Med*, **4**(2), 101–19.

86 Drake CL, Roehrs T, Roth T (2003). Insomnia causes, consequences, and therapeutics: an overview. *Depress Anxiety*, **18**(4), 163–76.

87 Molnar MZ, Szentkiralyi A, Lindner A, et al. (2007). Restless legs syndrome and mortality in kidney transplant recipients. *Am J Kidney Dis*, **50**(5), 813–20.

88 Iliescu EA, Coo H, McMurray MH, et al. (2003). Quality of sleep and health-related quality of life in haemodialysis patients. *Nephrol Dialy Transplant*, **18**(1), 126–32.

89 Walker S, Fine A, Kryger MH (1995). Sleep complaints are common in a dialysis unit. *Am J Kidney Dis,* **26**(5), 751–6.

90 Devins GM, Edworthy SM, Paul LC, et al. (1993). Restless sleep, illness intrusiveness, and depressive symptoms in three chronic illness conditions: rheumatoid arthritis, end-stage renal disease, and multiple sclerosis. *J Psychosom Res*, **37**(2), 163–70.

91 Han S-Y, Yoon J-W, Jo S-K, et al. (2002). Insomnia in diabetic hemodialysis patients: Prevalence and risk factors by a multicenter study. *Nephron*, **92** (1), 127–32.

92 Sabbatini M, Minale B, Crispo A, et al. (2002). Insomnia in maintenance haemodialysis patients. *Nephrol Dialy Transplant*, **17** (5), 852–6.

93 Venmans BJ, van Kralingen KW, Chandi DD, et al. (1999). Sleep complaints and sleep disordered breathing in hemodialysis patients. *Netherlands J Med*, **54**(5), 207–12.

94 Holley JL, Nespor S, Rault R (1992). A comparison of reported sleep disorders in patients on chronic hemodialysis and continuous peritoneal dialysis. *Am J Kidney Dis*, **19**(2), 156–61.

95 Locking-Cusolito H, Huyge L, et al. (2001). Sleep pattern disturbance in hemodialysis and peritoneal dialysis patients. *Nephrol Nurs J*, **28**(1), 40–4.

96 Stepanski E, Faber M, Zorick F, et al. (1995). Sleep disorders in patients on continuous ambulatory peritoneal dialysis. *J Am Soc Nephrol*, **6**(2), 192–7.

97 Kimmel PL, Emont SL, Newmann JM, et al. (2003). ESRD patient quality of life: symptoms, spiritual beliefs, psychosocial factors, and ethnicity. *Am J Kidney Dis*, **42**(4), 713–21.

98 Shayamsunder AK, Patel SS, Jain V, et al. (2005). Sleepiness, sleeplessness, and pain in end-stage renal disease: distressing symptoms for patients. *Semin Dial*, **18**(2), 109–18.

99 Hanly P (2004). Sleep apnea and daytime sleepiness in end-stage renal disease. *Semin Dialy*, **17**(2), 109–14.

100 Iliescu EA, Yeates KE, Holland DC (2004). Quality of sleep in patients with chronic kidney disease. *Nephrol Dial Transplant*, **19**(1), 95–9.

101 Jhamb M, Weisbord SD, Steel JL, et al. (2008). Fatigue in patients receiving maintanence dialysis: a review of definitions, measures and contributing factors. *Am J Kidney Dis*, **52**(2), 353–65.

102 Chang WK, Hung KY, Huang JW, et al. (2001). Chronic fatigue in long-term peritoneal dialysis patients. *Am J Nephrol*, **21**(6), 479–85.

103 Heiwe S, Clyne N, Dahlgren MA (2003). Living with chronic renal failure: patients' experiences of their physical and functional capacity. *Physiother Res Int*, **8**(4), 167–77.

104 Weisbord SD, Fried L, Mor MK, et al. (2007). Renal provider recognition of symptoms in patients on maintenance hemodialysis. *Clin J Am Soc Nephrologists*, **2** (5), 960–7.

105 Parfrey PS, Vavasour HM, Gault MH (1988). A prospective study of health status in dialysis and transplant patients. *Transplant Proceed*, **20**(6), 1231–2.

106 Davison SN, Jhangri GS, Johnson JA (2006). Cross-sectional validity of a modified Edmonton symptom assessment system in dialysis patients: a simple assessment of symptom burden. *Kidney Int*, **69**(9), 1621–5.

107 Weisbord SD, Fried LF, Arnold RM, et al. (2004). Development of a symptom assessment instrument for chronic hemodialysis patients: the Dialysis Symptom Index. *J Pain Symp Manag*, **27**(3), 226–40.

108 Murphy EL, Murtagh FE, Carey I, et al. (2009). Understanding symptoms in patients with advanced chronic kidney disease managed without dialysis: use of a short patient-completed assessment tool. *Nephron Clin Pract*, **111**(1), c74–80.

109 Bruera E, Kuehn N, Miller MJ, et al. (1991). The Edmonton Symptom Assessment System (ESAS): a simple method for the assessment of palliative care patients. *J Palliat Care*, **7**(2), 6–9.

110 Jaeschke R, Singer J, Guyatt GH (1990). A comparison of seven-point and visual analogue scales. Data from a randomized trial. *Control Clin Trials*, **11**(1), 43–51.

111 Portenoy RK, Thaler HT, Kornblith AB, et al. (1994). The Memorial Symptom Assessment Scale: an instrument for the evaluation of symptom prevalence, characteristics and distress. *Eur J Cancer*, **30A**(9), 1326–36.

112 Chang VT, Hwang SS, Feuerman M, et al. (2000). The memorial symptom assessment scale short form (MSAS-SF). *Cancer*, **89**(5), 1162–71.

113 Aspinal F, Hughes R, Higginson IJ (2002). *A user's guide to the Palliative care Outcome Scale*. King's College London: Palliative Care & Policy Publications.

114 Higginson IJ, Hart S, Silber E, et al. (2006). Symptom prevalence and severity in people severely affected by multiple sclerosis. *J Palliat Care*, **22**(3), 158–65.

115 Daut RL, Cleeland CS, Flanery RC (1983). Development of the Wisconsin Brief Pain Questionnaire to assess pain in cancer and other diseases. *Pain*, **17**(2), 197–210.

116 Melzack R (1975). The McGill Pain Questionnaire: major properties and scoring methods. *Pain*, **1**(3), 277–99.

117 Beck AT, Steer RA (1984). Internal consistencies of the original and revised Beck Depression Inventory. *J Clin Psychol*, **40**(6), 1365–7.

118 Majeski CJ, Johnson JA, Davison SN, et al. (2007). Itch Severity Scale: a self-report instrument for the measurement of pruritus severity. *Br J Dermatol*, **156**(4), 667–73.

119 Allen RP, Burchell BJ, Macdonald B, et al. (2009). Validation of the self-completed Cambridge-Hopkins questionnaire (CH-RLSq) for ascertainment of restless legs syndrome (RLS) in a population survey. *Sleep Med*, **4** (2), 121–32.

120 Bailie GR, Mason NA, Bragg-Gresham JL, et al. (2004). Analgesic prescription patterns among hemodialysis patients in the DOPPS: potential for underprescription. *Kidney Int*, **65**(6), 2419–25.

121 Davison SN (2003). Pain in hemodialysis patients: prevalence, cause, severity, and management. *Am J Kidney Dis*, **42**(6), 1239–47.

122 Launay-Vacher V, Karie S, Fau JB, et al. (2005). Treatment of pain in patients with renal insufficiency: the World Health Organization three-step ladder adapted. *J Pain*, **6**(3), 137–48.

123 Murtagh FE, Chai MO, Donohoe P, et al. (2007). The use of opioid analgesia in end-stage renal disease patients managed without dialysis: recommendations for practice. *J Pain Palliat Care Pharmacother*, **21**(2), 5–16.

124 National LCP Steering Group (2009). National LCP Renal Symptom Control Guidelines. Liverpool; 2008. www.mcpcil.org.uk/liverpool_care_pathway. Accessed on 12th March 2009

125 Muscaritoli M, Molfino A, Chiappini MG, et al. (2007). Anorexia in hemodialysis patients: the possible role of des-acyl ghrelin. *Am J Nephrol*, **27**(4), 360–5.

126 Bossola M, Tazza L, Giungi S, et al. (2006). Anorexia in hemodialysis patients: an update. *Kidney Int*, **70**(3), 417–22.

127 Kalantar-Zadeh K, Block G, McAllister CJ, et al. (2004). Appetite and inflammation, nutrition, anemia, and clinical outcome in hemodialysis patients. *Am J Clin Nutr*, **80**(2), 299–307.

128 Burrowes JD, Larive B, Chertow GM, et al. (2005). Self-reported appetite, hospitalization and death in haemodialysis patients: findings from the Hemodialysis (HEMO) Study. *Nephrol Dial Transplant*, **20**(12), 2765–74.

129 Akpele L, Bailey JL (2004). Nutrition counseling impacts serum albumin levels. *J Ren Nutr*, **14**(3), 143–8.

130 Suri RS, Nesrallah GE, Mainra R, et al. (2006). Daily hemodialysis: a systematic review. *Clin J Am Soc Nephrol*, **1**(1), 33–42.

131 Booth S, Farquhar M, Gysels M, et al. (2006). The impact of a breathlessness intervention service (BIS) on the lives of patients with intractable dyspnea: a qualitative phase 1 study. *Palliat Support Care*, **4**(3), 287–93.

132 Booth S, Wade R, Johnson M, Kite S, et al. (2004). The use of oxygen in the palliation of breathlessness. A report of the expert working group of the Scientific Committee of the Association of Palliative Medicine. *Resp Med*, **98**(1), 66–77.

133 Jennings AL, Davies AN, Higgins JP, et al. (2001). Opioids for the palliation of breathlessness in terminal illness. *Cochrane Datab Sys Rev*, (4), CD002066.

134 Jennings AL, Davies AN, Higgins JP, et al. (2002). A systematic review of the use of opioids in the management of dyspnoea. *Thorax*, **57**(11), 939–44.

135 Lee BO, Lin CC, Chaboyer W, et al. (2007). The fatigue experience of haemodialysis patients in Taiwan. *J Clin Nurs*, **16**(2), 407–13.

136 O'Sullivan D, McCarthy G (2007). An exploration of the relationship between fatigue and physical functioning in patients with end stage renal disease receiving haemodialysis. *J Clin Nurs*, **16**(11C), 276–84.

137 Brunier G, Graydon J (1992). The relationship of anemia, nonspecific uremic symptoms, and physical activity to fatigue in patients with end stage renal disease on hemodialysis. *ANNA J*, **19**(2), 157.

138 Ross SD, Fahrbach K, Frame D, et al. (2003). The effect of anemia treatment on selected health-related quality-of-life domains: a systematic review. *Clin Ther*, **25**(6), 1786–805.

139 Schmelz M, Schmidt R, Bickel A, et al. (1997). Specific C-receptors for itch in human skin. *J Neurosci*, **17**(20), 8003–8.

140 Lugon JR (2005). Uremic pruritus: a review. *Hemodial Int*, **9**(2), 180–8.

141 Duque MI, Thevarajah S, Chan YH, et al. (2006). Uremic pruritus is associated with higher kt/V and serum calcium concentration. *Clin Nephrol*, **66**(3), 184–91.

142 Kimmel M, Alscher DM, Dunst R, et al. (2006). The role of micro-inflammation in the pathogenesis of uraemic pruritus in haemodialysis patients. *Nephrol Dialy Transplant*, **21**(3), 749–55.

143 Yosipovitch G, Greaves MW, Schmelz M (2003). Itch. *Lancet*, **361**(9358), 690–4.

144 Ikoma A, Steinhoff M, Stander S, et al. (2006). The neurobiology of itch. *Nat Rev Neurosci*, **7**(7), 535–47.

145 Dawn AG, Yosipovitch G (2006). Butorphanol for treatment of intractable pruritus. *J Am Acad Dermatol*, **54**(3), 527–31.

146 Wikstrom B, Gellert R, Ladefoged SD, et al. (2005). Kappa-opioid system in uremic pruritus: multicenter, randomized, double-blind, placebo-controlled clinical studies. *J Am Soc Nephrol*, **16**(12), 3742–7.

147 Keithi-Reddy SR, Patel TV, Armstrong AW, et al. (2007). Uremic pruritus. *Kidney Int*, **72**(3), 373–7.

148 Morton CA, Lafferty M, Hau C, et al. (1996). Pruritus and skin hydration during dialysis. *Nephrol Dial Transplant*, **11**(10), 2031–6.

149 Okada K, Matsumoto K (2004). Effect of skin care with an emollient containing a high water content on mild uremic pruritus. *Therap Apher Dialy*, **8**(5), 419–22.

150 Wasik F, Szepietowski J, Szepietowski T, et al. (1996). Relief of uraemic pruritus after balneological therapy with a bath oil containing polidocanol. *J Dermat Treat*, **7**, 231–3.

151 Szepietowski JC, Reich A, Szepietowski T (2005). Emollients with endocannabinoids in the treatment of uremic pruritus: discussion of the therapeutic options. *Therap Apher Dialy*, **9**(3), 277–9.

152 Tarng DC (1996). Hemodialysis-related pruritus: a double-blind, placebo-controlled, crossover study of capsaicin 0.025% cream. *Nephron*, **72**(4), 617–22.

153 Breneman DL, Cardone JS, Blumsack RF, et al. (1992). Topical capsaicin for treatment of hemodialysis-related pruritus. *J Am Acad Dermat*, **26**(1), 91–4.

154 Pauli-Magnus C, Klumpp S, Alscher DM, et al. (2000). Short-term efficacy of tacrolimus ointment in severe uremic pruritus. *Periton Dialy Int*, **20** (6), 802–3.

155 Kuypers DR, Claes K, Evenepoel P, et al. (2004). A prospective proof of concept study of the efficacy of tacrolimus ointment on uraemic pruritus (UP) in patients on chronic dialysis therapy. *Nephrol Dialy Transplant*, **19**(7), 1895–901.

156 Duque MI, Yosipovitch G, Fleischer AB, Jr., et al. (2005). Lack of efficacy of tacrolimus ointment 0.1% for treatment of hemodialysis-related pruritus: a randomized, double-blind, vehicle-controlled study. *J Am Acad Dermat*, **52**(3 Pt 1), 519–21.

157 Gilchrest BA, Rowe JW, Brown RS, et al. (1979). Ultraviolet phototherapy of uremic pruritus. Long-term results and possible mechanism of action. *Ann Intern Med*, **91**(1), 17–21.

158 Gilchrest BA, Rowe JW, Brown RS, et al. (1977). Relief of uremic pruritus with ultraviolet phototherapy. *N Engl J Med*, **297**(3), 136–8.

159 Blachley JD, Blankenship DM, Menter A, et al. (1985). Uremic pruritus: skin divalent ion content and response to ultraviolet phototherapy. *Am J Kidney Dis*, **5**(5), 237–41.

160 Russo GE, Spaziani M, Guidotti C, et al. (1986). Pruritus in chronic uremic patients in periodic hemodialysis. Treatment with terfenadine (an antagonist of histamine H1 receptors). *Minerva Urol Nefrol*, **38**(4), 443–7.

161 Francos GC, Kauh YC, Gittlen SD, et al. (1991). Elevated plasma histamine in chronic uremia. Effects of ketotifen on pruritus. *Int J Dermatol*, **30**(12), 884–9.

162 Gunal AI, Ozalp G, Yoldas TK, et al. (2004). Gabapentin therapy for pruritus in haemodialysis patients: a randomized, placebo-controlled, double-blind trial. *Nephrol Dialy Transplant*, **19**(12), 3137–9.

163 Naini AE, Harandi AA, Khanbabapour S, et al. (2007). Gabapentin: a promising drug for the treatment of uremic pruritus. *Saudi J Kidney Dis Transplant*, **18**(3), 378–81.

164 Murphy M, Reaich D, Pai P, et al. (2003). A randomized, placebo-controlled, double-blind trial of ondansetron in renal itch. *Brit J Dermatol*, **148**(2), 314–17.

165 Ashmore SD, Jones CH, Newstead CG, et al. (2000). Ondansetron therapy for uremic pruritus in hemodialysis patients. *Am J Kidney Dis*, **35**(5), 827–31.

166 Layegh P, Mojahedi MJ, Malekshah PE, et al. (2007). Effect of oral granisetron in uremic pruritus. *Ind J Dermatol Venereol Leprol*, **73**(4), 231–4.

167 Peer G, Kivity S, Agami O, et al. (1996). Randomised crossover trial of naltrexone in uraemic pruritus. *Lancet*, **348**(9041), 1552–4.

168 Pauli-Magnus C (2000). Naltrexone does not relieve uremic pruritus: results of a randomized, double-blind, placebo-controlled crossover study. *J Am Soc Nephrol*, **11**(3), 514–19.

169 Andersen LW, Friedberg M, Lokkegaard N (1984). Naloxone in the treatment of uremic pruritus: a case history. *Clin Nephrol*, **21**(6), 355–6.

170 Twycross R, Greaves MW, Handwerker H, et al. (2003). Itch: scratching more than the surface. *QJM-An Int J Med*, **96**(1), 7–26.

171 Silva SR (1994). Thalidomide for the treatment of uremic pruritus: a crossover randomized double-blind trial. *Nephron*, **67**(3), 270–3.

172 Allen R (2004). Dopamine and iron in the pathophysiology of restless legs syndrome (RLS). *Sleep Med*, **5**(4), 385–91.

173 O'Keeffe ST, Noel J, Lavan JN (1993). Restless legs syndrome in the elderly. *Postgrad Med J*, **69**(815), 701–3.

174 Takaki J, Nishi T, Nangaku M, et al. (2003). Clinical and psychological aspects of restless legs syndrome in uremic patients on hemodialysis. *Am J Kidney Dis*, **41**(4), 833–9.

175 Telarovic S, Relja M, Trkulja V (2007). Restless legs syndrome in hemodialysis patients: association with calcium antagonists. A preliminary report. *Euro Neurol*, **58**(3), 166–9.

176 Silber MH, Ehrenberg BL, Allen RP, et al. (2004). An algorithm for the management of restless legs syndrome. *Mayo Clin Proc*, **79**(7), 916–22.

177 Trenkwalder C, Stiasny K, Pollmacher T, et al. (1995). L-dopa therapy of uremic and idiopathic restless legs syndrome: a double-blind, crossover trial. *Sleep*, **18**(8), 681–8.

178 Walker SL, Fine A, Kryger MH (1996). L-DOPA/carbidopa for nocturnal movement disorders in uremia. *Sleep*, **19**(3), 214–18.

179 Sandyk R, Bernick C, Lee SM, et al. (1987). L-dopa in uremic patients with the restless legs syndrome. *Int J Neurosci*, **35**(3-4), 233–5.

180 Pellecchia MT, Vitale C, Sabatini M, et al. (2004). Ropinirole as a treatment of restless legs syndrome in patients on chronic hemodialysis: an open randomized crossover trial versus levodopa sustained release. *Clin Neuropharmacol*, **27**(4), 178–81.

181 Miranda M, Kagi M, Fabres L, et al. (2004). Pramipexole for the treatment of uremic restless legs in patients undergoing hemodialysis. *Neurology*, **62**(5), 831–2.

182 Pieta J, Millar T, Zacharias J, et al. (1998). Effect of pergolide on restless legs and leg movements in sleep in uremic patients. *Sleep*, **21**(6), 617–22.

183 Read DJ, Feest TG, Nassim MA (1981). Clonazepam: effective treatment for restless legs syndrome in uraemia. *Brit Med J*, **283**(6296), 885–6.

184 Micozkadioglu H, Ozdemir FN, Kut A, et al. (2004). Gabapentin versus levodopa for the treatment of restless legs syndrome in hemodialysis patients: An open-label study. *Ren Fail*, **26**(4), 393–7.

185 Thorp ML, Morris CD, Bagby SP (2001). A crossover study of gabapentin in treatment of restless legs syndrome among hemodialysis patients. *Am J Kidney Dis*, **38**(1), 104–8.

Dialysis Symptom Index

The University of Pittsburgh Medical Center

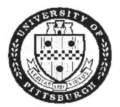

VA Pittsburgh Healthcare System

Patient Id: _____

Today's Date: _____

Code: _____

Interviewer Id: _____

Instructions

Below is a list of physical and emotional symptoms that people on dialysis may have. For each symptom, please indicate if you had the symptom during the past week by circling "yes" or "no." If "yes", please indicate how much that symptom bothered you by circling the appropriate number.

During the past week: Did you experience this symptom?		If "yes": How much did it bother you?				
		Not At All	A Little Bit	Some- what	Quite a Bit	Very Much
1. Constipation	NO					
	YES →	1	2	3	4	5
2. Nausea	NO					
	YES →	1	2	3	4	5
3. Vomiting	NO					
	YES →	1	2	3	4	5
4. Diarrhea	NO					
	YES →	1	2	3	4	5
5. Decreased appetite	NO					
	YES →	1	2	3	4	5
6. Muscle cramps	NO					
	YES →	1	2	3	4	5
7. Swelling in legs	NO					
	YES →	1	2	3	4	5
8. Shortness of breath	NO					
	YES →	1	2	3	4	5
9. Lightheadedness or dizziness	NO					
	YES →	1	2	3	4	5
10. Restless legs or difficulty keeping legs still	NO					
	YES →	1	2	3	4	5

During the past week: Did you experience this symptom?		Not At All	A Little Bit	Some-what	Quite a Bit	Very Much
			If "yes": *How much did it bother you?*			
11. Numbness or tingling in feet	NO					
	YES →	1	2	3	4	5
12. Feeling tired or lack of energy	NO					
	YES →	1	2	3	4	5
13. Cough	NO					
	YES →	1	2	3	4	5
14. Dry mouth	NO					
	YES →	1	2	3	4	5
15. Bone or joint pain	NO					
	YES →	1	2	3	4	5
16. Chest pain	NO					
	YES →	1	2	3	4	5
17. Headache	NO					
	YES →	1	2	3	4	5
18. Muscle soreness	NO					
	YES →	1	2	3	4	5
19. Difficulty concentrating	NO					
	YES →	1	2	3	4	5
20. Dry skin	NO					
	YES →	1	2	3	4	5
21. Itching	NO					
	YES →	1	2	3	4	5
22. Worrying	NO					
	YES →	1	2	3	4	5

During the past week: Did you experience this symptom?		*If "yes": How much did it <u>bother</u> you?*				
		Not At All	A Little Bit	Some -what	Quite a Bit	Very Much
23. Feeling nervous	NO					
	YES →	1	2	3	4	5
24. Trouble falling asleep	NO					
	YES →	1	2	3	4	5
25. Trouble staying asleep	NO					
	YES →	1	2	3	4	5
26. Feeling irritable	NO					
	YES →	1	2	3	4	5
27. Feeling sad	NO					
	YES →	1	2	3	4	5
28. Feeling anxious	NO					
	YES →	1	2	3	4	5
29. Decreased interest in sex	NO					
	YES →	1	2	3	4	5
30. Difficulty becoming sexually aroused	NO					
	YES →	1	2	3	4	5

The Patient Outcome Scale symptom module (renal version)

Ref No:	Date: __/__/__

Questionnaire POS-S (renal) – patient version

Below is a list of symptoms, which you may or may not have experienced.
Please put a tick in the box to show how each of these symptoms has affected how you have been feeling **over the last week.**

	Not at all, no effect	Slightly – but not bothered to be rid of it	Moderately – limits some activity or concentration	Severely – activities or concentration markedly affected	Overwhelmingly – unable to think of anything else
Pain	❑	❑	❑	❑	❑
Shortness of breath	❑	❑	❑	❑	❑
Weakness or lack of energy	❑	❑	❑	❑	❑
Nausea (feeling like you are going to be sick)	❑	❑	❑	❑	❑
Vomiting (being sick)	❑	❑	❑	❑	❑
Poor appetite	❑	❑	❑	❑	❑
Constipation	❑	❑	❑	❑	❑
Mouth problems	❑	❑	❑	❑	❑
Drowsiness	❑	❑	❑	❑	❑
Poor mobility	❑	❑	❑	❑	❑
Itching	❑	❑	❑	❑	❑
Difficulty sleeping	❑	❑	❑	❑	❑
Restless legs or difficulty keeping legs still	❑	❑	❑	❑	❑
Feeling anxious	❑	❑	❑	❑	❑
Feeling depressed	❑	❑	❑	❑	❑
Changes in skin	❑	❑	❑	❑	❑
Diarrhoea	❑	❑	❑	❑	❑
Any other symptoms?	❑	❑	❑	❑	❑
....	❑	❑	❑	❑	❑
....	❑	❑	❑	❑	❑

Which symptom has affected you the most? ....

Which symptom, if any, has improved the most? ....

Ref No:

Date: __/__/__

Questionnaire POS-S (renal) – staff version

Below is a list of symptoms which the patient may or may not have experienced. Please record how these symptoms have affected the patient in the table below. Put a tick in the box to show how you think they have affected how they have been feeling **over the last week.**

	Not at all, no effect	Slightly – but not bothered to be rid of it	Moderately – limits some activity or concentration	Severely – activities or concentration markedly affected	Overwhelmingly – unable to think of anything else
Pain	❑	❑	❑	❑	❑
Shortness of breath	❑	❑	❑	❑	❑
Weakness or lack of energy	❑	❑	❑	❑	❑
Nausea (feeling like you are going to be sick)	❑	❑	❑	❑	❑
Vomiting (being sick)	❑	❑	❑	❑	❑
Poor appetite	❑	❑	❑	❑	❑
Constipation	❑	❑	❑	❑	❑
Mouth problems	❑	❑	❑	❑	❑
Drowsiness	❑	❑	❑	❑	❑
Poor mobility	❑	❑	❑	❑	❑
Itching	❑	❑	❑	❑	❑
Difficulty sleeping	❑	❑	❑	❑	❑
Restless legs or difficulty keeping legs still	❑	❑	❑	❑	❑
Feeling anxious	❑	❑	❑	❑	❑
Feeling depressed	❑	❑	❑	❑	❑
Changes in skin	❑	❑	❑	❑	❑
Diarrhoea	❑	❑	❑	❑	❑
Any other symptoms?	❑	❑	❑	❑	❑
....	❑	❑	❑	❑	❑
....	❑	❑	❑	❑	❑

Which symptom has affected the patient the most? ....

Which symptom, if any, has improved the most? ....

Chapter 8

Management of pain in renal failure

Sara N Davison, E Joanna Chambers, and
Charles J Ferro

*Even thinking of pain is like tapping at a high voltage wire with
the back of your finger to see if it's live.*

8.1 Introduction

Pain has been defined by the International Association for the Study of Pain as "an unpleasant
sensory and emotional experience associated with actual or potential tissue damage, or described
in terms of such damage".[1] This definition reminds us of the emotional associations of pain
including fear and depression. There are numerous potential causes for pain in the patient with
chronic kidney disease (CKD); the experience of pain will, however, be unique to each individual
as pain is a subjective experience and can only be described and measured by that individual.
The term 'total pain' – first used by Cicely Saunders[2] to describe cancer pain – emphasizes the
contribution of psychological, spiritual, and social factors to the experience of pain. This concept
is equally applicable to the CKD patient who has pain. A unidimensional approach to pain
management is likely to be unsuccessful, until the whole person, in the context of their disease
and personal life, is taken into account.[3]

> *It seems to me that pain in itself, though a pretty nasty piece of work, wouldn't have half the street cred if it
> wasn't like all bullies joined at the hip with that cringing lickspittle, fear.*

8.2 Incidence and types of pain

A growing body of literature clearly demonstrates that pain is common in patients with CKD.
[4–6] In fact, the number and severity of pain and other symptoms reported by end-stage renal
disease (ESRD) patients, whether they be treated with dialysis or managed conservatively (without
dialysis), is similar to that reported by cancer patients hospitalized in palliative care settings.[6–8]
Approximately 50% of ESRD patients experience chronic pain, with as many as 82% reporting
this pain as moderate to severe in intensity. Pain in ESRD is also often experienced in the context
of numerous other symptoms such as anorexia, fatigue, nausea, insomnia, pruritus, anxiety, and
depression. In North America, approximately 20–25% of dialysis patients die following withdrawal
of dialysis, the second leading cause of death for this group of patients.[9] In this subset of patients,
up to 50% are known to have significant pain as well as other distressing symptoms as they
die.[4,10–12]

Pain in patients with CKD includes most of the same types of pain experienced by cancer patients, namely nociceptive, somatic and visceral, neuropathic, and possibly complex regional pain syndromes. Pain in CKD may be due to the primary renal disease (e.g. polycystic kidney disease), concurrent co-morbidity (e.g. diabetic neuropathy, peripheral vascular disease), or disease consequent upon renal failure (e.g. calciphylaxis, bone pain from renal osteodystrophy, dialysis-related amyloid arthropathy). Pain may also result from the treatment of ESRD. Painful chronic infections such as osteomyelitis and discitis are complications seen from central lines. Arteriovenous fistulae can lead to painful ischaemic neuropathies, including the 'steal syndrome' in which blood that would normally flow to the palmar arch is diverted by the creation of an arteriovenous fistula. Patients on peritoneal dialysis often contend with recurrent pain due to abdominal distension, lower back strain, and recurrent peritonitis, while those on haemodialysis may experience recurrent cramps or headaches.[4,13,14] Patients frequently experience more than one type of pain,[4] a not unexpected finding in view of the diverse causes of pain in these patients. Despite improvements in dialysis technology and the care of the renal patient, the incidence of chronic pain appears to be increasing and probably reflects an ageing dialysis population with greater co-morbidity. Unfortunately, pain in CKD remains underrecognized,[15] undertreated,[16] and presents significant challenges to the patient and the nephrology team throughout the patient's illness.

8.2.1 Health-related quality of life

Pain carries only two messages to the sufferer 'You are broken. Mend or die.'

Pain is a multidimensional phenomenon with physical and psychosocial components. It is widely recognized that chronic pain is associated with psychological distress, depressive disorders, impairment of interpersonal relationships, excessive use of the healthcare, and substantial limitations in work, family, social life, and health-related quality of life.[17–22] Recent research has confirmed the tremendous psychosocial burden of pain in CKD patients[23] and supports the increasing awareness that patients' perceptions of symptom burden – and, in particular, chronic pain – may be more important than objective clinical assessments in determining health-related quality of life.[24–26] Dialysis patients with chronic pain are 2.3 times more likely to suffer from insomnia and depression than patients without chronic pain[27] and chronic pain may be a factor in considerations of withdrawal from dialysis. [27,28] Large studies in dialysis patients have demonstrated that symptom burden, including chronic pain, accounted for 29–34% of the impairment in physical health-related quality of life and 39–46% of the impairment in mental health-related quality of life.[7,29] The lack of significant association between clinical and dialysis-related parameters and health-related quality of life reinforces the relative importance from the patient's perspective of pain and other symptoms.

The relationship between pain and quality of life is complex and not entirely clear. Pain may increase anxiety and impair function affecting both social activities and work. A reduction in both of these can further contribute to low mood or depression. In CKD, pain is often experienced in the context of multiple, complex symptoms and end-of-life issues which may interfere markedly with psychological, social, and physical coping strategies. This concept is fundamental to the term "total pain" as stated in the introduction of this chapter. Effective clinical approaches to pain management are clearly essential if efforts to improve the health-related quality of life of these patients are to be successful.

8.2.2 Categories of pain

8.2.2.1 Nociceptive pain

Tissue damage in the skin, muscle, and other tissues causes stimulation of sensory receptors with electrical discharge to the spinal cord along mainly Aδ and C-fibres. Pain is characteristically felt at the site of damage and may be described using terms such as sharp or like a knife. This is the mechanism of joint pain in dialysis-related amyloid arthropathy. Visceral nociceptors may be stimulated in a similar way by chemical or mechanical irritation, experienced as a sharp pain from liver capsule distension in polycystic kidney and liver disease or a dull, poorly localized pain from gut ischaemia.

8.2.2.2 Neuropathic pain

Neuropathic pain results from damage to and changes in the nervous system resulting in either dysfunction or pathological change in the nerve – either at the site of damage or at the level of the dorsal horn. A complex series of changes can occur, leading to an increase in excitation. This is contributed to by a reduction in descending (noradrenergic and serotonergic) inhibitory pathways and an increased local activation of excitatory neurotransmitters and N-methyl-D-aspartate (NMDA) receptors. Common descriptors of neuropathic pain include burning, shooting, and stabbing. It may be felt at a site distant from its cause, e.g. in the distribution of a nerve. It may be associated with episodes of spontaneous pain, hyperalgesia, and allodynia. The presence of the latter is pathognomonic. The pain of peripheral neuropathy and phantom-limb pain belongs in this category. The majority of pains seen in patients with CKD are of mixed type, particularly those of ischaemia, calciphylaxis, carpal tunnel syndrome, and the steal syndrome.

Categorizing pain helps the physician choose an appropriate management strategy which may include both drug and non-drug therapies. Generally, nociceptive pain responds well to opioids whereas neuropathic pain may be poorly responsive or require doses for response that are associated with unacceptable toxicity. The handling of opioids by patients with CKD increases the likelihood of this toxicity occurring before useful pain relief. Diagnosing neuropathic pain reminds the physician to consider the use of adjuvant analgesics such as antidepressants and anticonvulsants where there is evidence for their efficacy.[30,31] Good descriptive studies of the types of pain seen in cancer have helped its management: the same is likely to be true for CKD.

8.2.3 Types of pain

8.2.3.1 Acute pain

Acute pain occurs following tissue damage and activation of nociceptors at the site of injury and is normally seen as serving an important protective physiological function. The dialysis patient may experience repeated episodes of acute pain during dialysis, such as headaches and muscle cramps, as well as short-lived, but severe, pain in other sites such as the abdomen. These may occur over long periods of time, though the patient will also be free from them for long periods. These recurring pains need distinguishing from chronic pain, as the management is different. The term recurrent pain has been used to describe this;[32] drawing attention to the fact that it increases the amount the illness intrudes on everyday life. In addition, anticipation of pain before each dialysis has an impact on quality of life and may increase the distress from the pain (see Case study 1).

Case study 1: To illustrate management of temporary, but excruciating, pain during dialysis

Y is a 31-year-old woman with a 13-year history of insulin-dependent diabetes. Both parents had diabetic nephropathy; her mother had succumbed to renal failure and her father had a renal transplant. Renal insufficiency was first diagnosed 4 years previously at routine screening during her first pregnancy, with further deterioration following the birth of her second child. Recently, admission was precipitated by extensive infected oedema of her anterior abdominal wall with full-thickness necrosis in the lateral margins of her abdominal apron. Daily haemodialysis, alternating with ultrafiltration, was started to reduce the fluid overload, together with antibiotic treatment.

Y had two pains. The first was across her anterior abdomen and was present at all times although eased at rest by tramadol 50 mg 8 hourly. Within minutes of starting dialysis, a second excruciating pain, described as such a strong burning pain she expected to smell burning, would occur across her abdomen, particularly in the 'apron', starting laterally and working medially. The pain lasted throughout dialysis and for approximately 30 min following completion. Anxiety about this pain dominated her feelings. She had been taking hydromorphone, first 1.3 mg, then 2.6 mg, and finally 3.9 mg during dialysis without benefit despite the dose being repeated.

Actions:

Day 1. Fentanyl 25 μg given subcutaneously (SC) prior to dialysis and available hourly as needed plus clonazepam 0.5 mg at night. This led to a better night's sleep but no real improvement in dialysis pain.

Day 2. Fentanyl 50 μg SC before dialysis and as needed (prn). There was some improvement, but by the time she received subsequent doses of fentanyl, she had already started to lose control over the pain. Clonazepam was increased to 1 mg at night and amitriptyline added, working up to a dose of 40 mg at night.

Day 6. Changed to short SC fentanyl infusion of 50 μg/h, starting 30 min before dialysis and running for 30 min after dialysis stopped. This was extremely effective and she was able to tolerate dialysis comfortably on this regimen. Since this episode it has been possible to stop the SC fentanyl regimen during dialysis as the infected, loculated fluid on her abdominal wall has been managed with plastic surgery. Her background pain control 3 months after this episode is with transdermal fentanyl.

8.2.3.2 Chronic pain

Chronic pain is usually initiated by tissue injury but is perpetuated by neurophysiological changes which take place within the peripheral and central nervous system leading to continuation of pain in the absence of the pain stimulus. The intensity of the pain may be out of proportion to the original injury or tissue damage. As pain persists, other factors, such as the psychosocial and spiritual distress relating to the disease or unrelated situations, can influence the experience of pain. Chronic pain is not defined by duration but rather by the experience of pain in the absence of persistent nociceptor damage. This pain has no recognized biological function. Pain perpetuated by continued physical damage from disease processes, such as dialysis-related amyloid arthropathy, are therefore better described as repetitive acute pain or recurrent pain,[32] although they are chronic in the sense of occurring over many years. Patients may, in addition, experience chronic pain as defined above and thus the total picture is complex with mixed categories.

8.2.3.3 Episodic, incident, paroxysmal, and breakthrough pain

These are terms used to describe pain that breaks through or occurs despite regular analgesic medication. Episodic pain can be defined as "a transitory exacerbation of pain experienced by the patient who has relatively stable and adequately controlled baseline pain".[33] It falls into two main categories: incident pain and paroxysmal pain. Incident pain occurs in relation to specific events, e.g. movement. Paroxysmal pain arises without obvious precipitators and is often neuropathic in nature. Breakthrough pain occurs when background medication is inadequate for continuous pain control so pain occurs towards the end of a dosing period. Management is discussed in section 8.5.3.

8.2.4 Barriers to adequate pain relief

Despite what appears to be an increasing prevalence of chronic pain, analgesic use in ESRD has decreased over the last few years. The Dialysis Outcomes and Practice Patterns Study (DOPPS) compared analgesic use in 1997 to that in 2000 for 3749 dialysis patients in 142 United States facilities.[34] The percentage of patients using any analgesic decreased from 30% to 24%. Narcotic use decreased from 18% to <15% and paracetamol use decreased from 11% to 6%. Seventy-four percent of patients with pain that interfered with work had no analgesic prescription. These findings are consistent with other reports where 35% of haemodialysis patients with chronic pain were not prescribed analgesics despite the vast majority experiencing moderate or severe pain, and less than 10% were prescribed strong opioids.[4]

The high prevalence of unrelieved pain is not unique to CKD. Despite the availability of effective pain management interventions[31] and published guidelines for its management,[35] many patients with cancer have considerable pain and receive inadequate analgesia.[36] Inadequate pain assessment, reluctance of the patient to report pain, and lack of staff time and training in the basic principles of pain management have been identified as barriers to adequate pain management in cancer patients.[37] Many of these apply to CKD; however, the management of pain in CKD is more complex for several reasons:

Lack of recognition of the problem: Patients may under-report pain, assuming that pain is an integral part of their condition. Others may have cognitive dysfunction preventing effective communication. If pain is reported, it may not be acknowledged and managed effectively by the nephrology team as pain management may not have sufficient priority in dialysis units.

Lack of research/knowledge: There is a lack of a discrete medical literature that synthesizes pain management and nephrology. Studies of the pattern and types of pain seen in CKD are needed in addition to those evaluating the efficacy of analgesia with particular reference to toxicity, pharmacokinetic, and pharmacodynamic data.

Altered pharmacokinetics and pharmacodynamics of analgesics in CKD: The absorption and clearance of drugs are more complex in renal failure. CKD patients are much more likely to run into problems of opioid toxicity, such as confusion, myoclonus, and sedation (see later section on opioids).

Adverse effects of analgesics are common and may be mimicked by uraemic symptoms resulting in the inappropriate withdrawal of analgesics. Even after appropriate withdrawal or reduction they are often not restarted when the acute crisis resolves. In our experience, the most common presentation of opioid toxicity necessitating opioid switch in CKD patients is confusion and cognitive impairment, often precipitated by infection or an acute change in medical condition.

Co-morbid disease and an increase in susceptibility to adverse drug effects often limit the use of analgesics. Patients with CKD are frequently on multiple drugs, with the consequent increase in risk of adverse interactions between these drugs. For example, warfarin increases the risk of gastrointestinal bleeding associated with non-steroidal anti-inflammatory drugs (NSAIDS), some of which potentiate the action of warfarin itself by inhibiting its metabolism. In addition, there is known to be an increase in the non-nephrotoxic adverse effects of NSAIDS in patients with CKD, particularly relating to gastrointestinal bleeding.

Lack of training in pain management: Pain management has not been a focus of training in renal medicine, resulting in the lack of understanding of effective pain evaluation and management.

Many patients will have more than one cause for their pain: This makes the diagnosis and management of pain challenging. However, it is of clinical importance to try and distinguish the types or components of a patient's pain in order to treat them effectively.

Limb preservation: CKD patients may experience severe pain from ischaemic limbs for a considerable time in an effort to preserve a limb or defer high-risk surgery.

Adequate pain management in CKD will require:

◆ Recognition of the need to work collaboratively with other teams, including palliative care and pain-management teams.

◆ Better education in pain management of the nephrology team.

◆ Better understanding of renal-specific issues by palliative care and pain-management teams.

◆ Recognition of the spiritual and psychosocial aspects of pain.

◆ Increased study and understanding of the pharmacology of analgesics in patients with CKD.

8.2.5 **Evaluation of pain**

The principles of pain management in CKD are similar to those of managing acute and chronic pain in other conditions: to provide effective analgesia without undue or unacceptable toxicity. This requires regular assessment and recording of the intensity of pain, its effect on functioning and quality of life, and the impact of analgesic medications on these factors.

Evaluation starts at the bedside with a good pain history, documentation of sites, severity, and postulated causes of the pain (Table 8.1). It will include previous measures of pain relief, their

Table 8.1 Suggested contents of a pain history

Pain dimension	Relevant questions
Site of pain	Where do you feel this pain? Does it go anywhere else? Is there numbness or other strange sensation at the site of the pain?
Character of pain	Describe your pain. Is it dull, burning, or shooting?
History of pain	How long have you had it? How did it start? Did something appear to cause it or did it appear out of the blue?
Relieving factors	Does anything make it better, such as position, medication?
Accentuating factors	Does anything make it worse?
Pattern	Is there any pattern to the pain? Is it worse at any particular time of day?
Sleep disturbance	Does the pain prevent you getting to sleep? Does it wake you in the night?
Activities	Does the pain stop you doing things you would otherwise do?
Previous treatments	What have you used in the past for you pain? What was helpful/What was not helpful and why?

Adapted from: Relief of chronic malignant pain? Henry McQuay at http:www.jr2.ox.ac.uk/bandolier/booth/painpag/-wisdom/493HJM.html

effectiveness, and toxicity. It should also embrace the effects of the pain on social functioning and psychosocial and spiritual issues that may impact on the perception of the pain. Pain can be recorded either as pain intensity or pain relief using verbal or numerical scales. It has proved reliable to work on the principle that pain is what the patient says it is and he or she is the only person who can measure it. This can then safely be used as a measure of severity and gauge of effectiveness. It is also important to listen to the patient to validate the significance of their pain and suffering. This expression of understanding of their situation is an important part of the therapeutic intervention.

Pain measurement tools (PMTs) have been used extensively in cancer patients – both as research tools and for bedside evaluation of therapy. They range from simple unidimensional bedside tools that can be used by all physicians and nurses; such as visual analogue scales and verbal and numerical rating scales, to more sophisticated multidimensional tools such as the McGill Pain Questionnaire (MPQ),[38] or the Brief Pain Inventory (BPI)[39] which incorporate quality-of-life questions. Both of these multidimensional PMTs have been validated in cancer care across a wide variety of cultural and linguistic backgrounds.[40] The BPI uses numerical scales to score worst, least, average, and current pain. It covers medications, pain relief, and interference with mood, physical activity, and other functional areas. It is self-administered and easy to use. The MPQ is also self-administered. It asks the patient to specify pain experience using classes of word descriptors; sensory, affective, and evaluative.

More recently, there have been global symptom-assessment tools that were developed for use in patients with advanced cancer but have subsequently been adapted and validated for use in CKD patients: the modified Edmonton Symptom Assessment System (mESAS),[7,29] the Memorial Symptom Assessment Scale Short Form (MSAS-SF) – renamed the Dialysis Symptom Index (DSI)[5,41] – and most recently, the modified Patient Outcome Scale – symptom module (mPOSs).[6] An advantage of utilizing tools common to other end-of-life patient groups is that relevant and useful comparisons can be made. The mESAS is a simple, widely used tool that consists of visual analogue scales with a superimposed 0–10 scale for 10 commonly experienced symptoms in CKD, including pain. It has the advantage of being simple, quick, and easily understood by both staff and patients and can be successfully used in patients even as they approach death. The DSI looks at 31 common, and less common symptoms. The mPOSs assesses 17 common symptoms in CKD based on the degree symptoms affect activities and concentration.

8.3 Treatment strategy

Following assessment of the pain, a straightforward explanation of the postulated cause(s) and a proposed management plan should be given to the patient. It is important to give the patient achievable goals. Management may need to be staged, initially aiming for freedom from pain at rest and at night, progressing to relief of more difficult pain such as that which is movement related. It is important to the patient that the clinician is honest and does not raise unrealistic expectations. The patient should also be reassured that the clinician will continue to address the patient's pain-management needs if unsuccessful initially. Since relief of all pain is not always possible, an important treatment target can be that pain will be reduced sufficiently for it to cause less interference with the individual's desired lifestyle. Attention to psychosocial and spiritual issues must not be forgotten (see Case study 2). The incidence of depression in dialysis patients is known to be high and pain is also known to be associated with depression. [42] Appropriate pharmacological management should be instituted where indicated clinically.

Case study 2: Psychosocial issues matter

A 62-year-old West Indian had phantom-limb pain following amputation for peripheral vascular disease. Pain relief had been successfully achieved using a fentanyl 75 µg/h transdermal patch. Severe infection – without a change in the level of pain or other parameters – led to an episode of opioid toxicity, necessitating reversal of narcosis. Fentanyl was stopped but his pain returned. He described his pain as starting in his absent limb and spreading up his leg through the stump to his shoulders and head. Further questioning revealed that he had been living in a residential home away from his wife for several months since the amputation as essential alterations to his house had not been done. Analgesia was restarted at the bottom of the analgesic ladder with regular paracetamol and codeine if needed. At the same time, he was seen by the social worker to look at how to address the social problems. By the next day he reported his pain as improved without the need for any strong opioids, though later it increased again, while his psychosocial issues continued to be addressed. His analgesic requirements were titrated against pain until he achieved satisfactory pain control with a dose of modified-release morphine of 20 mg bid, which is one-quarter as potent as his original dose of fentanyl, and without the necessity to increase it further for several months.

8.3.1 Use of analgesics

In 1986, the first edition of Cancer Pain Relief was published by the World Health Organization (WHO). This publication proposed a method for relief of cancer pain – based on a small number of relatively inexpensive drugs, including morphine – and introduced the concept of the 'analgesic ladder' (Fig. 8.1). Field-testing in several countries demonstrated the usefulness and efficacy of this method in cancer patients.[35] The second edition, published in 1996,[3] takes into account many of the advances in understanding and practice that have happened since the publication of the first edition, but retained most of the original method. The groundwork for this revision was started in 1989, in the context of the meeting of a WHO Expert Committee on Cancer Pain Relief and Active Supportive Care.[43] These publications stress that pain management should be undertaken as part of comprehensive palliative care. Relief of other symptoms and of psychological,

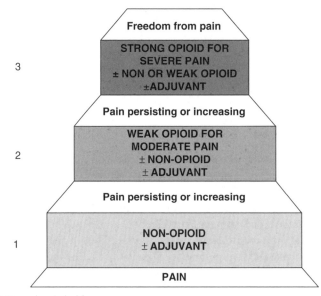

Fig. 8.1 The WHO analgesic ladder.

social, and spiritual problems is paramount. Attempting to relieve pain without addressing the patient's non-physical concerns is unlikely to be successful.[3] Since then these principles of pain management have become the basis for pain management in other areas of medicine, including ESRD.[44] They can be summarized by five phrases:

- 'by mouth'
- 'by the clock'
- 'by the ladder'
- 'for the individual'
- 'attention to detail'

8.3.1.1 'By mouth'

The key to safety is through use of the oral route and whenever possible, drugs should be given orally. Where ingestion or absorption of the medication is uncertain – as in dysphagia or vomiting, or the patient is too weak to swallow – analgesia must be given by an alternative route such as transdermal, subcutaneous, or rectal routes.

8.3.1.2 'By the clock'

Where pain is continuous, analgesics should be given regularly. Additional 'breakthrough' or 'rescue' medication should be available on an 'as needed' (prn) basis in addition to the regular dose. This enables the dose to be titrated against need according to the amount of extra opioid that has been required while monitoring toxicity.

8.3.1.3 'By the ladder'

Using the sequence of the WHO analgesic ladder (Fig. 8.1), initial analgesia is selected according to the severity of pain, starting at the lowest appropriate level. The drug should be used at its full tolerated dose before moving to the next level. Only one Step-2 opioid should be used at a time. If ineffective, it is unlikely that another drug from the same step will be effective and generally it is necessary to proceed to a Step-3 analgesic. Step-1 analgesics (NSAIDs and paracetamol) at full dose can be added to Step-2 or -3 drugs. Adjuvant analgesics can be added to all three steps for specific indications.

8.3.1.4 'For the individual'

There is no standard dose of strong opioids. The 'right dose' is the dose that relieves pain without causing unacceptable side effects. Opioids for mild to moderate pain have a dose limit in practice because of formulation (e.g. combined with aminosalicylic acid or paracetamol) or because of little increase in analgesia above standard doses together with a disproportionate increase in adverse effects at higher doses (e.g. codeine). Doses of opioids for moderate to severe pain have to be titrated against the patient's pain. Only the patient can measure the pain or quantify the side effects experienced. Evaluation and recording of benefit and toxicity is essential. The clinician must listen to and believe the patient. Sensitivity to different adverse effects is not predictable, and will vary between patients and within the same patient at different times. If an individual finds that a particular strong opioid causes unacceptable side effects, an alternative has to be sought.

8.3.1.5 'Attention to detail'

Pain changes over time, thus there is the need for on-going reassessment. The need for regular administration of pain-relief drugs should be explained to the patient. The first and last doses of the day should be linked to the patient's waking time and bedtime. Side effects should be explained and actively managed. All patients should have a laxative prescribed if on regular opioids and an antiemetic should be available. Written information about the drug, dosage, reason for using it, and possible side effects should accompany the prescription.

8.3.2 Choice of analgesic and dosing in chronic kidney disease

The choice of analgesic will depend on a number of factors including the nature and severity of the pain, the level of renal impairment, concomitant medication, and concurrent illnesses. Special consideration is needed when prescribing for patients with CKD and a basic knowledge of renal drug handling is required. The distinction between efficacy and toxicity is particularly narrow in the patient with CKD; certain principles help the clinician when managing the patient in pain. In view of the potential for severe and unpleasant toxicity, normal-release (short-acting) not modified-release (long-acting) preparations should ideally be used till stable pain relief has been achieved. Thus duration of toxicity, if it occurs, is for the shortest possible time. As discussed below, the duration of action of drugs may be extended, so the dosing interval may need to be increased; at least until the individual patient's response to the medication has been observed. In the acutely ill CKD patient, the changing clinical condition frequently leads to changes in the effect the drug has on an individual. A particular dose of analgesia that had been effective and safe may lead to acute toxicity in the presence of infection and need to be temporarily reduced or reversed. It is customary when titrating analgesia against requirement to add the previous days "breakthrough doses" to the regular background medication. However, some doses may be given to preempt known painful activity, such as washing. These are not true "breakthrough doses" but a necessary part of the regimen and their use will depend on the activity of the day; as such they should not be included in the next days increased dose.

8.3.2.1 Handling of drugs by the kidney

Many drugs and their metabolites are excreted in the kidney by glomerular filtration, tubular secretion, or both. Renal impairment thus has a significant effect on the clearance of these drugs, with potentially important clinical consequences. These are most obvious in patients with overt renal failure but more subtle forms of renal dysfunction may also be important and are extremely common, most notably as an accompaniment of ageing. Patients on dialysis are often prescribed multiple drugs.[45] Although, in theory, changes in dose and dosage interval of all drugs that are affected by renal impairment need to be considered, in practice, dose adjustment is important for relatively few specific drugs with a narrow therapeutic index or adverse effects related to drug or metabolite accumulation. Although renal impairment has its most important effects upon excretion, other aspects of pharmacokinetics (what the body does to the drug) – absorption, metabolism, distribution (including protein binding), and renal haemodynamics – may be affected, as may pharmacodynamics (what the drug does to the body).

The major determinant of alteration in dosage is the change in drug clearance. This can be predicted from measurements of creatinine clearance which can be estimated from the serum creatinine concentration using the Cockcroft–Gault formula.[46] In the UK and Canada, the Modification of Diet in Renal Disease formula (MDRD) is used routinely to provide clinicians with an estimated glomerular filtration rate (eGFR). Many recommendations in the Summaries of Product Characteristics produced by drug companies (UK) are, however, based on the creatinine clearance and not on eGFR. This may lead to both over and underdosing, but more commonly the former as the eGFR is least accurate in cachexia, extremes of age or body habitus.[47] In addition, tubular secretion of drugs[48] and changes in pharmacokinetics due to extra-renal factors[49] do not always change in parallel with GFR.

There are many handbooks that provide guidelines for the adjustment in dosage in renal impairment.[50–52] The data in these are derived from measurement or estimation of changes in clearance, half-life, and volume of distribution. The determination of these pharmacokinetic variables is very model-dependent and their application has limitations.[53–55] Consequently, these guidelines should be regarded only as useful approximations. A systematic comparison of four sources of drug information regarding adjustment of dose for renal function found scarce details of evidence for recommendations; variations in definition of renal failure; and differing recommendations for both dosage and dosing interval.[56] As a general principle, dosages of renally excreted drugs should be adjusted according to the patient's renal function (calculated as creatinine clearance or eGFR; with the initial dose determined using published guidelines and later adjustments based on response and adverse effects with monitoring of serum drug concentrations when appropriate and available.[57] Few drugs used in palliative care, however, are mentioned in these reviews, so reference needs to be made to the specialist palliative care literature. The evidence for advice given is usually however consensus, disease-oriented evidence, usual practice, expert opinion, or from case series.

8.3.2 Pharmacokinetics

Subcutaneous and intramuscular drug administration may be associated with reduced absorption in patients with renal failure or who are critically ill with shock and hypotension. Protein binding is affected by renal impairment resulting in increased plasma concentrations of a number of acidic compounds that compete with drugs for binding sites on albumin and other plasma proteins.[58,59] Serum albumin concentration is low in patients with nephrotic syndrome and may also decline in cachectic patients and in the elderly, reducing the number of drug-binding sites. As a consequence the proportion of free to bound drug is increased, and there are greater fluctuations in the free drug following the administration of each dose. This could be responsible for an increased susceptibility to adverse drug reactions.[60]

Drugs are excreted by the kidney either as the original (parent) drug or more polar (watersoluble) substances after metabolism in the liver. Uraemia may directly affect liver drug metabolism by affecting hepatic enzyme function.[61] Kidneys also contain many of the enzymes important in hepatic drug metabolism. In experimental uraemia, the metabolism of drugs such as morphine and paracetamol has been shown to be reduced in the diseased kidney.[61] These alterations in metabolism are minor in comparison to active metabolite retention as a direct consequence of renal impairment. Renal failure may also reduce drug activation. For example, the conversion of sulindac to its active sulphide metabolite is reduced in uraemia.[62] This has been invoked as a partial explanation for the lower incidence of side effects observed with sulindac compared with indomethacin.[63]

8.3.3 The World Health Organization analgesic ladder. Step 1: non-opioid analgesics +/− adjuvants

The non-opioid analgesics include acetylsalicylic acid (ASA, aspirin), other NSAIDs and paracetamol (acetaminophen). In most countries several NSAIDs will be available and the choice will depend on a number of factors including side effect profile, cost, and the physician's experience with the drug.

8.3.3.1 Non-steroidal anti-inflammatory drugs (NSAIDs)

NSAIDs, including ASA, inhibit prostaglandin synthesis by inhibition of cyclo-oxygenase, of which there are two main isoforms – cyclo-oxygenase-1 (COX-1) and COX-2. The primary renal prostaglandins in humans are prostaglandin E2 and I2, each of which is a vasodilator and natriuretic.[64] In addition to effects on renal blood flow, the prostaglandins also influence tubular ion transport directly. In healthy individuals the inhibition of cyclo-oxygenase has no detectable effects on renal function, but in patients with decreased effective circulating volume (e.g. patients with cardiac failure, nephrotic syndrome, liver disease, renal failure) the cyclo-oxygenase inhibitors cause a reduction in GFR that can be severe and irreversible.[65,66] They can also cause sodium and water retention, aggravating hypertension,[67–69] and hyperkalaemia. Inhibition of COX-1 reduces the production of thromboxane and thus impairs platelet aggregation. It also compromises the gastrointestinal mucosa by inhibiting the secretion of cytoprotective mucus. The effectiveness of selective COX-2 inhibitors as analgesics is comparable with COX-1 inhibitors such as naproxen, ibuprofen, and diclofenac.[70–72] The major limitation of NSAIDs is their gastrointestinal toxicity.[70] Selectivity for COX-2 reduces the risk for peptic ulceration, and appears to be the main advantage of members of this drug class. However, COX-2 selectivity does not appear to lessen the risk of other adverse effects associated with NSAIDs (most notably worsening renal function), and some studies have aroused significant suspicion that there might be an increased risk of myocardial infarction by a relative increase in thromboxane. Rofecoxib (Vioxx) was taken off the market in 2004 because of these concerns.[73,74]

Hypersensitivity occurs occasionally as an idiosyncratic reaction with NSAIDs. If it occurs, aspirin and NSAIDs should not be prescribed again.

Clinicians should be very cautious about use of NSAIDs for chronic pain in patients with CKD. Their use is best reserved for specific indications of acute pain, e.g. gout.

8.3.3.2 Paracetamol (acetaminophen)

Paracetamol is a long-established, non-prescription, antipyretic analgesic drug[75–77] with weak anti-inflammatory activity.[78] These effects are thought to be mediated by inhibition of prostaglandin synthesis, although the exact mechanism is still not clear.[78] In therapeutic doses, paracetamol has no other important pharmacological effects and does not adversely affect platelet function and haemostasis.[79]

Paracetamol is extensively metabolized in the liver. Some 2–5% of the dose is excreted unchanged in the urine.[79] The kinetics of paracetamol elimination have been investigated in patients with renal, hepatic, thyroid, and gastrointestinal disease. No clinically significant changes have been observed except in patients with severe acute and decompensated chronic liver disease in whom the half-life is considerably prolonged. In patients with CKD there is a marked accumulation of inactive paracetamol conjugates.[80] Paracetamol is also less likely to cause further deterioration in renal function than NSAIDs.[81]. It is generally considered safe to give paracetamol at full dose to patients with ESRD although there are concerns that chronic use may hasten the progression of CKD.[82]

8.3.4 The World Health Organization analgesic ladder. Step 2: opioid for mild to moderate pain +/− non-opioid +/− adjuvant

The WHO analgesic ladder divides opioids into those used for mild to moderate pain and those used for moderate to severe pain (Step 3). Lower doses of drugs used in Step 3 will have a similar analgesic effect as higher doses of those used in Step 2. When pain persists or increases despite non-opioid drugs a Step-2 analgesic should be started. These include codeine, dihydrocodeine, dextropropoxyphene, and tramadol.

8.3.4.1 Codeine

Codeine, a naturally occurring opium alkaloid produced by methylation of morphine, is a less potent analgesic than morphine with a ceiling effect.[83] It is metabolized in the liver to form morphine and norcodeine and conjugated to form glucuronides and sulphates of both codeine and its metabolites.[84] Its analgesic action is thought to be in part through binding to the μ- and κ-opioid receptors in addition to an effect from the morphine produced by metabolism.[85,86] The metabolites of codeine are renally excreted and accumulate in patients with renal impairment.[87–89] Serious dependence is probably very uncommon, and withdrawal symptoms are milder and develop more slowly than with morphine.

In normal subjects, codeine does not cause appreciable respiratory depression but does have antitussive[90] and constipating effects.[91] However, there have been several case reports of prolonged narcosis in patients with CKD.[89,92] Profound unconsciousness and respiratory depression, which can be delayed, has occurred after trivial doses. This appears to be an idiosyncratic phenomenon. In the authors' experience patients are often still distressed and in pain despite profound central nervous system depression. Some patients with CKD, however, are able to tolerate regular doses of codeine for a prolonged period without experiencing toxicity.

8.3.4.2 Dextropropoxyphene

Dextropropoxyphene is usually prescribed in combination with paracetamol.[93] Decreased elimination of dextropropoxyphene and its major pharmacologically active metabolite, norpropoxyphene, has been reported in patients with renal failure.[94] Norpropoxyphene accumulation is associated with central nervous system toxicity, respiratory depression, and cardiotoxicity.[95] Dextropropoxyphene is, therefore, not recommended for use in patients with severe CKD. It has been withdrawn from use in the UK, but is available as a prescription formulation with paracetamol in the US and either in pure form or combination in Australia.

8.3.4.3 Tramadol

Tramadol – a single-entity, centrally acting analgesic – exerts its analgesic actions through at least two complementary modes of action; agonism at the μ-opioid receptor and inhibition of noradrenaline and serotonin re-uptake.[96,97] It can be administered orally, rectally, or parenterally. Good results have been published for cancer pain in a number of studies[98] where it was shown to be effective in different types of moderate to severe pain, including neuropathic pain, although with a ceiling effect.[99] It has been suggested that tramadol induces fewer side effects for a given level of analgesia compared with traditional opioids.[99,100] Importantly, it does not appear to cause significant respiratory depression when recommended doses are used.[98,100–102] This has been attributed to the low affinity of tramadol for the μ-receptor which is 10 times less than codeine and 6000 times less than morphine.[101] Only 30% of the antinociceptive and analgesic actions of tramadol can be antagonized by naloxone.[103]

Tramadol is metabolized in the liver to O-desmethyl tramadol (M1) which has a higher affinity for the μ-opioid receptor than the parent drug,[104] but its slow production results in very low and clinically insignificant plasma levels. Ninety percent of tramadol and its metabolites are excreted in the urine, with 30% as unchanged tramadol.[105] In those with normal renal function the recommended dose of tramadol is 50–100 mg 4 times daily with a maximum dose of 400 mg a day. Adjustments are required in patients over 75 years of age and in those with renal or hepatic impairment.[106] Suggested dose adjustments are that patients with a creatinine clearance of <30 ml/min or who dialyse should receive a maximal daily dose of 200 mg;[106] and those whose clearance is <15 ml/min and who are not being dialysed should receive a maximum daily dose of 100 mg.

8.3.5 The World Health Organization analgesic ladder. Step 3: opioid for moderate to severe pain +/− non-opioid +/− adjuvant

8.3.5.1 Tolerance, dependence, and addiction – myths and fears

There are many myths surrounding the use of strong opioids. Tolerance is defined as the need for increasing doses of a drug in order to achieve the same pharmacological action. It can occur both to unwanted effects such as respiratory depression (see Case study 3) and nausea as well as to the desired pain relief. There are concerns regarding tolerance in the chronic pain-clinic population, although its incidence is unclear. However, studies of cancer patients with chronic pain taking oral morphine show that, after a period of dose titration, patients may continue on the same dose of morphine for many months without needing to increase the dose. The requirement for dose escalation is usually on account of progression of disease. In the authors' experience, tolerance is not commonly a problem in ESRD patients, likely because the pain seen in ESRD patients is disease related and more like that seen in the cancer patients than a pain clinic. Fear of tolerance or addiction should not stop the physician from providing adequate analgesia for his ESRD patients.

Physical dependence is characterized by withdrawal symptoms if treatment is stopped abruptly or if an antagonist is given. This does not, however, prevent dose reduction if pain is relieved by other means and in practice it does not prevent the effective use of opioids. If pain is relieved by other means, a gradual discontinuation of opioids will prevent withdrawal symptoms.[107] Following abrupt pain reduction, such as a nerve block, the dose will need to be reduced to prevent respiratory depression, but low, prn doses, may be required initially to treat withdrawal symptoms.[108]

Drug addiction is a behavioural pattern characterized by loss of control over use, continued use despite knowledge of harmful consequences, compulsion to use, and craving.[3] Short-term opioid treatment is associated with negligible addiction rates (0.03–5%).[109] In patients with chronic non-malignant pain who are screened for previous or current history of abuse or addictive behaviour, the incidence of addiction has been shown to be very low at 0.19%.[110] Studies have not been carried out in the ESRD population but in view of our knowledge of the causes, incidence, and severity of pain in this group of patients we should not be afraid of prescribing adequate analgesia for fear of addiction.

Case study 3: Tolerance to adverse effects

A 56-year-old, white, woman with polycystic kidney and liver disease had started haemodialysis at age 53. Eighteen months later she was admitted with severe liver pain, caused by infection in one of the cysts. Analgesia had been gradually increased until she was taking hydromorphone 1.3 mg every 4 h with only partial relief. A fentanyl 25-µg/h transdermal patch was started with excellent pain control at 24 h (when blood levels would still be rising). By 48 h she was toxic with falling oxygen saturation and the patch was removed. Subcutaneous fentanyl was then started at 50% of the 25-µg/h patch (i.e. 300 µg/24 h). This was supplemented with prn fentanyl 25 µg SC. By taking into account the previous day's prn doses,the dose in the SC syringe driver was gradually increased to 600 µg/24 h over 5 days. At this time, the transdermal patch was reintroduced at 25 µg/h without further toxicity. When pain subsequently escalated, the strong opioid dose was titrated upwards using hydromorphone 1.3 mg prn. She was later able to tolerate transdermal fentanyl at doses of 50 µg/h and then 75 µg/h without respiratory depression.

8.3.5.2 Initiating strong opioids

The initiation of strong opioids is triggered by the intensity of pain and not the life expectancy of a patient. The balance between toxicity and benefit with opioid administration for those with CKD or on dialysis is weighted heavily towards toxicity, hence the need for careful dose titration and use of some alternative strong opioids which may have a better efficacy to toxicity ratio. The onset of adverse side effects should trigger a reassessment of analgesic strategy and choice of strong opioid.

8.3.5.3 Morphine

Sir William Osler referred to morphine as 'God's own medicine' and is generally considered to be the 'drug of choice' for the treatment of severe pain in patients with normal renal function. It is the opioid against which all new drugs with suspected opioid activity are compared. There are three main opioid receptors: mu (µ), kappa (κ), and delta (δ). Morphine is a potent µ agonist and the µ-receptor, in addition to analgesia, is thought also to mediate some non-analgesic actions such as respiratory depression, euphoria, reduced gastrointestinal motility, and physical dependence.[111] Information about κ-receptor effects suggests that, in addition to analgesia, it mediates dysphoria and psychotomimetic effects,[112] while protecting against some of the unpleasant µ and δ effects.

Morphine has low oral bioavailability of 20–30% and undergoes extensive first-pass removal with considerable inter-individual variability. It is extensively metabolized by the liver with only 5–10% excreted unchanged in the urine. Despite this, liver disease does not appear to have a marked effect on morphine pharmacokinetics,[113] although the clearance of morphine has been found to be decreased in liver cirrhosis[114] with the consequent risk of accumulation with repeated administration.

Morphine-3-glucuronide (M3G) is the major metabolite (~45% of a dose). Morphine-6-glucuronide (M6G) is a quantitatively minor (5% of a dose) but a qualitatively more important metabolite[115] due to its actions, which are indistinguishable from those of morphine. When given systemically, M6G is approximately twice as potent an analgesic as morphine.[116] It plays a special role in morphine's effects accounting for a significant proportion of morphine's analgesic actions with chronic administration.[116–119] It is excreted by the kidney in direct relationship to creatinine clearance[120] and accumulates in renal failure,[121–126] probably explaining morphine's toxicity and long duration of action in patients with renal impairment.

In our experience, **chronic administration** of morphine is associated with significant and unpleasant toxicity and frequently not well tolerated by patients with severe CKD or on dialysis. It is our practice to use alternative strong opioids such as hydromorphone alfentanil and fentanyl when starting strong opioids for prolonged use in these patients (see Section 8.5.1.4).

8.3.5.4 Hydromorphone

Hydromorphone is a potent µ-receptor agonist. It is an effective analgesic approximately 5–7 times more potent than morphine following oral administration.[127] Studies suggest the parenteral potency is about 3 times that of morphine.[128] It has a similar side effect profile to morphine[129] although it may cause less pruritus, sedation, and nausea.[130] Hydromorphone is primarily metabolized in the liver to hydromorphone-3-glucuronide (H3G) with conjugates excreted in the urine.

A case study demonstrated an approximate fourfold increase in the ratio of H3G to hydromorphone in one patient with renal failure when compared with 18 cancer patients with normal renal function.[131] This led to the postulation that H3G may have been responsible for myoclonus or agitated delirium in 2 other patients in renal failure.[132] The patients in these two case studies were taking higher doses of hydromorphone than is common in UK practice (equivalent to ~ 1000–3000 mg oral morphine per 24 h).

To date, the only study to examine the pharmacokinetics and pharmacodynamics of hydromorphone in CKD[133] showed that hydromorphone did not substantially accumulate in 12 anuric haemodialysis patients, most likely due to the rapid conversion to H3G. These patients had been taking hydromorphone for a mean of 9 months with a mean daily dose of 20 mg. Conversely, H3G accumulated between dialysis treatments but appeared to be effectively removed during haemodialysis. Importantly, hydromorphone resulted in greater than a 65% reduction in pain over dosing intervals and no clinically significant opioid toxicity was observed. Interestingly, the accumulation of H3G between haemodialysis treatments appeared to be associated with greater sensory-type pain and reduced duration of analgesia. Despite the lack of clinical evidence for a role of M3G in opioid toxicity, these findings are suggestive for a role of H3G in antagonism of hydromorphone analgesia in patients with CKD. An important clinical implication is that while hydromorphone may be a safe, well-tolerated, and effective opioid for use in selected dialysis patients, it may not be as effective or as well tolerated in patients during the final days of life following withdrawal from dialysis or in patients with ESRD being managed conservatively without dialysis or yet to start dialysis.

A retrospective audit[134] and our own clinical experience in dialysis patients support the notion that hydromorphone is better tolerated than morphine when normal release preparations are used for titration to pain relief; followed by conversion to transdermal fentanyl if pain is continuous and stable. Careful dose titration, with monitoring for potential toxicity, has enabled many dialysis patients with continuous severe pain to take hydromorphone with adequate pain relief and without unacceptable toxicity (see case studies).

8.3.5.5 Methadone

Methadone is a synthetic effective opioid analgesic for the treatment of severe pain[135,136] with activity mainly at the μ receptor. In addition, there is some evidence that it is able to function as an NMDA receptor antagonist.[137] Clinically, its main use has been as a substitute opioid in the management of dependence. In addition, it is used as an alternative opioid in cancer pain,[138] where some clinicians believe it may be more effective for neuropathic pain than other strong opioids because of its NMDA receptor antagonism.

Methdone has high oral bioavailability and is extensively distributed in the tissues where it accumulates with repeated dosing. Thus, though it has a plasma half-life of 2–3 h, it has prolonged pharmacological action because of slow release from the reservoirs in the tissues, of up to 60 hours.[139,140] It is excreted mainly in the faeces, with metabolism into pharmacologically inactive metabolites primarily in the liver, although ~20% is excreted unchanged in the urine.[141] It does not appear to be removed by dialysis[142,143] but in anuric patients methadone is exclusively excreted in faeces with no accumulation in plasma. [142] These factors would suggest that methadone may be a safe, effective analgesic for use in patients with CKD, by those familiar with its use as attention to detail and careful monitoring are essential.[142]

8.3.5.6 Pethidine (Meperidine)

Pethidine is a synthetic opioid agonist, which is less potent and shorter-acting than morphine, with a similar side effect profile. When given by the oral route, pethidine is about 25% as potent as when given parenterally and has 12% of the potency of oral morphine in repeated doses.

It is metabolized in the liver mainly to norpethidine, which is pharmacologically active, and other inactive metabolites, with only 5% excreted in the urine unchanged.[144,145] Norpethidine is about half as potent as an analgesic but has twice the proconvulsive activity as its parent compound.[146] It is excreted in the urine[144] and accumulates in patients with renal impairment.[147] Pethidine is not recommended for use in chronic pain because of its short duration of action and need for frequent doses. In addition, accumulation of norpethidine can occur even in the presence of normal renal function with neuroexcitatory effects and risk of convulsions. Pethidine should be avoided in patients with renal failure.

8.3.5.7 Oxycodone

Oxycodone is a semi-synthetic opioid.[148] It has a similar analgesic and side effect profile to morphine,[149,150] with the possible exception of hallucinations, which may occur less commonly after oxycodone.[151] Oxycodone is a useful opioid in patients with normal renal function when an 'opioid switch' is required to improve analgesia with fewer adverse effects. In North America, low-dose oxycodone is often used as a Step-2 opioid. It is eliminated mainly by metabolism in the liver[152] to noroxycodone[153] and oxymorphone,[154] both of which were shown to accumulate in a single-dose study in patients prior to renal transplant.[155] Less than 10% of administered oxycodone is excreted unchanged in the urine.[156] Oxymorphone is a potent analgesic but its role in pain relief is unclear, although one study suggests it may contribute to some of its effect.[149] In a single case study, oxycodone and its metabolites were show to be reduced by dialysis, but without loss of analgesia.[157] However, a further case report detailed respiratory depression in a dialysis patient who received regular doses of oxycodone 5 mg/paracetamol 325 mg 6 times a day over 8 days for pain relief. The patient needed a 4-day naloxone infusion to reverse the opioid toxicity.[158] There are no long-term studies of chronic use in renal failure and the conflicting case reports mean there is insufficient evidence currently for a recommendation.

8.3.5.8 Fentanyl (see Case study 3)

Fentanyl is a potent synthetic μ-opioid receptor agonist with a short onset time and relatively short half-life (terminal half-life range: 1.5–6 h)[159] mainly because of rapid redistribution. Alfentanil and sufentanil are derived from fentanyl citrate.[159] Fentanyl is 50–100 times more potent and 1000 times more lipophilic than morphine.[160] These properties make it suitable for use in a transdermal delivery system.[161] Fentanyl causes less histamine release, has a lower incidence of constipation, and affords greater cardiovascular stability than morphine,[162] and can thus be a useful alternative when morphine's side effects hamper effective pain management.[160]

Fentanyl has poor oral bioavailability; it is therefore usually administered intravenously or transdermally, the latter is only suitable for stable pain or to provide background analgesia while dose titration takes place with a short-acting opioid. It is rapidly metabolized in the liver, with only 5–10% excreted unchanged in the urine.[163] Its metabolites are considered to be inactive. There does not appear to be any clinically significant accumulation of fentanyl when administered to patients with renal impairment.[162,164–166] The transdermal preparation, therefore, has a role to play in the management of continuous stable pain after titration with a short-acting opioid such as hydromorphone in dialysis patients. However, it should be remembered that a subcutaneous depot forms under a transdermal patch so a patient will continue to receive fentanyl for up to 24 h following removal of the patch in the event of pain relief by an alternative means or the advent of toxicity (see Case study 4).

Within palliative care, fentanyl has been used quite extensively by the subcutaneous route and the authors have found it particularly useful in patients with renal impairment, where toxicity, such as myoclonus or agitation, has been experienced with morphine but pain is still present. Continuous subcutaneous doses of between 100 and 250 µg/24 h, equivalent to less than half that in the smallest patch (delivering 12 µg/h) have been found to be effective starting doses. Even lower doses have been effective in patients with concomitant severe liver impairment. The use of subcutaneous fentanyl boluses prn to titrate the dose against need enable pain control to be achieved. (See End of Life guidelines Chapter 15.)

Case study 4: Prolonged opioid toxicity following cessation of transdermal fentanyl for a reduction in pain intensity

Z was 61 when he was first diagnosed with multiple myeloma. Over the following 2 years he received many courses of chemotherapy until his disease became refractory to treatment and he was maintained on supportive therapy including regular bisphosphonate infusions. He had been dialysis dependent due to the multiple myeloma since its diagnosis. Pain had been a consistent feature of his illness with only a partial response from palliative radiotherapy. Each course had taken 4–5 weeks before onset of relief of pain. His analgesia had been titrated upwards using oral hydromorphone and transdermal fentanyl so that by 6 months from diagnosis he required fentanyl 125 µg/h transdermally to achieve acceptable pain control.

He remained on this dose of fentanyl for the next 16 months, at which time he developed severe pain in his wrists due to diffuse infiltration with myeloma, demonstrated on magnetic resonance imaging (MRI) scan. He received further palliative radiotherapy and over the following 4 weeks his fentanyl was increased to 200 µg/h. Five weeks following radiotherapy, a course of dexamethasone was started as an adjuvant analgesic, and a week later – while attending his regular dialysis – he became increasingly drowsy and collapsed with a respiratory rate of six breaths per minute followed by apnoea. His fentanyl patches were removed and he was given naloxone with a good response but this was not sustained and it was necessary to maintain him on a naloxone infusion for the following 24 h. Over the next 48 h, he gradually awoke, though he experienced opioid withdrawal symptoms, with crampy abdominal pain, diarrhoea, shaking, and a new feeling of distress. These symptoms were treated with short-acting opioids, benzodiazepines, and loperamide.

One month later, his pain was managed with regular paracetamol and tramadol 50 mg prn. His sudden reduction in pain was likely due to the combination of radiotherapy and steroids. With pain no longer acting as a physiological antagonist to the opioid, he developed opioid toxicity, resulting in respiratory depression. The elimination plasma half-life for transdermal fentanyl is almost 24 h resulting in the need for continuous reversal of narcosis following removal of the transdermal patch.

8.3.5.9 Alfentanil

Alfentanil – a derivative of fentanyl – is approximately a quarter as potent an analgesic as fentanyl. [159] It is extensively metabolized in the liver to inactive compounds and its clearance may be reduced in patients with hepatic dysfunction. Its pharmacokinetic profile differs from fentanyl by having a smaller volume of distribution and a shorter terminal half-time in plasma leading to less accumulation than with fentanyl.[159] When doses greater than 600 µg/24 h of fentanyl are required, alfentanil can be administered more easily by subcutaneous infusion[167] because of its greater solubility, leading to a smaller total volume required; this also favours its use for intranasal or buccal administration for breakthrough pain.[168] Its short half-life means that titration may be difficult but is an advantage when additional analgesia is required for short periods such as dressing change; when either the subcutaneous or buccal route may be appropriate.

8.3.5.10 Buprenorphine

Buprenorphine is a semi-synthetic opioid with a long duration of action.[169] It is between 30 and 60 times as potent as oral morphine when given sublingually.[169,170] It is a partial agonist at the μ-opioid receptor[170,171] and an antagonist at the κ-opioid receptor.[172] Despite this – within the analgesic range of less than 10 mg/24 h – it behaves as a full agonist at the μ-opioid receptor and can have an additive effect to morphine and other μ agonists. For effects other than analgesia, a ceiling effect has been demonstrated at doses of 16–32 mg, well in excess of the analgesic range. Because of the avidity with which buprenorphine binds to the μ-opioid receptor, it might be difficult to antagonize with opioid antagonists.[173]

Buprenorphine is metabolized by the liver[174] with little unchanged drug found in the urine. [175] The two major metabolites – buprenorphine-3-glucuronide (B3G) and norbuprenorphine – are excreted in the urine and accumulate in patients with renal failure, although the parent compound does not.[175] B3G is inactive with no analgesic properties. Norbuprenorphine is a less potent analgesic at the μ receptor than buprenorphine; the clinical relevance of which is thought to be limited as it does not readily cross the blood brain barrier.(176) Whether this remains the situation for the uraemic patient who will experience increased sensitivity to drugs acting on the central nervous system is unknown. Norbuprenorphine is also a more potent respiratory depressant than buprenorphine in rats.[177] Again, its significance is unknown in humans.

Buprenorphine is an effective, long-acting opioid analgesic with an apparent ceiling effect on respiration. It can be administered effectively sublingually or via a transdermal patch. Given these properties and the minimal changes in kinetics in renal failure, it may be a potentially useful analgesic for use in patients with CKD, although until there are longer term studies the authors remain cautious about recommending it. [178]

Care should be taken when it is used in conjunction with benzodiazepines as there may be synergy as evidence by deaths in opioid addicts who were using buprenorphine and were found at post mortem to have also taken benzodiazepines.[179,180] In a study looking at buprenorphine and its metabolite norbuprenorphine pre and post dialysis in 10 patients who could tolerate the drug, buprenorphine levels were shown not to be reduced by dialysis over a 1-week period. Norbuprenorphine was only detectable <0.05 ng/ml in three patients. The median buprenorphine dose was 52.5 μg/h. Regrettably, we are not told the number of patients who could not tolerate buprenorphine and were therefore excluded from the study and there are no data from longer term use.[181]

8.3.5.11 Adverse effects of strong opioids (Table 8.2)

Adverse effects of strong opioids are sufficiently common to prevent effective analgesia and should be vigorously managed. Constipation is persistent and nearly universal while nausea and vomiting occur in approximately 50% of people, wearing off in most after 7–10 days. The central nervous system effects occur most frequently on initiating strong opioids and when escalating the dose. Patients should be warned of this, as there may be improvement after a few days at a stable dose. Respiratory depression is rare in patients taking strong opioids for pain if oral, short-acting preparations are used and the dose titrated against effect and toxicity. Pain is said to be the physiological antagonist of opioids. The use of long-acting, slow-release, or parenteral preparations in CKD patients is more likely to be associated with narcosis and respiratory depression. However, when the clinical condition and the pain is stable, the strong opioids least likely to cause toxicity can be used in long-acting preparations such as transdermal fentanyl. Hallucinations are a very distressing adverse effect and should be managed either by dose reduction with co-administration of haloperidol, if needed, or by switching to an alternative opioid, if possible. Patients should be informed of the steps that can be taken to prevent or treat adverse effects (see section 8.4.2).

Table 8.2 Adverse effects of strong opioids

1	Occur with sufficient severity in a substantial minority to prevent successful analgesia, and with an increased incidence in patients with renal failure
2	Include the following common symptoms: Gastrointestinal: nausea and vomiting, constipation Autonomic nervous system: dry mouth, itching, sweating Central nervous system: drowsiness, cognitive impairment, hallucinations, delirium, respiratory depression, myoclonus
3	Striking interindividual variability in sensitivity to adverse effects
4	Ageing associated with altered pharmacokinetics and generally lower doses are required
5	Tolerance to some adverse effects appears to occur after some days
6	Explanation to the patient and vigorous management (see text) essential

8.3.6 **Naloxone**

Naloxone is the first competitive opioid antagonist to be developed that is devoid of agonist activity. It is more potent at the μ receptor than at other opioid receptors.[182] Its observed effects are related to antagonism of endogenous or exogenous opioids and it produces no effects when administered in clinical doses to healthy subjects. When administered to those in pain who have not received exogenous opioids, some studies have demonstrated a biphasic response dependent on the dose used, with low doses producing analgesia and higher doses hyperalgesia. [183,184] Naloxone will reverse all the effects of exogenous opioids, i.e. analgesia, respiratory depression, pupillary constriction, delayed gastric emptying, dysphoria, coma, and convulsions in addition to the analgesia produced by transcutaneous electrical nerve stimulation, acupuncture, and placebo response.[185]

Naloxone is mainly metabolized by conjugation in the liver with little excreted unchanged in urine.[68] No dosage alteration is required in renal impairment. However, it should be remembered that prolonged dosing may be needed to counteract the accumulation of opioid metabolites in renal failure patients.

Naloxone may be administered by the intravenous, intramuscular, or subcutaneous routes. In opioid overdose, 5–10 μg/kg is the usual initial intravenous dose and may be repeated at 2–3-min intervals until the desired response is seen. At least 2 mg should be used to constitute an adequate trial in overdose of unknown cause. If no response is seen following 50 μg/kg, then the diagnosis of opioid overdose should be seriously questioned. The duration of action of long-lasting opioids such as methadone or those administered by the transdermal route where there may be a depot of the drug remaining under the skin, may outlast that of an intravenous dose of naloxone so patients should be carefully monitored for signs of returning opioid depression. Intravenous infusions have been used to overcome this problem starting at 2.5 μg/kg hourly and adjusted according to response (see Case study 4).

8.3.7 **Cannabinoids**

Some ESRD patients may be unable to tolerate a sufficient dose of opioid to provide effective analgesia, as they may worsen overall symptom burden by exacerbating other symptoms, particularly cognitive impairment and sleepiness or less commonly nausea, vomiting, anorexia, and pruritus and therefore fail to improve overall health-related quality of life. Cannabinoids may play a role in these selected patients.

Cannabinoids such as delta-9-tetrahydrocannabinol (THC) and cannabidiol (CBD) appear to have therapeutic potential for the treatment of intractable pain (neuropathic, inflammatory, and visceral) in a range of medical conditions.[186] The principal pharmacological effects of THC include analgesia, muscle relaxant, antiemetic, appetite stimulant, and psychoactive effects. There is now a buccal spray available that combines THC in a 1:1 ratio with CBD which has analgesic, anticonvulsant, muscle relaxant, anxiolytic, neuroprotective, antioxidant, and, importantly, antipsychotic activity. Health Canada has approved this buccal spray as adjunctive treatment for the symptomatic relief of neuropathic pain in multiple sclerosis and more recently for cancer patients with intractable neuropathic and visceral pain.

Cannabinoids are metabolized rapidly in the liver by the cytochrome P_{450} enzyme system and there is the possibility for drug interactions with analgesics such as fentanyl, adjuvant therapies such as amitriptyline, and immunosuppressive therapy with cyclosporine or tacrolimus. THC is metabolized to 11-hydroxy-tetrahydrocannabinol (11-OH-THC), a psychoactive metabolite. 11-OH-THC is excreted renally (~13%) and in the faeces (~53%). CBD is extensively metabolized in the liver and more than 33 metabolites have been identified in the urine. All cannabinoids have a large volume of distribution as they are highly lipid soluble and accumulate in fatty tissue. They are also highly protein bound. As a result, they are unlikely to be removed effectively by haemodialysis. Since the nature of these metabolites has not been fully elucidated, should they accumulate in CKD, the clinical relevance is unclear.

There are no data of cannabis-based medicine in ESRD but tolerability and safety data of cannabinoids, especially buccal THC:CBD, in other chronically ill populations over a period of 4 weeks to 2 years indicate it may be better tolerated than conventional therapies for many symptoms in some patients.[186–188] There is also no evidence to suggest tolerance to their therapeutic effects,[188] unlike with the use of opioids in chronic pain. For intractable pain, a trial of cannabis-based medicine may be warranted, although close observation will be required as data and clinical experience in ESRD are lacking.

8.3.8 **Alternative routes for administration of analgesics** (Table 8.3)

Most patients are able to take strong opioids by mouth. However, it is often necessary to make use of alternative routes for a number of reasons including vomiting, end-of-life weakness, bowel obstruction, and severe adverse effects with oral administration. The transmucosal route may be a useful alternative for rapid effect with short duration of action (see Table 8.3). When opioids are associated with unacceptable toxicity or failure of pain relief, the spinal route may be indicated, often in conjunction with local anaesthetic agents[189] or clonidine,[190] for neuropathic pain. The availability of the expertise necessary for their use may vary from centre to centre.

8.3.8.1 Topical analgesia

The potential toxicity of analgesics in patients with renal failure makes the possibility of using drugs topically where applicable very attractive. Most drugs appear to act locally rather than through local systemic absorption, thus there is reduced risk of toxicity.

Topical opioids: In the presence of inflammation, peripheral opioid receptors are recruited very rapidly and have been identified on peripheral cutaneous sensory nerves.[191] The effect of intra-articular morphine is probably mediated in this way, a theory that is supported by the fact that it can be reversed by naloxone. The presence of inflammation appears to be essential for the

Table 8.3 Alternative routes for analgesic administration

Route	Indications	Advantages	Disadvantages and contraindications	Suitable drugs	Additional comments
Per rectum	Oral intake not possible. Poor absorption. End of life drowsiness	Simple, effective. Suitable for home use	Immunocompromised patients, diarrhea, incontinence	Paracetamol, morphine, oxycodone, NSAIDs	Consider patient preference
Subcutaneous	Reduced or no oral intake. End of life drowsiness or weakness	Simple, non-invasive, effective, portable, safe for home use, cheap	Very low platelets. Widespread edema	Morphine, diamorphine, hydromorphone (not UK), methadone, fentanyl, alfentanil	Can be combined with other drugs if needed (e.g. antiemetics). Continuous infusion preferable to intermittent dosing
Intramuscular	Rapid pain relief required	Simple	Painful	Morphine, hydromorphone, methadone, pethidine	Only use if subcutaneous route not possible or intravenous route not appropriate
Intravenous	Rapid pain relief required	Rapid effect. Rapid dose titration	Requires higher level of trained staff. Not suitable for repeated home use.	As for subcutaneous	
Transdermal	Stable pain. Suitable for strong opioid	Simple. Infrequent patch change	Risk of increased absorption with pyrexia or sweating. Depot of preparation remains under the skin after patch removed.	Fentanyl, buprenorphine	Lowest patch size may contain too high a dose for initiation. Depot beneath the skin remains when patch removed
Transmucosal e.g. buccal, intranasal or sublingual	Breakthrough analgesia in conscious patient	Simple. Patient may finely control breakthrough analgesia required	Dry mouth may hinder use of Actiq but newer preparations now available	Fentanyl, buprenorphine, alfentanil	Dose needs individual titration
Spinal (epidural/intrathecal)	Severe adverse effects or pain poorly responsive to opioids	Pain relief with few adverse effects	Expensive. Special expertise. Infection	Opioids, local anaesthetics	Selective availability

efficacy of topical morphine.[192] The use of a number of opioids has been described, including morphine, diamorphine, and fentanyl. The opioid is added to a suitable medium, frequently a commercial hydrogel containing carboxymethylcellulose polymer (Intrasite) and spread on the ulcerated area once or twice a day at dressing changes. Benefit appears to occur shortly after the first application and may last 12 or more hours; the evidence currently is only from case reports. [192,193]

Topical NSAIDs: It has been shown in a systematic review that topically applied NSAIDs can provide effective pain relief,[194] and do not appear to be associated with serious side effects. Where pain is present in joints or non-ulcerated skin, this may be a useful alternative to oral administration.

Topical capsaicin: Capsaicin is an alkaloid from chillies that can deplete substance P, which is thought to be associated with the transmission of painful stimuli in local sensory nerve endings. A meta-analysis showed that one in four patients with diabetic neuropathy and one in three patients with osteoarthritis treated with capsaicin, significantly benefited.[195] Though not as effective as anticonvulsants, it has lower toxicity.

8.3.8.2 Transmucosal opioids

The use of buccal or intranasal strong opioids is well established for managing episodes of pain that are known to be of short duration. Oral dosing can take a long time to relieve pain; a rapid effect of onset is commonly obtainable only with parenteral or transmucosal administration. [196] The intravenous route is not always feasible and can be particularly difficult to manage in a patient's own home.

Transmucosal preparations should have a rapid onset and a short duration of action. Transmucosal administration is only suitable for opioids of high solubility such as buprenorphine, fentanyl, sufentanil, and methadone. Transmucosal preparations of these drugs are available (sufentanil and methadone not in the UK). The bioavailability of nasal fentanyl and alfentanil is 65% and 71%, respectively.[197,198] There is a rapid rise in plasma concentrations with a T^{max} of 5 and 9 min for fentanyl and alfentanil, respectively.[197,198] Similar profiles are to be expected from the buccal route. This pharmacokinetic profile makes the use of the transmucosal route attractive for breakthrough pain or for short periods when an increase in pain is expected. [199] Studies of oral transmucosal fentanyl and the newer preparations have shown that this approach produces a faster onset of pain relief than oral morphine and have shown a large margin of safety,[196] presumably related to short duration of action and liver clearance. There is no dose relationship between the regular opioid dose and the breakthrough dose of transmucosal fentanyl citrate required to produce pain relief,[196] so the breakthrough dose will need to be individually titrated. A wide range of doses of these preparations are available for this purpose. The use of shorter acting preparations should reduce side effects and increase patient control. Problems with transmucosal administration include the bitter taste of most opioids and the difficulty in knowing how much drug is absorbed rather than being swallowed reflexively. However, transmucosal opioids are increasingly being used in the management of breakthrough pain in cancer.

8.3.8.3 Transdermal opioids

The lipophylic nature of fentanyl and buprenorphine make them suitable for delivery transdermally. They have a slow onset of action and time to steady-state plasma drug concentrations and are therefore not suitable for acute pain management. However, when analgesic requirements are known or the patient has more chronic pain where titration over many days is acceptable then they have a role to play. The availability of very low doses of buprenorphine transdermally in the UK (minimum 5 µg/h, which is equivalent to approximately 10–12 mg/24 h oral morphine) means that patients can be started on very modest doses of Step-3 analgesia this way. The lowest-dose fentanyl patch delivers 12 μg/h and is equivalent to approximately 30–60 mg/24 h oral morphine. Opioid-naïve patients may experience toxicity at this dose so it is advised to initiate opioids with a short-acting drug such as hydromorphone and switch to the patch when the equivalent morphine dose is tolerated, continuing to titrate with hydromorphone if higher dose are required. It is important to remember that a depot of the drug remains under the skin after patch removal and, if respiratory depression needs to be reversed, then an infusion of naloxone for up to 24 h is likely to be required.

8.4 Adjuvant drugs

An adjuvant drug can be defined as any drug that has a primary indication other than pain, but is analgesic in some situations.[33] It has also come to mean drugs used in combination with analgesics either to enhance their action or manage their side effects such as antiemetics and laxatives. This is not strictly within the definition and thus it may be necessary to use an alternative classification:

- Drugs with a primary indication other than pain management (e.g. antidepressants, corticosteroids).
- Drugs to treat the adverse effects of analgesics (e.g. antiemetics, laxatives, psychotropics).
- Drugs to treat concomitant psychological disturbances such as insomnia, anxiety, and depression (e.g. night sedatives, anxiolytics, antidepressants).

8.4.1 Pain syndromes requiring adjuvant drugs

8.4.1.2 Neuropathic pain (Table 8.4)

Many patients with CKD experience neuropathic pain or mixed neuropathic and nociceptive pain. For **pure neuropathic pain,** adjuvant drugs are often used alone or with analgesics from Step 1 or 2 of the WHO analgesic ladder. For **severe mixed pains** they can be used with analgesics from all three steps of the WHO analgesic ladder. Where the pain appears to be sensitive to a weak opioid, continuing on to Step 3 may give added benefit and should be tried. Strong opioids should be titrated upwards in the normal way until maximum or optimal pain relief is achieved or toxicity prohibits further increase. It is important when making changes to do so to one drug at a time so efficacy and causes of toxicity can be accurately determined.

Tricyclic antidepressants (TCA) and anticonvulsants are the two classes of drugs for which there is most evidence of efficacy in neuropathic pain. Although antidepressants have been used in the UK for over 30 years to manage neuropathic pain, no antidepressant has a product license for this indication. A systematic review of their use found that TCAs were effective in reducing neuropathic pain.[200] The NNT for at least 50% pain relief compared with placebo in diabetic neuropathy was 3 with a similar number (2.9) for anticonvulsants.[201] Both these classes of drugs have important side effects. Minor adverse events occur in about one-third of patients. One in 22 patients stopped TCA treatment and one in eight stopped anticonvulsants on account of them. Selective serotonin re-uptake inhibitors (SSRIs) appear to be less effective than adjuvant analgesics but have fewer adverse reactions.[200]

It is suggested that the analgesic mechanism of action of anticonvulsants is similar to that which reduces the risk of seizure, through blocking use-dependent sodium channels (e.g. carbamazepine) or the facilitation of γ-aminobutyric acid (GABA) inhibition (e.g. sodium valproate). Although anticonvulsants are widely used in the treatment of chronic neuropathic pain,[30]

Table 8.4 Adjuvant drugs in neuropathic pain

Class of drug		Renal handling	Side-effects		Contraindications	Dose schedule	Comments
			Commonly occurring	**Less common but important**			
Tricyclic antidepressants (TCAs)	Amitriptyline	Metabolized in the liver (cytochrome P-450) <5% excreted unchanged in the urine. Unaffected by dialysis	Antihistaminic: sedation. Anticholinergic: dry mouth, blurred vision, constipation, urinary retention. Central effects: fatigue, dizziness, weakness, tremor, confusion, postural hypotension	Conduction disturbances, especially tachyarrythmias, Weight gain. Reduced libido	Glaucoma. Concurrent MAOIs. Recent myocardial infarction. Multiple drug interactions	10–25mg nocte, increasing every few days to relief or toxicity (rarely need to use more than 75mg)	Lowers seizure threshold. Dose alteration not usually necessary in renal failure, though may be poorly tolerated
Anticonvulsants	Carbamazepine	Metabolized by liver. Induces microsomal enzymes	Anorexia, nausea, vomiting, ataxia, headaches, dizziness, drowsiness, visual disturbance – may improve with continued treatment	Fluid overload due to antidiuretic action. Interaction possible with:warfarin, oral contraceptive pill, dextropropoxyphene, clonazepam, some SSRIs, haloperidol, tramadol and possibly TCAs	Concurrent MAOIs	200mg daily increasing weekly to effectiveness or toxicity or a maximum dose of 1600mg	Effect may occur within 2–3 days. Plasma concentrations reduced by other anticonvulsants.
	Valporic acid	Metabolized by the liver and eliminate via the kidneys	Gastric irritation, nausea, tremor, ataxia, drowsiness, weight gain	Liver toxicity	Acute liver disease, family history of severe hepatic dysfunction, porphyria	200mg daily increasing by 200mg to pain control or a maximum dose of 1000mg	Well tolerated. Interaction with other anticonvulsants

(Continued)

Table 8.4 (continued) Adjuvant drugs in neuropathic pain

Class of drug		Renal handling	Side-effects		Contraindications	Dose schedule	Comments
			Commonly occurring	**Less common but important**			
	Gabapentin	Excreted unchanged by the kidney. Accumulates in renal impairment	Drowsiness, dizziness, ataxia, fatigue, myoclonus. Need to watch closely for signs of toxicity	Instability of blood glucose in diabetics. Antacids reduce absorption	Lactation	Creatinine clearance <15ml/Min 300mg q.o.d HD 200–300mg after each 4h dialysis	Withdraw dose gradually over 1 week. Licensed (UK) for treatment of neuropathic pain
	Pregabalin	Excreted unchanged by the kidney. Accumulates in renal impairment	Dizziness, drowsiness, may resolve over time			Depends on creatinine clearance Extra dose after dialysis	Partial removal by haemodialysis
	Clonazepam	Metabolism by cytochrome CYP3A pathway	Sedation Respiratory depression			0.5–1mg nocte, gradual increase to a maximum of 2mg daily	Simple to administer. Can be given PO or SC.
Oral local anaesthetic agents	e.g. Mexiletine		Nausea, ataxia, tremor, dizziness, confusion	Cardiac conduction defects	History of cardiac disease	See text	Should be used with great caution, consult pain specialist
NMDA receptor antagonists	e.g Ketamine	See text					Consult specialist physician
Topical agents	e.g. Capsaicin	See text					

surprisingly few trials show analgesic effectiveness.[202] There is no evidence that anticonvulsants are effective for acute pain.[203] Gabapentin and pregabalin are the only anticonvulsants licensed for use in neuropathic pain in the UK and the former is increasingly being used for its management. However, the evidence suggests that gabapentin is not superior to carbamazepine,[201] although it may have fewer adverse effects or drug interactions. However, unlike gabapentin, carbamazpine requires no dose alteration in CKD.

Ketamine is a dissociative anaesthetic agent, often used for short painful procedures in children or where there is limited availability of anesthetists.[204] It is a potent NMDA receptor antagonist[205] and has potent analgesic actions at subanaesthetic doses.[204] Ketamine may have a role in severe, intractable neuropathic pain, or for short painful procedures, but should be used only by an experienced practitioner.

Oral local anaesthetics may have a role in severe, resistant neuropathic pain. Some such as mexilitine work by blocking sodium channels. However, all carry the risk of cardiac rhythm disorders and should only be administered and monitored by those experienced in their use.

8.4.1.3 Musculoskeletal pain (Table 8.5)

Benzodiazepines,[30] particularly diazepam, has antispasticity efficacy and if carefully titrated may be useful for the pain of muscle spasm, particularly associated with back pain from disc or other spinal lesions, such as osteoporotic fracture. Clonazepam[206] also has some evidence for use in neuropathic pain. It is easy to administer with a once daily oral or subcutaneous nocturnal dose and may be substituted for other neuropathic agents in patients unable to swallow at the end of life and in whom it is considered important to continue an agent for neuropathic pain. Subcutaneous midazolam may be helpful at the end of life for agitation and distress, and thus indirectly help pain control. As its active metabolite can accumulate in the elderly, care should be taken with prolonged use and doses kept low.

Antispasticity activity has been shown for baclofen,[207] a stimulant of GABA receptors, and also for tizanidine – an α_2-agonist.[208] These drugs may be tried where muscle spasm is thought to play an important part in the aetiology of pain.

8.4.1.4 Nerve compression and raised intracranial pressure (Table 8.5)

Corticosteroids have a role in the management of pain associated with nerve compression and headache associated with raised intracranial pressure. For these indications dexamethasone is usually recommended in preference to prednisolone due to its greater potency and reduced mineralocorticoid activity. It has good oral bioavailability and a long duration of action so can be given once daily. Dose reduction is not usually necessary in renal failure.

The dose of dexamethasone for nerve root compression is initially 6–12 mg daily, reducing after 7–10 days to as low a dose as can be used to maintain relief. For raised intracranial pressure, doses of up to 16 mg daily will be needed initially, again with gradual dose reduction to prevent the long-term adverse effects relating to its glucocorticoid, mineralocorticoid, and immunosuppressant effects. In the US and Canada, higher doses – for a shorter period of time – are used with a daily dose of 40 mg of dexamethasone being fairly standard. If used in conjunction with an NSAID, the risk of peptic ulceration is greatly increased.

8.4.1.5 Renal colic – stones (Table 8.5)

NSAIDs may be particularly useful in some pain syndromes such as renal colic.[209] Acute ureteral obstruction by a stone can increase renal pressure leading to a release of prostaglandins causing vasodilation of the afferent arterioles and inhibition of antidiuretic hormone. This results in diuresis and a further increase in renal pressure establishing a vicious cycle leading to renal colic.

Table 8.5 Adjuvant drugs

Class of drug	Indication	Drug name	Dose adjustment in renal failure	Adverse effects and contraindications	Suggested dose range	Comment
Corticosteroids	Nerve root compression. Raised intracranial pressure	Dexamethasone	No dose change normally necessary	See text	8–16mg daily after food	See text
Benzodiazepines	Muscle spasm	Diazepam	Start with small doses; increased sensitivity	Drowsiness, weakness	2–10mg daily	
Benzodiazepines	Myoclonus agitation	Midazolam	As above	Sedation at high doses. Tolerance if given over long periods	Dose rapidly titrated, usual range 2.5–7.5mg SC hourly. Continuous infusion, 10–30mg/24h	Rapid effect after SC administration. Can be repeated hourly if needed for optimal benefit. If several doses needed advise 24-h infusion
Skeletal muscle relaxants	Muscle spasm, hic-cups	Baclofen	Renally cleared, dose reduction if necessary	Sedation, nausea	5mg 0.d/b.i.d. titrated up to a maximum of 10mg t.i.d	Must discontinue by gradual dose reduction to avoid serious side effects
Alpha-2 agonist	Muscle spasm	Tizanidine	Low initial dose advised	Drowsiness	2mg o.d. initially with slow titration up to 36mg daily in divided doses	Contraindicated in hepatic dysfunction
Alpha-2 agonist	Neuropathic pain	Clonidine		Somnolence, orthostatic hypotension, dry mouth		Consult pain specialist. Can be given orally, transdermally, or epidurally
Antimalarial	Noctural cramps	Quinine		Tinnitus, headaches	200–300mg nocte	Can take 4 weeks for maximum benefit
NSAIDS	Renal colic	See text	See text			
Anticholinergic	Bowel colic or excess secretions	Hyoscine butylbromide	No dose change normally necessary	Dry mouth	20mg SC prn or as 24-h infusion 60–160 mg/24-h	Does not cross blood-brain barrier, so not sedative

Thus, NSAIDs would be seem to be an ideal choice in managing pain from kidney stones. Studies have shown that they are as effective as opioids in providing pain relief from kidney stones. [209,210] Care must be exercised in those in whom renal function is being preserved.

8.4.1.6 Colic – bowel obstruction (Table 8.5)

Hyoscine butylbromide (scopolamine butylbromide) has a useful role in the management of severe bowel colic, particularly where it is associated with bowel obstruction.[211] It can provide effective pain relief without the toxicity of opioids.[212] As it is poorly absorbed,[213] it has to be given parenterally. This can be done either by subcutaneous (intermittent or continuous), intramuscular, or intravenous injections; continuous subcutaneous infusions are probably the least invasive means with optimal efficacy. Subcutaneous injections of octreotide – a somatostatin analogue – have also been shown to be effective in controlling gastrointestinal symptoms of bowel obstruction.[211,214]

8.4.2 Drugs to manage opioid side effects

8.4.2.1 Antiemetics

Antiemetics are needed by 50–75% of patients on strong opioids, some of whom may have additional causes for nausea and vomiting. This may result in patients not taking medication or interfere with drug absorption, thus hampering successful pain management. Effective management with appropriate antiemetics is therefore important. A methodical approach will enhance this:

- Postulate the cause.
- Select an appropriate antiemetic.
- Give it regularly by most suitable route at full dose.
- Prescribe a rescue antiemetic, either further doses of the same drug if not at maximum dose, or complementary drug.
- Assess effectiveness and review the cause of vomiting and route and absorption of drug before changing or adding additional drugs.

In the authors' experience, if parenteral antiemetics are necessary, a continuous subcutaneous infusion may be more effective than intermittent boluses.

Opioids are thought to cause nausea and vomiting either by stimulation of the chemoreceptor trigger zone or by delayed gastric emptying; thus an appropriate first choice antiemetic is either haloperidol[215] or metoclopramide.[216] Cyclizine – a histamine antagonist with antimuscarinic activity – is also a useful general-purpose antiemetic.[217] It blocks the prokinetic action of meto-clopramide so the two drugs should not be used concurrently. (See also Chapter 7, Table 7.2.)

8.4.2.2 Haloperidol

Haloperidol,[215,218] used both as an antiemetic and for relief of hallucinations caused by strong opioids is predominantly a dopamine antagonist with some action at histamine H1 receptors. It is extensively metabolized, mainly in the liver, but also in the brain and other tissues.[219] Around 1% is excreted in the urine and renal failure has very little effect on its pharmacokinetics so no dosage adjustment is usually necessary. However, in the authors' experience, smaller doses are often effective in dialysis patients. Liver-enzyme inducers (e.g. rifampicin) increase the elimination of haloperidol and the dose may need to be increased by up to 50%. It is absolutely contraindicated in patients with closed-angle glaucoma[220] and should be used with caution in patients with epilepsy as it lowers the seizure threshold.[221]

Parkinson's disease can be exacerbated by it,[220] and caution should be exercised in patients at risk of cardiac arrhythmias as they can be precipitated.[222,223] Haloperidol can be prescribed on a regular or as-required basis. It is the antiemetic recommended in the UK Liverpool Care Pathway for end-of-life care for renal patients at reduced doses.[224]

8.4.2.3 Metoclopramide

Metoclopramide is a prokinetic agent having effects on the upper gastrointestinal tract to increase lower oesophageal sphincter pressure, gastric emptying, and gastric–duodenal coordination. [225] Its effects on the gut may result from a local action on acetycholine release or be in part related to its actions within the central nervous system, which are mediated primarily via dopamine receptor antagonism.[225] This latter action can result in adverse effects including acute dystonia, akathisia, parkinsonism, tardive dyskinesia, and hyperprolactinaemia.[225]

Metoclopramide is extensively metabolized but the major route of elimination is the urine. [225] In patients with CKD the clearance is approximately half of that found in normal subjects. [226] It should therefore be used at 50% of the recommended dose in patients with normal renal function because of the increased risk of extrapyramidal side effects.

8.4.2.4 Cyclizine

Cyclizine is an antihistaminic antiemetic with antmuscarinic effects.[217] The same oral and parenteral doses can be used. Its main disadvantages are due to its sedating and antimuscarinic effects, particularly dry mouth, already common in ESRD patients. There are no studies on its use in renal failure, so it should be used with care, although in clinical practice dose reduction has not been found to be necessary.[52] Cyclizine, can cause hypotension and tachyarrythmias so should be used with care in patients with cardiac problems.

8.4.2.5 5-hydroxytryptamine 3 (5-HT3) receptor antagonists

This group of drugs was developed specifically for the management of chemotherapy-induced vomiting, for which there is evidence of benefit, as well as for anaesthetic and radiation-induced vomiting.[227–230] Dosage reduction is not necessary in renal impairment with ondansetron. [231] Since some,[232] but not a randomized controlled trial,[233] studies have shown an improvement in uraemic pruritus with regular use of ondansetron, consideration could be given to using this agent if nausea and uraemic pruritus are a problem in the same patient.

8.4.2.6 Levomepromazine

Levomepromazine is a broad-spectrum antiemetic, with dopamine, 5-HT2, and α_1-receptor antagonist properties. It is very sedating and associated with postural hypotension at antipsychotic doses (100–200 mg daily) but has recently been used extensively at low doses (5–12.5 mg daily) as an antiemetic in palliative care patients.[234] It has approximately 50% oral bioavailability. Essentially, the complete drug is metabolized in the liver, although the activity of the metabolites is not fully quantified. Excretion of the metabolites is mainly in the urine and faeces.

8.4.3 Laxatives

As a general rule, a laxative should be prescribed when an opioid is started. Opioids reduce gut mobility and increase electrolyte and water absorption from faeces. Thus most patients need the regular use of a peristaltic stimulant such as senna, and a faecal softener such as sodium docusate, although alternatively a macrogol which acts as an osmotic laxative may be effective. The dose of laxative required will differ between patients, who, if severely constipated, may require rectal measures first. In the uncommon situation where constipation is solely caused by opioids, the subcutaneous μ-opioid receptor antagonist methylnaltrexone rapidly induces laxation in patients with advanced illness and opioid-induced constipation.[235]

8.4.4 Psychotropic drugs

Psychotropic drugs have an important role in managing psychological morbidity that may accompany CKD and may also be used to reduce the side effects of analgesics. Haloperidol is the most important – used to alleviate hallucinations and to help the vivid and often unpleasant dreams that can be associated with strong opioids.

The concurrent use of two or more drugs that act on the central nervous system is likely to produce a greater sedative effect in ill and malnourished renal patients. The starting dose of any psychotropic drug is likely to be less than that used for physically healthy patients.

8.4.5 Non-drug measures for pain relief

8.4.5.1 Transcutaneous nerve stimulation (TENS) and acupuncture

The gate theory of pain[236] provides the rationale for TENS. There is little published evidence that TENS is effective in the treatment of acute pain, although it can be effective in patients with chronic pain.[237] However, there are few robust studies with which to judge efficacy in specific situations.[238] Attention to detail (e.g. electrode placement) makes considerable difference to the its efficacy.[239] It may have a useful role in neuropathic pain where efficacy of drugs is reduced by the potential for toxicity.

The data that acupuncture is effective in the management of chronic pain are equivocal or contradictory.[240,241] Theories for its mode of action in pain relief include the production of endorphins and other neurohumoral mechanisms for which there is some evidence, particularly in animal models. It is not routinely available in mainstream medicine, but where conventional medicine has failed to relieve symptoms and the patient wishes, it can be explored and used if effective. It is not affected by renal function so its side effect profile remains favourable!

8.4.5.2 Physiotherapy and variants

Despite a lack of evidence for the benefits of physiotherapy and manipulation for pain management,[242] many people will try these methods of pain relief where conventional methods have been unsuccessful. Physiotherapists are usually members of pain-management teams, to which patients may be referred with chronic pain. Physiotherapy programmes, particularly in the bed-bound or those with markedly reduced mobility, may improve overall well-being and thus pain relief.

For chronic back pain, a six-session course in the Alexander technique combined with an exercise prescription has been shown in a randomized controlled trial to be effective at 12 months in terms of reduction in disability and pain scores.[243] Spinal manipulation has also been shown to be a cost-effective addition to "best care" for **back pain** in general practice.[244] These therapies may provide pain relief for individual patients so a trial of therapy where conventional medicine has not relieved symptoms may be indicated.

8.4.5.3 Psychological treatments

Psychological factors are central to the experience of pain, and their management is essential for the delivery of effective analgesia,[245] especially for patients on dialysis who are known to have a high incidence of psychological illness, particularly anxiety and depression.[246,247]

Psychological treatments – when used as an adjunct – may enhance the efficacy of pharmacological measures and improve quality of life, although this may be difficult to prove.

8.4.6 Specific pain syndromes in renal patients

The principles of pain management discussed above are common to all causes of pain. However, there are a number of painful syndromes which are encountered almost exclusively in renal patients. These conditions may require very specific measures that will almost certainly involve very specialized skills in pain management and possibly surgery. The three examples given below are not intended to be an exhaustive list but have been chosen as illustrative example of difficult problems.

8.4.6.1 Autosomal dominant polycystic kidney disease (ADPKD)

> The pain of bursting renal cysts: 'A quaint little pain this one, it actually had an almost exact time scale of 45 minutes start to finish. Always the same it would proceed thus: vague sensation in the pit of the stomach, not unakin to the feeling of butterflies. Within 5 minutes I would have taken the defensive position. I would then oscillate between trying to relax and losing it to full blown panic. The pain would grow worse as I knew it would, panic would rise as I knew it would, and for the next 30 minutes I would be in (literally) unbearable pain'

Acute and chronic pain are common in patients with autosomal dominant polycystic kidney disease (ADPKD).[248] It is by far the most common of genetic conditions causing ESRD.[249] ADPKD patients may suffer complications such as infected cysts, cyst rupture/haemorrhage, and nephrolithiasis, causing severe acute pain.[248,250] Patients with ADPKD are also frequently afflicted by chronic pain syndromes. Chronic back pain is a common problem caused by increased abdominal girth leading to increased lumbar lordosis that accelerates degenerative change in the spine. As in the general population, the problem of back pain is complex and requires a thorough evaluation to determine the exact cause, which will then need to be treated appropriately. Pain also occurs as a result of compression of cysts on surrounding tissues, traction on the pedicle of the kidney, and distension of the renal capsule. Liver cysts can become massive and often cause more disabling pain than the renal cysts. This appears to be especially true of multiparous women.

In addition to the usual pain-relief measures discussed in the previous sections there are physical/invasive measures that have been used to control resistant pain related to ADPKD. Autonomic (coeliac) plexus blockade,[250] spinal cord stimulation by implantable electrodes,[251] neuraxial opioids, and local anaesthetics – often given by continuous infusion[252] – have been used in problematic cases. Surgical management including cyst decortication and marsupialization, renal denervation, and nephrectomy have been used with some success.[250] Surgical liver fenestration and combined liver resection–fenestration techniques have been used with some success.[253] Liver transplantation has also been tried when all other measures at pain control have failed.[254]

8.4.6.2 Calciphylaxis (calcific uraemic arteriolopathy – CUA)

CUA refers to a relatively rare but serious disorder seen almost exclusively in dialysis patients. It is characterized by tissue ischaemia due to metastatic calcification of subcutaneous tissue and small arteries[255,256] resulting in areas of ischaemic necrosis that usually develop in the dermis, subcutaneous fat, and less often in muscle. Patients develop painful violaceous mottling of the skin (livedo reticularis) that can progress to painful, well-demarcated non-ulcerating plaques, which may be misdiagnosed as cellulitis.[69,257] If not treated, the majority will progress to ulcer and eschar formation that often become superinfected. Mortality is high (60–90%), with sepsis and ischaemic events as the main causes of death. Proximal lesions over the abdomen, thigh, or buttock have a poorer prognosis than lesions over the distal sites such as hands, fingers, and elbows or below the knees. These more distal lesions may mimic atherosclerotic peripheral vascular disease. The incidence of CUA appears to be increasing, due in part to the current practice of treating severe hyperparathyroidism with high doses of calcium and calcitriol. The rate has been reported as high as 4.5/100 patient-years in one Canadian centre.[257]

The high mortality and the severity of pain associated with CUA make referral to palliative care services important. The pain experienced may have both nociceptive and neuropathic features and a thorough history may guide the clinician to the drugs most likely to help. Sympathetic blockade has been reported as providing some benefit.[258] However, it is often very difficult to provide adequate pain relief even with expert help.[255] No definitive treatment regimens are available owing to unidentified clear pathogenetic mechanisms. Hyperbaric oxygen therapy has been reported to cure the cutaneous ulcers of CUA.[255,259] Supplemental oxygen therapy may help ulcer healing.[255] It is thought that the supplemental oxygen therapy may also improve the cutaneous hyperaesthesia related to nerve ischaemia.

8.4.6.3 Nephrogenic systemic fibrosis (NSF)

NSF – previously named nephrogenic fibrosis dermopathy (NFD) – is a recently recognized (1997) fibrosing disorder in dialysis and pre-dialysis patients that causes significant pain and disability.[260–262] It is characterized by an acute onset of hardening of the skin of the extremities and trunk (typically spares the face), papules and nodules with hyperpigmentation, and flexion contractures. Recently, it has been shown to also involve internal viscera. Patients typically describe pain and pruritus at the site of fibrosis. A skin biopsy is required to confirm the diagnosis. Histologically, the lesions are characterized by an increase in immature collagen and dermal mucin, prominent collagen bundles, an increase in dermal spindle-shaped cells, and a lack of inflammation.[263] The condition appears to be associated with the use of gadolinium-containing contrast agents for MRI and gadodiamide is now contraindicated in patients with a GFR <30 ml/min/1.73 m^2.[261,264] The pathophysiology remains to be elucidated. There is currently no consistently effective treatment for this unremitting disease. Treatments that have been tried include physical therapy, steroids, thalidomide, methotrexate, and psoralen plus ultraviolet A (PUVA). The pain may have features of both nociceptive and neuropathic pain, and a thorough history will be required to guide the clinician to the analgesics most likely to help.

Case study 5: Pain relief using one neuropathic agent and the step-wise titration of Step-3 analgesia

X is a 72-year-old man who lives alone. He had a right nephroureterectomy in 1990 for a transitional cell carcinoma of the ureter. Eleven years later, glomerulonephritis led to renal failure requiring dialysis, compli-cated by discitiis the following year. This was managed medically with intravenous antibiotics and drainage. Following treatment, rehabilitation was unsuccessful due to severe pain on movement and during dialysis. He required readmission to hospital for pain control.

His pain was a mixture of nociceptive pain in his back and neuropathic pain going down his leg. Prior to referral he had received tramadol 50 mg tid and paracetamol 1 g qid and had moved up the analgesic ladder to hydromorphone 2.6 mg 4 hourly at the time of referral. Although there was partial improvement, he still had a pain score of 5/10 at rest and 8/10 on movement or during dialysis. A stepwise approach was taken.

In hospital

A dose of fentanyl (25 μg/h) equivalent to the hydromorphone he had been taking was administered by transdermal patch. Hydromorphone 2.6 mg orally 2 hourly prn was continued for breakthrough pain.

There was some improvement when he used six prn doses in 24 h, so the fentanyl patch size was increased to 50 μg/h with a corresponding increase in the prn hydromorphone dose to 5.2 mg. The neuropathic element remained prominent so clonazepam 0.5 mg was started at night and increased to 1 mg after a few days, with benefit, although he was not yet pain free.

Able to return to rehabilitation unit

Over the following 2 months his analgesic requirements were monitored by a palliative care nurse at his dialysis visits. By increasing the patch size to account for prn doses of hydromorphone for breakthrough pain, a dose of fentanyl 125 μg/h was reached. When on 100 μg/h of fentanyl he was:

Able to return to his own home with considerable help

As the dose per hour of fentanyl increased there was a corresponding increase in the dose of hydromorphone used for breakthrough pain. As pain relief was achieved, fewer doses were needed and currently one dose of 7.8 mg at night is sufficient. **Twenty weeks from referral he was living independently,** had dispensed with delivered meals because he could cook his own, and his mobility had progressed to needing only a walking stick for help.

He is likely to have some back pain for the rest of his life. However, attending physicians should be alert to the risk of opioid toxicity with this long-acting opioid preparation should **his pain diminish**. As the long-acting drug is fentanyl, he is not thought to be at risk of toxicity due to retention of active metabolites, but the subcutaneous depot of fentanyl will remain a source of analgesia for at least 24 h following patch removal.

8.5 Suggested guidelines for using the World Health Organization analgesic ladder in patients with severe chronic kidney disease and end-stage renal disease

8.5.1 General points (see Case study 5)

- Assess the patient's pain.
- Choose an appropriate step.
- Give the drug regularly.
- Assess the response and toxicity.
- Adjust or move up a step as appropriate.

8.5.1.2 Step 1

- Non-opioid analgesic (paracetamol 1 g qid and/or NSAID for specific acute indications such as gout).
- Caution needed with NSAID use because of potential detrimental effects on residual renal function and increased toxicity.
- If NSAID to be used, consider selective COX-2 inhibitor or gastroprotection.
- Consider use of adjuvant drugs for specific indications.

8.5.1.3 Step 2. Pain persisting or increasing

- Non-opioid analgesic (paracetamol 1 g qid and/or NSAID for specific acute indications such as gout)
- Add tramadol 50 mg bd/qid up to a total daily dose of 200 mg for dialysis patients and 100 mg daily for conservatively managed patients **or**
- Consider adding codeine 30 mg up to a total daily dose of 120 mg (see text).

- Warn patient and monitor carefully for toxicity.
- Consider the use of adjuvant drugs for specific indications.

8.5.1.4 **Step 3. Pain persisting or increasing**

(i) Dialysis patients able to swallow oral medication

- Non-opioid analgesic (paracetamol 1 g qid and/or NSAID for specific acute indications such as gout).
- Stop codeine or tramadol and **substitute: Hydromorphone 1–1.3 mg 6 hourly and prn** (smallest available capsule in UK is 1.3 mg; 0.5-mg capsules are available in the USA and Canada allowing for lower initial doses and more gradual dose titration).
- If tolerated, increase frequency to 4 hourly within 24 h if needed. Titrate dose upwards every 24–48 h according to the number of prn doses needed.
- If six or greater doses are required per 24 h stop regular hydromorphone and replace with TD fentanyl 12 µg/h. Continue using prn hydromorphone
- Continue dose titration upwards if needed, remembering to increase the dose of hydromorphone for breakthrough pain if the patch size increases (see Table 8.6).
- Monitor carefully for toxicity: myoclonus, sedation, or agitation.

(ii) Conservatively managed patients able to swallow oral medication

- Non-opioid analgesic (paracetamol 1 g qid and/or NSAID for specific acute indications such as gout).
- Stop tramadol and **substitute** hydromorphone 1–1.3 mg 6 hourly (caution with prolonged use at this dose; aim for maintenance with TD fentanyl or consider low dose buprenorphine)
- Monitor carefully for toxicity and switch to TD fentanyl 12 µg/h if 4–6 doses hydromorphone used consistently each 24 h
- Or start transdermal buprenorphine 5 µg/h; review and monitor carefully

Alternatives include:

- **Normal-release morphine 2.5–5 mg 4–6 hourly and prn.** Then, as for hydromorphone, with close monitoring. The appearance of toxicity varies but is likely to increase with the duration

Table 8.6 Strengths of transdermal fentanyl: to show breakthrough dose of hydromorphone

Fentanyl patch Strength (µg/h)	24-h fentanyl dose (µg)	4-hourly oral morphine (mg)	4-hourly oral hydromorphone (mg)
12	300	*	*
25	600	<20	<2.6
50	1200	25–35	2.6–3.9
75	1800	40–50	5.2
100	2400	55–65	6.5–7.8
125	3000	70–80	9.1

*no information from drug company

of treatment, and can be reduced by converting to transdermal fentanyl if the dose reaches 20 mg qid or above.

◆ **Methadone**. This should only be used by those experienced in the management of chronic pain with methadone. There are several ways of switching a patient to methadone; it is suggested the physician becomes familiar with one method and uses it consistently. One technique is to stop all other opioids before switching to methadone; this will usually require inpatient monitoring. An alternative approach is to start patients on a low dose (e.g. 1 mg tid) and titrate upwards as needed every few days with gradual reduction of previous opioid. Hydromorphone should be available for breakthrough pain. Monitor carefully for signs of toxicity.

(iii) Patient unable to swallow
Patient in continuous pain:
◆ Start 24 h SC fentanyl or alfentanil in syringe driver.
◆ Initial dose depends on previous analgesic use, pain intensity, and size/frailty of patient.
◆ In the opioid-naïve patient, SC fentanyl 100–150 µg/24 h with 12.5–25 µg prn are safe starting doses or SC alfentanil 400–600 µg/24 h with 40–60 µg prn for breakthrough pain.
◆ Adjust dose in the syringe driver accordingly depending on toxicity or number of prn doses required.
◆ In those already taking strong opioids by mouth, convert to the appropriate-size fentanyl patch.
◆ Use additional prn SC fentanyl at 1/10th the 24-h dose until therapeutic blood levels are reached and for titration.
◆ Alternatively, convert to a 24-h SC fentanyl or alfentanil syringe driver with prn drug available, adjusting the dose as above (see Table 8.6 for approximate equivalent doses).
◆ See also end of life guidelines Chapter 15.

Patient in intermittent pain:
◆ Use as needed SC fentanyl 12.5–25 µg.
◆ If more than three doses needed in 24 h, consider setting up continuous 24-h infusion.
◆ Alfentanil can be substituted for fentanyl at appropriate doses if preferred. It is one-quarter as potent (see end-of-life guidelines, Chapter 15 for more detail).

8.5.2 Guidelines for starting a fentanyl patch
◆ A fentanyl patch can be started as treatment for stable pain, or to provide background pain relief while dose titration takes place once the first patch size is reached.
◆ The breakthrough dose of hydromorphone depends on the 24 h of opioid and can be calculated from Table 8.6.
◆ Apply patch; continue regular normal release strong opioid for first 12 h.
◆ Prescribe a normal-release strong opioid equivalent to the 4-hourly dose for breakthrough pain.

8.5.3 Breakthrough pain, incident or movement-related pain
A short-acting preparation that works quickly is required for dose titration, or prior to planned activity:
◆ For **patients who can swallow**: normal release hydromorphone at one-sixth of the 24-h dose.

- For **patients unable to swallow** or vomiting: if on fentanyl or alfentanil as 24-h SC infusion or fentanyl transdermally, then use the same drug, usually SC but the buccal or intranasal route can also be used.
- **Calculation of prn dose**: There is no formula for the dose needed to relieve breakthrough pain when using fentanyl. It is sensible to start with a low dose such as either 12.5 µg or 25 µg, depending on the pain and the patient. If pain is not relieved in 1 h, repeat the dose. If a second dose at 1 h is needed consistently, then increase the breakthrough dose accordingly. The breakthrough dose can be titrated upwards according to the response and background dose of fentanyl. It is suggested that a breakthrough dose of between one-tenth and one-sixth of the 24-h dose of alfentanil is appropriate but this too can be individually titrated.

8.5.4 Alternative routes for prn medication

- Oral transmucosal fentanyl. A hardened lozenge on a stick enabling the fentanyl to be delivered buccally. There is no association between background opioid dose and effective breakthrough so each patient has to go through a dose-titration exercise to find which lozenge size is effective. The patient must be able hold the lozenge against the buccal mucosa, which may be less easy if the mouth is dry.
- Nasal/buccal/sublingual fentanyl, alfentanil, and sufentanil. This route can be used for all three of these drugs. There is good bioavailability and clinically effective plasma concentrations are achieved in less than 10 min for all three.[168] Fentanyl buccal and Sublingual tablets are now available in the UK.

8.6 Summary

In this chapter we have described the problem of pain, which often goes unrecognized, and its treatment in patients with renal failure. We have also described some of the difficulties which contribute to poor management in these patients. We have described three examples of painful syndromes, almost exclusively confined to those with renal disease, to illustrate the importance of familiarity with these conditions as well as the need to seek further expert help and advice.

Using the WHO analgesic ladder as a template and basic pharmacological principles, we have described a simple method for the assessment and treatment of pain in renal failure patients.

There is much still to be learnt about the handling of opioids for those needing chronic administration. This approach is supported by recent reviews of the evidence available for analgesics used in patients with CKD.[265–267] Genetic differences probably explain, in part, the large variation in response, both therapeutic and toxic, between patients. This highlights the importance of a thorough patient assessment with repeated reassessments as well as an individualized plan.

Ethical case analysis

It has been said that the first ethical responsibility of the physician is to be technically competent in the treatment of patients. This competence includes proficiency in pain and symptom management. Dialysis patients report that pain is their most severe symptom, one of their most common, and the one symptom that they are most concerned about at the end of life. For these reasons, it is very important for a nephrologist to master the principles of pain assessment and management discussed in this chapter. As Case studies 1 and 2 in this chapter illustrate, pain may be more than physical. In this chapter, the authors describe the concept of 'total pain'. It includes not only physical stimuli but also psychological, social, and spiritual factors. In Case 1, both of the patient's parents had diabetic nephropathy, and her mother had died from it. The initiation of dialysis was associated with excruciating pain. It is certainly possible that some of this pain may have been other than physical in origin. The case history notes that 'anxiety about this pain dominated her feelings'.

Her treatment included not only gradually escalating doses of fentanyl but also an anxiolytic, clonazepam, and an antidepressant, amitriptyline. With time and increasing doses of all three medications, the patient's pain gradually subsided. Although it is entirely possible that her pain was due only to the treatment of the infected, loculated fluid on her abdominal wall by the plastic surgeons, it is also possible that her total pain subsided as she became accustomed to being on dialysis and less fearful about it. In Case 2, the patient's pain seemed to resolve when the social worker assisted him in addressing his social problems. This case again emphasizes the ethical responsibility for nephrologists to do a complete pain assessment with attention to psychosocial and spiritual matters as well as physical.

Acknowledgements

All quotations were contributed by Mr. Christopher Wilson-Gleave.

References

1 Merskey H, Bogduk N (1998). Classification of chronic pain. *Seattle: Int Assoc Study Pain Press*, 210.

2 Saunders C (1967). *The management of terminal illness*. London, Edward Arnold.

3 World Health Organization (1996). Cancer Pain Relief: With a guide to opioid availability. 2d ed. Geneva.

4 Davison SN (2003). Pain in hemodialysis patients: prevalence, cause, severity, and management. *Am J Kidney Dis*, **42**(6), 1239–47.

5 Weisbord SD, Fried LF, Arnold RM, et al. (2005). Prevalence, severity, and importance of physical and emotional symptoms in chronic hemodialysis patients. *J Am Soc Nephrol*, Aug, **16**(8), 2487–94.

6 Murphy EL, Murtagh FE, Carey I, et al. (2008). Understanding symptoms in patients with advanced chronic kidney disease managed without dialysis: use of a short patient-completed assessment tool. *Nephron Clin Pract*, Dec 16, **111**(1), c74–80.

7 Davison SN, Jhangri GS, Johnson JA (2006). Cross-sectional validity of a modified Edmonton symptom assessment system in dialysis patients: a simple assessment of symptom burden. *Kidney Int*, May, **69**(9), 1621–5.

8 Saini T, Murtagh FE, Dupont PJ, et al. (2006). Comparative pilot study of symptoms and quality of life in cancer patients and patients with end stage renal disease. *Palliat Med*, Sep, **20**(6), 631–6.

9 US Renal Data System (2007). National Institutes of Health, National Institute of Diabetes and Digestive and Kidney Diseases. USRDS 2007 Annual Data Report: Atlas of Chronic Kidney Disease and End-Stage Renal Disease in the United States. Bethesda, MD.

10 Cohen LM, Germain MJ, Poppel DM, et al. (2000). Dying Well after discontinuing the life support treatment of dialysis. *Arch Intern Med*, **160**(16), 2513–18.

11 Chater S, Davison SN, Germain MJ, et al. (2006). Withdrawal from dialysis: a palliative care perspective. *Clin Nephrol*, Nov, **66**(5), 364–72.

12 Germain MJ, Cohen LM, Davison SN (2007). Withholding and withdrawal from dialysis: what we know about how our patients die. *Semin Dial*, May, **20**(3), 195–9.

13 Binik YM, Baker AG, Devins GM, et al. (1982). Pain, control over treatment, and compliance in dialysis and transplant patients. *Kidney Int*, **21**(6), 840–8.

14 Parfrey PS, Vavasour HM, Bullock HM, et al. (1988). Clinical features and severity of non specific symptoms in dialysis patients. *Nephron*. **50**, 121–8.

15 Weisbord SD, Fried LF, Mor MK, et al. (2007). Renal provider recognition of symptoms in patients on maintenance hemodialysis. *Clin J Am Soc Nephrol*, Sep, **2**(5), 960–7.

16 Bailie GR, Mason NA, Johnson CA, et al. (2001). Analgesic use among hemodialysis (HD) patients: Potential for drug related problems [Abstract]. *J Am Soc Nephrol*, **12**, 320A.

17 Ferrell BR, Wisdom C, Wenzl C (1989). Quality of life as an outcome variable in the management of cancer pain. *Cancer*, **63**(11 Suppl), 2321–7.

18 Becker N, Bondegaard TA, Olsen AK, et al. (1997). Pain epidemiology and health related quality of life in chronic non-malignant pain patients referred to a Danish multidisciplinary pain center. *Pain*, **73**(3), 393–400.

19 Skevington SM (1998). Investigating the relationship between pain and discomfort and quality-of-life using the WHOQOL. *Pain*, **76**, 395–406.

20 Wang XS, Cleeland CS, Mendoza TR, et al. (1999). The effects of pain severity on health related quality of life: a study of Chinese cancer patients. *Cancer*, **86**(9), 1848–55.

21 Poulos A (2001). Pain, mood disturbance, and quality of life in patients with multiple myeloma. *Oncol Nurs Forum*, **28**(7), 1163–71.

22 Nie J, Liu S, Di L (2000). Cancer pain and its influence on cancer patients' quality of life. *Zhonghua Zhong Liu Za Zhi*, **22**(5), 432–4.

23 Davison SN (2007). Chronic kidney disease: psychosocial impact of chronic pain. *Geriatrics*, Feb, **62**(2), 17–23.

24 Kimmel PL, Emont SL, Newmann JM, et al. (2003). ESRD patient quality of life: symptoms, spiritual beliefs, psychosocial factors, and ethnicity. *AJKD*, **42**(4), 713–21.

25 Valderrabano F, Jofre R, Lopez-Gomez JM (2001). Quality of life in end-stage renal disease patients. *Am J Kidney Dis*, **38**(3), 443–64.

26 Patel SS, Shah VS, Peterson RA, et al. (2002). Psychosocial variables, quality of life, and religious beliefs in ESRD patients treated with hemodialysis. *Am J Kidney Dis*, **40**(5), 1013–22.

27 Davison SN, Jhangri GS (2005). The impact of chronic pain on depression, sleep, and the desire to withdraw from dialysis in hemodialysis patients. *J Pain Symp Manag*, Nov, **30**(5), 465–73.

28 Bajwa K, Szabo E, Kjellstrand CM (1996). A Prospective study of risk factors and decision making in discontinuation of dialysis. *Arch Intern Med,* **156**(22), 2571–7.

29 Davison SN, Jhangri GS, Johnson JA (2006). Longitudinal validation of a modified Edmonton symptom assessment system (ESAS) in haemodialysis patients. *Nephrol Dialy Transplant*, Nov, **21**(11), 3189–95.

30 McQuay H, Carroll D, Jadad AR, et al. (1995). Anticonvulsant drugs for management of pain: a systematic review. *BMJ*, Oct 21, **311**(7012), 1047–52.

31 McQuay H, Moore A (1998). *An evidence based resource for pain relief*. Oxford, Oxford University Press.

32 Devins GM, Armstrong SJ, Mandin H, et al. (1990). Recurrent pain, illness intrusiveness, and quality of life in end-stage renal disease. *Pain*, Sep, **42**(3), 279–85.

33 Doyle D, Hanks Gw, MacDonald N (1997). *Textbook of palliative medicine*. Oxford, Oxford University Press.

34 Bailie GR, Mason NA, Bragg-Gresham JL, et al. (2004). Analgesic prescription patterns among hemodialysis patients in the DOPPS: potential for under prescription. *Kidney Int*, **65**(6), 2419–25.

35 Zech DFJ, Grond S, Lynch J, et al. (1995). Validation of World Health Organization Guidelines for cancer pain relief: a 10-year prospective study. *Pain*, **63**, 65–76.

36 Cleeland C, Gonin R, Hatfield AK, Edmonson JH, Blum RH, Stewart JA, et al. Pain and its treatment in outpatients with metastatic cancer. New England Journal of Medicine 1994 Mar 3;330:592-6.

37 Anderson KO, Mendoza TR, Valero V, et al. (2000). Minority cancer patients and their providers: Pain management attitudes and practice. *Cancer*, **88**(8), 1929–38.

38 Melzack R (1975). The McGill Pain Questionnaire: Major properties and scoring methods. *Pain*, **1**, 277–99.

39 Daut RL, Cleeland ES, Flanery RC (1983). Development of the Wisconsin Brief Pain Questionnaire to assess pain in cancer and other diseases. *Pain*, **17**, 197–210.

40 Caraceni A, Cherny N, Fainsinger R, et al. (2002). Pain Measurement tools and methods in clinical research in palliative care: Recommendations of an expert working group of the European Association of Palliative Care. *J Pain Symp Manag*, **23**(3), 239–55.

41 Weisbord SD, Fried LF, Arnold RM, et al. (2004). Development of a symptom assessment instrument for chronic hemodialysis patients: the Dialysis Symptom Index. *J Pain Symp Manag*, Mar, **27**(3), 226–40.

42 Dworkin RH, Gitlin MJ (1991). Clinical aspects of depression in chronic pain patients. *Clin J Pain*, **7**(2), 79–94.

43 World Health Organization (1990). Cancer Pain Relief and Palliative Care. Geneva, World Health Organization.

44 Barakzoy AS, Moss AH (2006). Efficacy of the world health organization analgesic ladder to treat pain in end-stage renal disease. *J Am Soc Nephrol*, Nov, **17**(11), 3198–203.

45 Anderson RJ, Melikian DM, Gambertoglio JG, et al. (1982). Prescribing medication in long-term dialysis units. *Arch Intern Med*, Jul, **142**(7), 1305–8.

46 Cockcroft DW, Gault MH (1976). Prediction of creatinine clearance from serum creatinine. *Nephron*, **16**(1), 31–41.

47 Melloni C, Peterson ED, Chen AY, et al. (2008). Cockcroft–Gault versus modification of diet in renal disease: importance of glomerular filtration rate formula for classification of chronic kidney disease in patients with non-ST-segment elevation acute coronary syndromes. *J Am Coll Cardiol*, Mar, 11, **51**(10), 991–6.

48 Reidenberg MM (1985). Kidney function and drug action. *N Engl J Med*, Sep 26, **313**(13), 816–8.

49 Gibaldi M (1977). Drug distribution in renal failure. *Am J Med*, Apr, **62**(4), 471–4.

50 British National Formulary (2002). British Medical Association and Royal Pharmaceutical Society of Great Britain.

51 Aronoff GR, Berns JS, Brier M, et al. (1998). *Drug prescribing in renal failure*. 4th ed. American College of Physicians, Philadelphia, PA.

52 Ashley C, Bunn R (1999). *The renal drug handbook*. Radcliffe Medical Press, 1999.

53 Chennavasin P, Brater DC (1981). Nomograms for drug use in renal disease. *Clin Pharmacokinet*, May, **6**(3), 193–214.

54 Michael KA, Mohler JL, Blouin RA, et al. (1985). Failure of creatinine clearance to predict gentamicin half-life in a renal transplant patient with diabetes mellitus. *Clin Pharm*, Sep, **4**(5), 572–5.

55 Maderazo EG, Sun H, Jay GT (1992). Simplification of antibiotic dose adjustments in renal insufficiency: the DREM system. *Lancet*, Sep 26, **340**(8822), 767–70.

56 Vidal L, Shavit M, Fraser A, et al. (2005). Systematic comparison of four sources of drug information regarding adjustment of dose for renal function. *BMJ*, Jul 30, **331**(7511), 263.

57 Munar MY, Singh H (2007). Drug dosing adjustments in patients with chronic kidney disease. *Am Fam Physician*, May, 15, **75**(10), 1487–96.

58 Gulyassay PF, Depner TA (1983). Impaired binding of drugs and ligands in renal diseases. *Am J Kidney Dis*, **2**, 578–601.

59 Vanholder R, van Landschoot N, de Sweet R, et al. (1988). Drug protein binding in chronic renal failure: evaluation of nine drugs. *Kidney Int*, **33**, 996–1004.

60 Lewis GP, Jusko WJ, Burke CW (1971). Prednisolone side-effects and serum protein levels. *Lancet*, **2**, 778–80.

61 Gibson TP (1986). Renal disease and drug metabolism: an overview. *Am J Kidney Dis*, **8**, 7–17.

62 Gibson TP, Dobrinska MR, Estwhistle LA, et al. (1987). Biotransformation of sulindac in end-stage renal disease. *Clin Pharm Therapeut*, **42**, 82–8.

63 Berg KJ, Talseth T (1985). Acute renal effects of sulindac and indomethacin in chronic renal failure. *Clin Pharmacol Ther*, Apr, **37**(4), 447–52.

64 Hart D, Lifschitz MD (1987). Renal physiology of the prostaglandins and the effects of nonsteroidal anti-inflammatory agents on the kidney. *Am J Nephrol*, **7**(5), 408–18.

65 Kleinknecht D, Landais P, Goldfarb B (1986). Analgesic and non-steroidal anti-inflammatory drug-associated acute renal failure: a prospective collaborative study. *Clin Nephrol*, Jun, **25**(6), 275–81.

66 Shankel SW, Johnson DC, Clark PS, et al. (1992). Acute renal failure and glomerulopathy caused by nonsteroidal anti-inflammatory drugs. *Arch Intern Med*, May, **152**(5), 986–90.

67 Minuz P, Barrow SE, Cockcroft JR, et al. (1990). Effects of non-steroidal anti-inflammatory drugs on prostacyclin and thromboxane biosynthesis in patients with mild essential hypertension. *Brit J Clin Pharmacol*, Oct, **30**(4), 519–26.

68 Weinstein S, Pfeffer M, Schor J, et al. (1971). Metabolites of naloxone in human urine. *J Pharm Sci*, Oct, **60**(10), 1567–8.

69 Farrell B, Godwin J, Richards S, et al. (1991). The United Kingdom transient ischaemic attack (UK-TIA) aspirin trial: final results. *J Neurol Neurosurg Psychiat*, Dec, **54**(12), 1044–54.

70 Bombardier C, Laine L, Reicin A, et al. (2000). Comparison of upper gastrointestinal toxicity of rofecoxib and naproxen in patients with rheumatoid arthritis. VIGOR Study Group. *N Engl J Med*, Nov, 23, **343**(21), 1520–8.

71 Lanas A (2002). Clinical experience with cyclooxygenase-2 inhibitors. *Rheumatology* (Oxford), Apr, **41** Supp 1, 16–22.

72 Silverstein FE, Faich G, Goldstein JL, et al. (2000). Gastrointestinal toxicity with celecoxib vs nonsteroidal anti-inflammatory drugs for osteoarthritis and rheumatoid arthritis: the CLASS study: A randomized controlled trial. Celecoxib Long-term Arthritis Safety Study. *JAMA*, Sep, 13, **284**(10), 1247–55.

73 Chen YF, Jobanputra P, Barton P, et al. (2008). Cyclooxygenase-2 selective non-steroidal anti-inflammatory drugs (etodolac, meloxicam, celecoxib, rofecoxib, etoricoxib, valdecoxib and lumiracoxib) for osteoarthritis and rheumatoid arthritis: a systematic review and economic evaluation. *Health Technol Assess*, Apr, **12**(11), 1–278, iii.

74 Rostom A, Moayyedi P, Hunt R, Canadian Association of Gastroenterology Consensus Group (2009). Systematic Review: Canadian Consensus guidelines on long-term NSAID therapy and the need for gastroprotection: benefits versus risks. *Aliment Pharmacol Ther*, Mar 1; **29**(5), 481–96. Epub 2008 Nov 27.

75 Eden AN, Kaufman A (1967). Clinical comparison of three antipyretic agents. *Am J Dis Child*, Sep, **114**(3), 284–7.

76 Brewer EJ, Jr. (1968). A comparative evaluation of indomethacin, acetaminophen and placebo as antipyretic agents in children. *Arthritis Rheum*, Oct, **11**(5), 645–51.

77 Skjelbred P, Lokken P (1979). Paracetamol versus placebo: effects on post-operative course. *Eur J Clin Pharmacol*, Feb 19, **15**(1), 27–33.

78 Botting R (2000). Paracetamol-inhibitable COX-2. *J Physiol Pharmacol*, Dec, **51**(4 Pt 1), 609–18.

79 Koch-Weser J (1976). Drug therapy. Acetaminophen. *N Engl J Med*, Dec, 2, **295**(23), 1297–300.

80 Forrest JA, Clements JA, Prescott LF (1982). Clinical pharmacokinetics of paracetamol. *Clin Pharmacokinet*, Mar, **7**(2), 93–107.

81 Prescott LF (1982). Analgesic nephropathy: a reassessment of the role of phenacetin and other analgesics. *Drugs*, Jan, **23**(1–2), 75–149.

82 Fored CM, Ejerblad E, Lindblad P, et al. (2001). Acetaminophen, aspirin, and chronic renal failure. *N Engl J Med*, Dec, 20, **345**(25), 1801–8.

83 Lasagna L (1964). The Clinical Evaluation of Morphine and its Substitutes as Analgesics. *Pharmacol Rev*, Mar, **16**, 47–83.

84 Boerner U (1975). The metabolism of morphine and heroin in man. *Drug Metab Rev*, **4**(1), 39–73.

85 Desmeules J, Gascon MP, Dayer P, et al. (1991). Impact of environmental and genetic factors on codeine analgesia. *Eur J Clin Pharmacol*, **41**(1), 23–6.

86 Sindrup SH, Poulsen L, Brosen K, et al. (1993). Are poor metabolisers of sparteine/debrisoquine less pain tolerant than extensive metabolisers? *Pain*, Jun, **53**(3), 335–9.

87 Barnes JN, Williams AJ, Tomson MJ, et al. (1985). Dihydrocodeine in renal failure: further evidence for an important role of the kidney in the handling of opioid drugs. *Brit Med J (Clin Res Ed)*, Mar, 9, **290**(6470), 740–2.

88 Guay DR, Awni WM, Findlay JW, et al. (1988). Pharmacokinetics and pharmacodynamics of codeine in end-stage renal disease. *Clin Pharmacol Ther*, Jan, **43**(1), 63–71.

89 Davies G, Kingswood C, Street M (1996). Pharmacokinetics of opioids in renal dysfunction. *Clin Pharmacokinet*, Dec, **31**(6), 410–22.

90 Empey DW, Laitinen LA, Young GA, et al. (1979). Comparison of the antitussive effects of codeine phosphate 20 mg, dextromethorphan 30 mg and noscapine 30 mg using citric acid-induced cough in normal subjects. *Eur J Clin Pharmacol*, **16**(6), 393–7.

91 Bradshaw MJ, Harvey RF (1982). Antidiarrhoeal agents. Clinical pharmacology and therapeutic use. *Drugs*, Nov, **24**(5), 440–51.

92 Barnes JN, Goodwin FJ (1983). Dihydrocodeine narcosis in renal failure. *Brit Med J (Clin Res Ed)*, Feb, 5, **286**(6363), 438–9.

93 Messick RT (1979). Evaluation of acetaminophen, propoxyphene, and their combination in office practice. *J Clin Pharmacol*, Apr, **19**(4), 227–30.

94 Gibson TP, Giacomini KM, Briggs WA, et al. (1980). Propoxyphene and norpropoxyphene plasma concentrations in the anephric patient. *Clin Pharmacol Ther*, May, **27**(5), 665–70.

95 Nickander RC, Emmerson JL, Hynes MD, et al. (1984). Pharmacologic and toxic effects in animals of dextropropoxyphene and its major metabolite norpropoxyphene: a review. *Hum Toxicol*, Aug, **3** Suppl, 13S–36S.

96 Raffa RB, Friderichs E, Reimann W, et al. (1992). Opioid and nonopioid components independently contribute to the mechanism of action of tramadol, an 'atypical' opioid analgesic. *J Pharmacol Exp Therapeut*, Jan, 1, **260**(1), 275–85.

97 Raffa RB, Friderichs E, Reimann W, et al. (1993). Complementary and synergistic antinociceptive interaction between the enantiomers of tramadol. *J Pharmacol Exp Ther*, Oct, **267**(1), 331–40.

98 Radbruch L, Grond S, Lehmann KA (1996). A risk-benefit assessment of tramadol in the management of pain. *Drug Saf*, Jul, **15**(1), 8–29.

99 Desmeules JA (2000). The tramadol option. *Eur J Pain*, **4** Suppl A, 15–21.

100 Scott LJ, Perry CM (2000). Tramadol: a review of its use in perioperative pain. *Drugs*, Jul, **60**(1), 139–76.

101 Bamigbade TA, Langford RM (1998). Tramadol hydrochloride: an overview of current use. *Hosp Med*, May, **59**(5), 373–6.

102 Shipton EA (2000). Tramadol – present and future. *Anaesth Intensive Care*, Aug, **28**(4), 363–74.

103 Desmeules JA, Piguet V, Collart L, et al. (1996). Contribution of monoaminergic modulation to the analgesic effect of tramadol. *Brit J Clin Pharmacol*, Jan, **41**(1), 7–12.

104 Sevcik J, Nieber K, Driessen B, et al. (1993). Effects of the central analgesic tramadol and its main metabolite, O-desmethyltramadol, on rat locus coeruleus neurones. *Brit J Pharmacol*, Sep, **110**(1), 169–76.

105 Lintz W, Erlacin S, Frankus E, et al. (1981). Biotransformation of tramadol in man and animal (author's transl). *Arzneimittelforschung*, **31**(11), 1932–43.

106 Gibson TP (1996). Pharmacokinetics, efficacy, and safety of analgesia with a focus on tramadol HCl. *Am J Med*, Jul, 31, **101**(1A), 47S–53S.

107 Messahel FM, Tomlin PJ (1981). Narcotic withdrawal syndrome after intrathecal administration of morphine. *Brit Med J (Clin Res Ed)*, Aug, 15, **283**(6289), 471–2.

108 Cousins MJ, Cherry DA (1988). Acute and chronic pain: use of spinal opiods. *Neural blockade in clinical anesthesia and management of pain*, pp. 955–1029. Philadelphia, PA, Lippincott Williams & Wilkins.

109 Ballantyne JC, LaForge KS (2007). Opioid dependence and addiction during opioid treatment of chronic pain. *Pain*, Jun, **129**(3), 235–55.

110 Fishbain DA, Cole B, Lewis J,et al. (2008). What percentage of chronic nonmalignant pain patients exposed to chronic opioid analgesic therapy develop abuse/addiction and/or aberrant drug-related behaviors? A structured evidence-based review. *Pain Med*, May, **9**(4), 444–59.

111 Narita M, Funada M, Suzuki T (2001). Regulations of opioid dependence by opioid receptor types. *Pharmacol Ther*, Jan, **89**(1), 1–15.

112 Gutstein HB, Akil H (2001). Opioid analgesics and antagonists, in Hardman JG, Limbird LE, Gilman AG (eds) *Goodman and Gilman's the pharmacological basis of therapeutics*, pp. 569–619, 10th ed. New York, McGraw-Hill.

113 Patwardhan RV, Johnson RF, Hoyumpa A, Jr., et al. (1981). Normal metabolism of morphine in cirrhosis. *Gastroenterology*, Dec, **81**(6), 1006–11.

114 Tegeder I, Lotsch J, Geisslinger G (1999). Pharmacokinetics of opioids in liver disease. *Clin Pharmacokinet*, Jul, **37**(1), 17–40.

115 Yeh SY, Gorodetzky CW, Krebs HA (1977). Isolation and identification of morphine 3- and 6-glucuronides, morphine 3,6-diglucuronide, morphine 3-ethereal sulfate, normorphine, and normorphine 6-glucuronide as morphine metabolites in humans. *J Pharm Sci*, Sep, **66**(9), 1288–93.

116 Osborne R, Joel S, Trew D, et al. (1988). Analgesic activity of morphine-6-glucuronide. *Lancet*, Apr, 9, **1**(8589), 828.

117 Osborne R, Joel S, Trew D, et al. (1990). Morphine and metabolite behavior after different routes of morphine administration: demonstration of the importance of the active metabolite morphine-6-glucuronide. *Clin Pharmacol Ther*, Jan, **47**(1), 12–19.

118 Portenoy RK (1990). Chronic opioid therapy in nonmalignant pain. *J Pain Symp Manag*, **5**, S46–62.

119 Portenoy RK, Khan E, Layman M, et al. (1991). Chronic morphine therapy for pain for cancer pain: plasma and cerebrospinal fluid morphine and morphine-6-glucuronide concentrations. *Neurology*, **41**, 1457–61.

120 Portenoy RK, Foley KM, Stulman J, et al. (1991). Plasma morphine and morphine-6-glucuronide during chronic morphine therapy for cancer pain: plasma profiles, steady-state concentrations and the consequences of renal failure. *Pain*, Oct, **47**(1), 13–19.

121 Sawe J, Odar-Cederlof I (1987). Kinetics of morphine in patients with renal failure. *Eur J Clin Pharmacol*, **32**(4), 377–82.

122 Sear JW, Hand CW, Moore RA, et al. (1989). Studies on morphine disposition: Influence of renal failure on kinetics of morphine and its metabolites. *Brit J Anaesth*, **62**, 28–32.

123 Chauvin M, Sandouk P, Scherrmann JM, et al. (1987). Morphine pharmacokinetics in renal failure. *Anesthesiology*, **66**, 327–31.

124 Osborne RJ, Joel SP, Slevin ML (1986). Morphine intoxication in renal failure: the role of morphine-6-glucuronide. *Brit Med J (Clin Res Ed)*, Jun, 14, **292**(6535), 1548–9.

125 Wolff J, Bigler D, Christensen CB, et al. (1988). Influence of renal function on the elimination of morphine and morphine glucuronides. *Eur J Clin Pharmacol*, **34**(4), 353–7.

126 Hanna MH, D'Costa F, Peat SJ, et al. (1993). Morphine-6-glucuronide disposition in renal impairment. *Brit J Anaesth*, **70**, 511–14.

127 Bruera E, Sloan P, Mount B, et al., for the Canadian Palliative Care Clinical Trials Group (1996). A randomized, double-blind, double-dummy, crossover trial comparing the safety and efficacy of oral sustained-releae hydromorphone with immediate-release hydromorphone in patients with cancer pain. *J Clin Oncol*, **14**, 1713–17.

128 Dunbar PJ, Chapman CR, Buckley FP, et al. (1996). Clinical analgesic equivalence for morphine and hydromorphone with prolonged PCA. *Pain*, **68**, 265–70.

129 Quigley C (2002). Hydromorphone for acute and chronic pain. *Cochrane Database Syst Rev CD003447*.

130 Sarhill N, Walsh D, Nelson KA (2001). Hydromorphone: pharmacology and clinical applications in cancer patients. *Support Care Cancer*, **9**, 84–96.

131 Babul N, Darke AC, Hagen N (1995). Hydromorphone metabolite accumulation in renal failure. *J Pain Symp Manag*, **10**(3), 184–6.

132 Fainsinger R, Schoeller T, Boiskin M, et al. (1993). Palliative care round: cognitive failure and coma after renal failure in a patient receiving captopril and hydromorphone. *J Palliat Care*, **9**(1), 53–5.

133 Davison SN, Mayo P (2008). Pain management in chronic kidney disease: the pharmacokinetics and pharmacodynamics of hydromorphone and hydromorphone-3-glucuronide in hemodialysis patients. *J Opioid Manag*, **4**(6), 335, 339–6, 344.

134 Lee MA, Leng ME, Tiernan EJ (2001). Retrospective study of the use of hydromorphone in palliative care patients with normal and abnormal urea and creatinine. *Palliat Med*, **15**, 26–34.

135 Morrison JD, Loan WB, Dundee JW (1971). Controlled comparison of of the efficacy of fourteen preparations in the relief of post-operative pain. *BMJ*, **2**, 287–90.

136 Gourlay GK, Cherry DA, Cousins MJ (1986). A comparative study of the efficacy and pharmacokinetics of oral methadone and morphine in the treatment of severe pain in patients with cancer pain. *Pain*, **25**, 297–312.

137 Davies AM, Inturrisi J (1999). d-Methadone blocks morphine tolerance and N-methyl-D-aspartate-induced hyperalgesia. *J Pharmacol Exp Ther*, **289**, 1048–53.

138 Bruera E, Neumann CM (1999). Role of methadone in the management of pain in cancer patients. *Oncology*, **13**, 1275–88.

139 Fainsinger R, Schoeller T, Bruera E (1993). Methadone in the management of cancer pain: a review. *Pain*, Feb, **52**(2), 137–47.

140 Dole VP, Kreek MJ (1973). Methadone plasma level: sustained by a resevoir of drug. *Proc Natl Acad Sci*, **70**, 10–15.

141 Pohland A, Boaz HE, Sullivan HR (1971). Synthesis and identification of metabolites resulting from the biotransformation of d,l-methadone in man and in the rat. *J Med Chem*, **14**, 194–7.

142 Kreek MJ, Schecter AJ, Gutjahr CL, et al. (1980). Methadone use in patients with chronic renal disease. *Drug Alcohol Depend*, **5**, 197–205.

143 Furlan V, Hafi A, Dessalles MC, et al. (1999). Methadone is poorly removed by haemodialysis. *Nephrol Dialy Transplant*, **14**(1), 254–5.

144 Mather LE, Meffin LE (1978). Clinical pharmacokinetics pethidine. *Clin Pharmacokin*, **3**, 352–68.

145 MacDonald AD, Wolfe AG, Gergel F (1946). Analgesic actions of pethidine derivatives and related compunds. *Brit J Pharmacol*, **1**, 4–14.

146 Miller JW, Anderson HH (1954). The effect of N-demethylation on certain pharmacologic actions of morphine, codeine and meperidine in the mouse. *J Pharmacol Exp Ther*, **112**, 191–6.

147 Szeto HH, Inturrisi CE, Houde R, et al. (1977). Accumulation of normeperidine, an active metabolite of meperidine, in patients with renal failure or cancer. *Ann Intern Med*, **86**(6), 738–41.

148 Ripamonti C, Dickerson ED (2001). Strategies for the treatment of cancer pain in the new millennium. *Drugs*, **61**(7), 955–77.

149 Kalso E, Vainio A, Mattila MJ, et al. (1990). Morphine and oxycodone in the management of cancer pain: plasma levels determined by chemical and radioreceptor assays. *Pharmacol Toxicol*, Jan, 10, **67**(4), 322–8.

150 Rischitelli DG, Karbowicz SH (2002). Safety and efficacy of controlled-release oxycodone: a systematic literature review. *Pharmacotherapy*, Jul, **22**(7), 898–904.

151 Poyhia R, Vainio A, Kalso E (1993). A review of oxycodone's clinical pharmacokinetics and pharmacodynamics. *J Pain Symp Manag*, Feb, **8**(2), 63–7.

152 Leow KP, Smith MT, Watt JA, et al. (1992). Comparative oxycodone pharmacokinetics in humans after intravenous, oral, and rectal administration. *Ther Drug Monit*, Dec, **14**(6), 479–84.

153 Weinstein SH, Gaylord JC (1979). Determination of oxycodone in plasma and identification of a major metabolite. *J Pharm Sci*, Apr, **68**(4), 527–8.

154 Baselt R, Stewart C (1978). Determination of oxycodone and a major metabolite in urine by electron-caputre GLD. *J Anal Toxicol*, **2**, 107–9.

155 Kirvela M, Lindgren L, Seppala T, et al. (1996). The pharmacokinetics of oxycodone in uremic patients undergoing renal transplantation. *J Clin Anesth*, Feb, **8**(1), 13–18.

156 Poyhia R, Seppala T, Olkkola KT, et al. (1992). The pharmacokinetics and metabolism of oxycodone after intramuscular and oral administration to healthy subjects. *Brit J Clin Pharmacol*, Jun, **33**(6), 617–21.

157 Lee MA, Leng M, Cooper RM (2005). Measurements of plasma oxycodone, noroxycodone and oxymorphone levels in a patient with bilateral nephrectomy who is undergoing haemodialysis. *Palliat Med*, May, **19**(3), 259–60.

158 Foral PA, Ineck JR, Nystrom KK (2007). Oxycodone Accumulation in a Hemodialysis Patient. *Southern Med J*, Feb, **100**(2), 212–14.

159 Clotz MA, Nahata MC (1991). Clinical uses of fentanyl, sufentanil, and alfentanil. *Clin Pharm*, Aug, **10**(8), 581–93.

160 Paix A, Coleman A, Lees J, et al. (1995). Subcutaneous fentanyl and sufentanil infusion substitution for morphine intolerance in cancer management. *Pain*, **63**, 263–9.

161 Zech DFJ, Grond SUA, Lynch J, et al. (1992). Transdermal fentanyl and initial dose-finding with patient-controlled analgesia in cancer pain. A pilot study with 20 terminally ill cancer patients. *Pain*, **50**, 293–301.

162 Koren G, Crean PGGV, Klein J, et al. (1984). Pharmacokinetics of fentanyl in children with renal disease. *Res Commun Chem Pathol Pharmacol*, **46**(3), 371–9.

163 McClain DA, Hug CC, Jr. (1980). Intravenous fentanyl kinetics. *Clin Pharmacol Ther*, **28**, 106–14.

164 Koehntop DE, Rodman JH (1997). Fentanyl pharmacokinetics in patients undergoing renal transplantation. *Pharmacotherapy*, **17**(4), 745–52.

165 Bower S (1982). Plasma protein binding of fentanyl: The effect of hyperlipoproteinaemia and chronic renal failure. *J Pharmacy Pharmacol*, **34**, 102–6.

166 Mercadante S, Caligara M, Sapio M, et al. (1997). Subcutaneous fentanyl infusion in a patient with bowel obstruction and renal failure. *J Pain Symp Manag*, **13**, 241–4.

167 Geerts P, Noorduin H, Vanden BG, et al. (1987). Practical aspects of alfentanil infusion. *Eur J Anaesthesiol Suppl*, **1**, 25–9.

168 Dale O, Hjortkjaer R, Kharasch ED (2002). Nasal administration of opioids for pain management in adults. *Acta Anaesthesiol Scand*, Aug, **46**(7), 759–70.

169 McQuay H, Moore RA, Bullingham REE (1986). Bubrenorphine kinetics, in Foley KM, Inturrisi CE (eds) *Opioid analgesics in the management of clinical pain*, pp. 271–8. New York, Raven Press.

170 Martin WR, Eades CG, Thompson JA, et al. (1976). The effects of morphine- and nalorphine- like drugs in the nondependent and morphine-dependent chronic spinal dog. *J Pharmacol Exp Ther*, Jun, **197**(3), 517–32.

171 Lewis JW (1985). Buprenorphine. *Drug Alcohol Depend*, Feb, **14**(3–4), 363–72.

172 Arner S, Meyerson BA (1988). Lack of analgesic effect of opioids on neuropathic and idiopathic forms of pain. *Pain*, Apr, **33**(1), 11–23.

173 Bullingham RE, McQuay HJ, Moore RA, et al. (1981). An oral buprenorphine and paracetamol combination compared with paracetamol alone: a single dose double-blind postoperative study. *Brit J Clin Pharmacol*, Dec, **12**(6), 863–7.

174 Armstrong SC, Cozza KL (2003). Pharmacokinetic drug interactions of morphine, codeine, and their derivatives: theory and clinical reality, Part II. *Psychosomatics*, Nov, **44**(6), 515–20.

175 Hand CW, Sear JW, Uppington J, et al. (1990). Buprenorphine disposition in patients with renal impairment: single and continuous dosing, with special reference to metabolites. *Brit J Anaesth*, Mar, **64**(3), 276–82.

176 Ohtani M, Kotaki H, Sawada Y, et al. (1995). Comparative analysis of buprenorphine- and norbuprenorphine-induced analgesic effects based on pharmacokinetic-pharmacodynamic modeling. *J Pharmacol Exp Therapeut*, Feb, 1, **272**(2), 505–10.

177 Ohtani M, Kotaki H, Nishitateno K, et al. (1997). Kinetics of respiratory depression in rats induced by buprenorphine and its metabolite, norbuprenorphine. *J Pharmacol Exp Ther*, Apr, **281**(1), 428–33.

178 Budd K, Chambers J, Dahan A, et al. (2009). Guidance about prescribing in palliative care, in Twycross R, Wilcock A, Mortimer, (eds) Palliative Care Formulary (website).

179 Elkader A, Sproule B (2005). Buprenorphine: clinical pharmacokinetics in the treatment of opioid dependence. *Clin Pharmacokinet*, **44**(7), 661–80.

180 Megarbane B, Hreiche R, Pirnay S, et al. (2006). Does high-dose buprenorphine cause respiratory depression? possible mechanisms and therapeutic consequences. *Toxicol Rev*, **25**(2), 79–85.

181 Filitz J, Griessinger N, Sittl R, et al. (2006). Effects of intermittent hemodialysis on buprenorphine and norbuprenorphine plasma concentrations in chronic pain patients treated with transdermal buprenorphine. *Eur J Pain*, Nov, **10**(8), 743–8.

182 Osterlitz HW, Watt AJ (1968). Kinetic parameters of narcotic agonists and antagonists, with particular reference to N-allylnoroxymorphone (naloxone). *Brit J Pharmacol Chemother*, Jun, **33**(2), 266–76.

183 Levine JD, Gordon NC, Fields HL (1979). Naloxone dose dependently produces analgesia and hyperalgesia in postoperative pain. *Nature*, Apr, 19, **278**(5706), 740–1.

184 Lasagna L (1965). Drug interaction in the field of analgesic drugs. *Proc R Soc Med*, Nov, **58**(11 Part 2), 978–83.

185 Kenyon JN, Knight CJ, Wells C (1983). Randomised double-blind trial on the immediate effects of naloxone on classical Chinese acupuncture therapy for chronic pain. *Acupunct Electrother Res*, **8**(1), 17–24.

186 Blake DR, Robson P, Ho M, et al. (2006). Preliminary assessment of the efficacy, tolerability and safety of a cannabis-based medicine (Sativex) in the treatment of pain caused by rheumatoid arthritis. *Rheumatology* (Oxford), Jan, **45**(1), 50–2.

187 Rog DJ, Nurmikko TJ, Friede T, et al. (2005). Randomized, controlled trial of cannabis-based medicine in central pain in multiple sclerosis. *Neurology*, Sep, 27, **65**(6), 812–19.

188 Rog DJ, Nurmikko TJ, Young CA (2007). Oromucosal Delta 9-tetrahydrocannabinol/cannabidiol for neuropathic pain associated with multiple sclerosis: an uncontrolled, open-label, 2-year extension trial. *Clin Ther*, Sep, **29**(9), 2068–79.

189 Mercadante S (1999). Problems of long-term spinal opioid treatment in advanced cancer patients. *Pain*, Jan, **79**(1), 1–13.

190 Uhle EI, Becker R, Gatscher S, et al. (2000). Continuous intrathecal clonidine administration for the treatment of neuropathic pain. *Stereotact Funct Neurosurg*, **75**(4), 167–75.

191 Stein C, Machelska H, Schafer M (2001). Peripheral analgesic and antiinflammatory effects of opioids. *Z Rheumatol*, Dec, **60**(6), 416–24.

192 Twillman RK, Long TD, Cathers TA, et al. (1999). Treatment of painful skin ulcers with topical opioids. *J Pain Symp Manag*, Apr, **17**(4), 288–92.

193 Back IN, Finlay I (1995). Analgesic effect of topical opioids on painful skin ulcers. *J Pain Symp Manag*, Oct, **10**(7), 493.

194 Moore RA, Tramer MR, Carroll D, et al. (1998). Quantitative systematic review of topically applied non-steroidal anti-inflammatory drugs. *BMJ*, Jan, 31, **316**(7128), 333–8.

195 Zhang WY, Li Wan PA (1994). The effectiveness of topically applied capsaicin. A meta-analysis. *Eur J Clin Pharmacol*, **46**(6), 517–22.

196 Mercadante S, Villari P, Ferrera P, et al. (2007). Transmucosal fentanyl vs intravenous morphine in doses proportional to basal opioid regimen for episodic-breakthrough pain. *Brit J Cancer*, Jun, 18, **96**(12), 1828–33.

197 Striebel H, Kr+ñmer J, Luhmann I, et al. (1993). Pharmakokinetische Studie zur intranasalen Gabe von Fentanyl. *Der Schmerz*, Jun, 1, **7**(2), 122–5.

198 Schwagmeier R, Boerger N, Meissner W, et al. (1995). Pharmacokinetics of intranasal alfentanil. *J Clin Anaesth*, Mar, **7**(2), 109–13.

199 Duncan A (2002). The use of fentanyl and alfentanil sprays for episodic pain. *Palliat Med*, Oct, **16**(6), 550.

200 McQuay HJ, Tramer M, Nye BA, et al. (1996). A systematic review of antidepressants in neuropathic pain. *Pain*, Dec, **68**(2–3), 217–27.

201 Wiffen PA, Collins S, McQuay H, et al. (2000). Anticonvulsant drugs for acute and chronic pain. *Cochrane Database Syst Rev*, 2, CD001133.

202 Perakyla A (1991). Hope work in the care of seriously ill patients. *Qualitat Health Res*, **1**(4), 407–33.

203 Wiffen PA (2000). CSMHea. Anticonvulsant drugs for acute and chronic pain. *Cochrane Database Syst Rev*, 2.

204 Fallon MT, Welsh J (1996). The role of ketamine in pain control. *Eur J Palliat Care*, **3**, 143–6.

205 Oye I (1998). Ketamine analgesia, NMDA receptors and the gates of perception. *Acta Anaesthesiol Scand*, Aug, **42**(7), 747–9.

206 Sindrup SH, Jensen TS (2002). Pharmacotherapy of trigeminal neuralgia. *Clin J Pain*, Jan, **18**(1), 22–7.

207 Young RR, Delwaide PJ (1981). Drug therapy: spasticity (second of two parts). *N Engl J Med*, Jan, 8, **304**(2), 96–9.

208 Groves L, Shellenberger MK, Davis CS (1998). Tizanidine treatment of spasticity: a meta-analysis of controlled, double-blind, comparative studies with baclofen and diazepam. *Adv Ther*, Jul, **15**(4), 241–51.

209 Hetherington JW, Philp NH (1986). Diclofenac sodium versus pethidine in acute renal colic. *Brit Med J (Clin Res Ed)*, Jan, 25, **292**(6515), 237–8.

210 Oosterlinck W, Philp NH, Charig C, et al. (1990). A double-blind single dose comparison of intramuscular ketorolac tromethamine and pethidine in the treatment of renal colic. *J Clin Pharmacol*, **30**(4), 336–41.

211 Mystakidou K, Tsilika E, Kalaidopoulou O, et al. (2002). Comparison of octreotide administration vs conservative treatment in the management of inoperable bowel obstruction in patients with far advanced cancer: a randomized, double-blind, controlled clinical trial. *Anticancer Res*, Mar, **22**(2B), 1187–92.

212 Ventafridda V, Ripamonti C, Caraceni A, et al. (1990). The management of inoperable gastrointestinal obstruction in terminal cancer patients. *Tumori*, Aug, 31, **76**(4), 389–93.

213 Hellstrom K, Rosen A, Soderlund K (1970). The gastrointestinal absorption and the excretion of H3-butylscopamine (hyoscine butylbromide) in man. *Scand J Gastroenterol*, **5**(7), 585–92.

214 Mercadante S, Ripamonti C, Casuccio A, et al. (2000). Comparison of octreotide and hyoscine butylbromide in controlling gastrointestinal symptoms due to malignant inoperable bowel obstruction. *Support Care Cancer*, May, **8**(3), 188–91.

215 Critchley P, Plach N, Grantham M, et al. (2001). Efficacy of haloperidol in the treatment of nausea and vomiting in the palliative patient: a systematic review. *J Pain Symp Manag*, Aug, **22**(2), 631–4.

216 Pinder RM, Brogden RN, Sawyer PR, et al. (1976). Metoclopramide: a review of its pharmacological properties and clinical use. *Drugs*, **12**(2), 81–131.

217 Dundee JW, Loan WB, Morrison JD (1975). A comparison of the efficacy of cyclizine and perhenazine in reducing the emetic effects of morphine and pethidine. *Brit J Clin Pharmacol*, Feb, **2**(1), 81–5.

218 Davis MP, Walsh D (2000). Treatment of nausea and vomiting in advanced cancer. *Support Care Cancer*, Nov, **8**(6), 444–52.

219 Pakes GE (1982). Haloperidol: pharmacokinetic properties, in Johnson P (ed.) *Haloperidol decanoate in the treatment of chronic schizophrenia*, pp. 41–7. New York, Adis Press.

220 Shader RI, Dimascio A (1970). *Psychotropic drugs side effects: chemical and theoretical perspectives.* Baltimore: Williams and Wilkins,

221 Pisani F, Oteri G, Costa C, et al. (2002). Effects of psychotropic drugs on seizure threshold. *Drug Saf*, **25**(2), 91–110.

222 Metzger E, Friedman R (1993). Prolongation of the corrected QT and torsades de pointes cardiac arrhythmia associated with intravenous haloperidol in the medically ill. *J Clin Psychopharmacol*, Apr, **13**(2), 128–32.

223 Di Salvo TG, O'Gara PT (1995). Torsade de pointes caused by high-dose intravenous haloperidol in cardiac patients. *Clin Cardiol*, May, **18**(5), 285–90.

224 DH Renal NSF team and Marie Curie Palliative Care Institute (2008). Guidelines for Liverpool Care Pathway prescribing in advanced kidney disease. National LCP Renal Steering Group 2008 January 5 [cited 2008 Dec 22];

225 Harrington RA, Hamilton CW, Brogden RN, et al. (1983). Metoclopramide. An updated review of its pharmacological properties and clinical use. *Drugs*, May, **25**(5), 451–94.

226 Bateman DN, Gokal R, Dodd TR, et al. (1981). The pharmacokinetics of single doses of metoclopramide in renal failure. *Eur J Clin Pharmacol*, **19**(6), 437–41.

227 Marty M, Pouillart P, Scholl S, et al. (1990). Comparison of the 5-hydroxytryptamine3 (serotonin) antagonist ondansetron (GR 38032F) with high-dose metoclopramide in the control of cisplatin-induced emesis. *N Engl J Med*, Mar, 22, **322**(12), 816–21.

228 Baber N, Palmer JL, Frazer NM, et al. (1992). Clinical pharmacology of ondansetron in postoperative nausea and vomiting. *Eur J Anaesthesiol Suppl*, Nov, **6**, 11–18.

229 Priestman TJ (1989). Clinical studies with ondansetron in the control of radiation-induced emesis. *Eur J Cancer Clin Oncol*, **25** Suppl 1, S29–33.

230 Roberts JT, Priestman TJ (1993). A review of ondansetron in the management of radiotherapy-induced emesis. *Oncology*, May, **50**(3), 173–9.

231 Wilde MI, Markham A (1996). Ondansetron. A review of its pharmacology and preliminary clinical findings in novel applications. *Drugs*, Nov, **52**(5), 773–94.

232 Balaskas EV, Bamihas GI, Karamouzis M, et al. (1998). Histamine and serotonin in uremic pruritus: effect of ondansetron in CAPD-pruritic patients. *Nephron*, **78**(4), 395–402.

233 Ashmore SD, Jones CH, Newstead CG, et al. (2000). Ondansetron therapy for uremic pruritus in hemodialysis patients. *Am J Kidney Dis*, May, **35**(5), 827–31.

234 Twycross RG, Barkby GD, Hallwood PM (1997). The use of low dose levomepromazine in the management of nausea and vomiting. *Prog Palliative Care*, **5**, 49–53.

235 Thomas J, Karver S, Gooney GA, et al. (2008). Methylnaltrexone for opioid induced constipation in advanced illness. *N Engl J Med*, May 29, **358**(22), 2332–43.

236 Melzack R, Wall PD (1965). Pain mechanisms: a new theory. *Science*, Nov, 19, **150**(699), 971–9.

237 Rushton DN (2002). Electrical stimulation in the treatment of pain. *Disabil Rehabil*, May, 20, **24**(8), 407–15.

238 Brosseau L, Milne S, Robinson V, et al. (2002). Efficacy of the transcutaneous electrical nerve stimulation for the treatment of chronic low back pain: a meta-analysis. *Spine*, Mar, 15, **27**(6), 596–603.

239 Johnson MI, Ashton CH, Thompson JW (1992). Long term use of transcutaneous electrical nerve stimulation at Newcastle Pain Relief Clinic. *J R Soc Med*, May, **85**(5), 267–8.

240 Linde K, Vickers A, Hondras M, et al. (2001). Systematic reviews of complementary therapies - an annotated bibliography. Part 1: acupuncture. *BMC Complement Altern Med*, **1**, 3.

241 Kaptchuk TJ (2002). Acupuncture: theory, efficacy, and practice. *Ann Intern Med*, Mar, 5, **136**(5), 374–83.

242 Furlan AD, Brosseau L, Imamura M, et al. (2002). Massage for low back pain. *Cochrane Database Syst Rev*, 2, CD001929.

243 Little P, Lewith G, Webley F, et al. (2008). Randomised controlled trial of Alexander technique lessons, exercise, and massage (ATEAM) for chronic and recurrent back pain. *Brit J Sports Med*, Dec, **42**(12), 965–8.

244 UK BEAM Trial Team United Kingdom back pain exercise and manipulation (UK BEAM) randomised trial: cost effectiveness of physical treatments for back pain in primary care (2004). *BMJ*, Dec, 11, **329**(7479), 1381.

245 Eccleston C (2001). Role of psychology in pain management. *Brit J Anaesth*, Jul, **87**(1), 144–52.

246 Wuerth D, Finkelstein SH, Ciarcia J, et al. (2001). Identification and treatment of depression in a cohort of patients maintained on chronic peritoneal dialysis. *Am J Kidney Dis*, May, **37**(5), 1011–17.

247 Kimmel PL (2001). Psychosocial factors in dialysis patients. *Kidney Int*, **59**(4), 1599–613.

248 Steinman TI (2000). Pain management in polycystic kidney disease. *Am J Kidney Dis*, Apr, **35**(4), 770–2.

249 Gabow PA (1990). Autosomal dominant polycystic kidney disease–more than a renal disease. *Am J Kidney Dis*, Nov, **16**(5), 403–13.

250 Bajwa ZH, Gupta S, Warfield CA, et al. (2001). Pain management in polycystic kidney disease. *Kidney Int*, Nov, **60**(5), 1631–44.

251 Meglio M, Cioni B, Rossi GF (1989). Spinal cord stimulation in management of chronic pain. A 9-year experience. *J Neurosurg*, Apr, **70**(4), 519–24.

252 Staats PS (1999). Neuraxial infusion for pain control: when, why, and what to do after the implant. *Oncology* (Williston Park), May, **13**(5 Suppl 2), 58–62.

253 Soravia C, Mentha G, Giostra E, et al. (1995). Surgery for adult polycystic liver disease. *Surgery*, Mar, **117**(3), 272–5.

254 Swenson K, Seu P, Kinkhabwala M, et al. (1998). Liver transplantation for adult polycystic liver disease. *Hepatology*, Aug, **28**(2), 412–15.

255 Wilmer WA, Magro CM (2002). Calciphylaxis: emerging concepts in prevention, diagnosis, and treatment. *Semin Dial*, May, **15**(3), 172–86.

256 Mathur RV, Shortland JR, el-Nahas AM (2001). Calciphylaxis. *Postgrad Med J*, Sep, **77**(911), 557–61.

257 Fine A, Zacharias J (2002). Calciphylaxis is usually non-ulcerating: risk factors, outcome and therapy. *Kidney Int*, Jun, **61**(6), 2210–7.

258 Green JA, Green CR, Minott SD (2000). Calciphylaxis treated with neurolytic lumbar sympathetic block: case report and review of the literature. *Reg Anesth Pain Med*, May, **25**(3), 310–12.

259 Wilmer WA, Voroshilova O, Singh I, et al. (2001). Transcutaneous oxygen tension in patients with calciphylaxis. *Am J Kidney Dis*, Apr, **37**(4), 797–806.

260 Morbidity and Mortality Weekly Report Centers for Disease Control and Prevention. Public Health Dispatch: Fibrosing Skin Condition Among Patients with Renal Disease – United States and Europe, 1997–2002. Morbidity and Mortality Weekly Report 2002 Jan, **185**1(2), 25–26. Available from: http://www.cdc.gov/mmwr/preview/mmwrhtml/mm5102a1.htm

261 Grobner T, Prischl FC (2007). Gadolinium and nephrogenic systemic fibrosis. *Kidney Int*, Aug, **72**(3), 260–4.

262 Introcaso CE, Hivnor C, Cowper S, et al. (2007). Nephrogenic fibrosing dermopathy/nephrogenic systemic fibrosis: a case series of nine patients and review of the literature. *Int J Dermatol*, May, **46**(5), 447–52.

263 Cowper SE, Su LD, Bhawan J, et al. (2001). Nephrogenic fibrosing dermopathy. *Am J Dermatopathol*, Oct, **23**(5), 383–93.

264 Marckmann P, Skov L, Rossen K, et al. (2006). Nephrogenic systemic fibrosis: suspected causative role of gadodiamide used for contrast-enhanced magnetic resonance imaging. *J Am Soc Nephrol*, Sep, **17**(9), 2359–62.

265 Dean M (2004). Opioids in renal failure and dialysis patients. *J Pain Symp Manag*, **28**(5), 497–504.

266 Davison SN (2007). The prevalence and management of chronic pain in end stage renal disease. *J Palliat Med*, **10**(6), 1277–87.

267 Murtagh Fe CMDP (2007). The use of opioid analgesia in end-stage renal disease patients managed without dialysis: Recommendations for practice. *J Pain Palliat Care Pharmacotherap*, **21**(2), 5–16.

Chapter 9

Psychological and psychiatric considerations in patients with advanced renal disease

Daniel Cukor, Eileen M Farrell, Lewis M Cohen, and Paul L Kimmel

9.1 Introduction

The goal of this chapter is to outline the major psychological reactions to a chronic condition such as end-stage renal disease (ESRD), to suggest an approach to provide optimum holistic patient care, and to summarize treatment issues in the management of common co-morbid psychiatric disorders in patients with kidney disease.

9.2 In-depth case report

Mr. James[#] had recently transferred into the haemodialysis (HD) centre. He was a 55-year-old, black man who had had diabetes and hypertension for most of his adult life. He was moderately obese and was started on dialysis about 2 years ago. Mr. James had been employed as an airport security officer for over 20 years and took great pride in his job. When he first began dialysis he attempted to keep working, but after a year, he went on disability due to fatigue. Mr. James was married for the second time, and he had enjoyed a meaningful and romantic relationship with his wife. He had two adult children who lived in another city, and he enjoyed a comfortable but somewhat distant relationship with them. His social network was primarily comprised of people who he knew through his job at the airport.

Mr. James had been doing well on haemodialysis, attending all of his appointments, and eating appropriately. He had been receiving haemodialysis near his job site, but switched to a unit which was closer to his home. At his initial psychosocial evaluation by the social worker, he denied any psychiatric history or past substance abuse. He acknowledged that his life had changed significantly over the past year but denied any major problems. The nutritionist was concerned over an apparent change in Mr. James's interdialytic weight gain. His previous haemodialysis center had reported him to typically be within the desired range, but he was currently regularly overweight. The nurses noted that Mr. James's wife had visited him during his haemodialysis treatment, often bringing him a healthy home-cooked meal to enjoy after his long day at work. Recently, however, his wife was seldom seen around the dialysis center. At team rounds the nephrologist commented that she was concerned by Mr. James's slowly increasing blood pressure, and the team concluded a behavioural consultation was warranted.

[#] This case is an amalgam of several cases, and the names have been changed, to protect confidentiality.

The psychologist evaluated Mr. James with a focus on understanding the changes he had undergone in the past year and how they may have affected his mood and health. Mr. James had been functioning quite well before stopping work, and then the events of the last year lead to increasing depression and poorer health. Mr. James reported that ever since he began dialysis he had been experiencing erectile difficulty. He was unable to discuss this with his wife, whom he viewed as being disappointed in their lack of sexual activity. In an effort to avoid the nightly reminder of his impotence, Mr. James had begun to fall asleep watching television on the couch and would only return to his bed long after his wife was asleep. He awakened early in the morning, but did not feel refreshed. In conversation, Mr. James would persistently highlight his wife's younger age and his belief that she had not expected to care for him and his ailing health so soon after their marriage. Mr. James' change in sleep pattern allowed him to avoid his wife's company in the evening and also caused him to be somnolent during the day. He felt that his inability 'to be a man' represented a catastrophic loss both for him and his wife. This burden coupled with his daytime tiredness was more than he could bear while working, and he decided to stop his job. This decision further pushed Mr. James towards clinical depression, as he was now isolated from the majority of his social network. As opposed to his previous attitude that he could handle any of life's problems with a smile, he now felt that his problems were compounding so quickly that he was going to buckle under the load. The change in his economic situation forced his wife to return to work, something she had not done in the 10 years of their marriage. Mr. James felt further humiliated by his need to accept his wife's earnings. He had almost no daily activities except for medical appointments. He made no effort to help around the home during the day, and his irregular schedule led to him often skipping medication doses and eating poorly. His wife, who was now exhausted from work and disappointed in his lack of contribution around the home, made no effort to hide her frustration. The more she displayed her irritation, the more Mr. James felt paralysed by his unchangeable predicament.

A multidisciplinary conference was convened. The psychologist proposed a biopsychosocial formulation of Mr. James's situation and a corresponding treatment plan was developed collaboratively with him. The first part of the interventional plan was to have a joint session with Mr. James's wife to review the conceptualization. Mrs. James was quiet throughout the discussion of the proposed chain of events and at the end commented that she was surprised at how 'proud and stupid' her husband appeared to be. She agreed with much of the sequence of events but denied any resentment of the predicament – except for his attitude. Her view of the events was that her husband responded to his sexual difficulty with such ferocity that he totally distanced himself emotionally from her. She certainly missed the sexual contact, but missed the intimacy even more. She felt that she could no longer communicate with him, and that she was frustrated by her inability to help him. The session was cathartic for the couple and they both committed to being more open in their communication.

The other parts of the treatment plan were put into action and Mr. James discussed the appropriateness of sildenafil with his nephrologist who prescribed it with the suggestion of using it on non-dialysis days, to reduce the risk of hypotension. A referral to a sleep laboratory was initiated after the patient agreed to evaluation. Mr. James also began 'behavioural activation' – a series of exercises to get him to reengage in pleasurable activities despite his lack of desire. Particular attention was given to getting Mr. James to reconnect with his work friends. Simultaneously, Mr. James's beliefs about what it means to 'be a man' were challenged. After some time, he was able to redefine his role from being a 'provider' to that of a 'partner'. He no longer felt the need to be the one to meet his wife's needs, but was able to accept that his role might be to help her facilitate meeting those needs. Furthermore, he expanded his understanding of what a husband provides a wife beyond sex and money to include intimacy and support.

Following 6 months of treatment, Mr. James was enjoying a new modified lifestyle with his wife and friends that provided him with satisfaction and fulfillment. The sleep evaluation did not show evidence of sleep apnoea. It was concluded that any sleep disturbance he had could be associated with anxiety or depression. Through the use of sildenafil, he successfully reintroduced sex into his marriage. There were still days when Mrs. James would return from work feeling frustrated and resentful, but her mood was quickly tempered by the home-cooked meal and relaxing environment at home. Mr. James's medication and diet compliance improved and he began to feel better emotionally and physically.

9.3 Co-morbid mental health issues

There are a number of psychiatric disorders that can either develop or manifest during the course of chronic kidney disease (CKD) and dialysis treatment. Nephrologists frequently serve the mental health requirements of this population as well as coordinate primary and other secondary care in addition to their specialist role. There is growing evidence and recognition that to provide comprehensive care to CKD patients, focus must be directed towards their emotional state. In addition to the burden that each of these mental health issues places upon patients and their families, they may also complicate the medical course and require clinical attention.

9.3.1 Depression

9.3.1.1 Definition

Depression is considered to be the most common psychiatric complication of ESRD. In general terms, depression is defined as a mood state characterized by a sense of sadness with related emotional, cognitive, and behavioural symptoms. These will differ with each individual but may include any or all of the following: anhedonia, sleep disturbances, fatigue, appetite changes, neurocognitive slowing, feelings of worthlessness, morbid thoughts, and possibly (though not necessarily) suicidal ideation and attempts. New cases of depression in ESRD patients can be conceptualized as reactive, in direct response to a change in the environment, especially if the patient has no history of prior depression.[1,2] Depression may take many forms and presentations depending on factors such as inherited susceptibility, social connectedness, personal reserves, and co-morbid conditions such as anxiety. It is often helpful to interview both the patient and family members, to obtain their perspective on the course of the illness.[3]

9.3.1.2 Prevalence/incidence

Depression can be difficult to accurately identify in ESRD populations due to the overlap of its core criteria with the symptoms produced by uraemia, progressive medical illness, and medication side effects.[1] Depression can be identified through clinical interview, self-report measures, or structured clinical interviews. The range of screening instruments used in ESRD populations includes the Beck Depression Inventory,[4] the Cognitive Depression Index,[5] the Hamilton Rating Scale for Depression,[6] the Zung Self-Rating Depression Scale,[7] the Short Form (SF-36) Health Survey,[8] the Center for Epidemiological Studies Depression Scale,[9] and items from the Kidney Disease Quality of Life Measure.[10] Structured interview instruments include the Diagnostic Interview Schedule,[11] Semi-structured Clinical Interview for the DSM-IV,[12] and the Patient Health Questionnaire.[13] Despite the different methods of assessment and the great diversity in ESRD populations, rough estimates suggest 10–20% of prevalent patients may have a diagnosable major depression,[14–16] and upwards of 30–40% may have significantly elevated levels of depressive affect.[1,16] There is also indication that depression may be a chronic, not just a transient state, for a sizable minority of patients. [17,18]

Suicidal ideation is one of the criteria for major affective disorders, and early findings of high suicide rates in dialysis patients were overestimates due to sampling bias and reaction to the then inferior and arduous dialytic delivery techniques. More recent studies show suicide to be less prevalent in contemporary ESRD populations, although the rate is still modestly higher than in the general population.[19–21] Alcohol dependence and hospitalization for substance abuse and mental illness were strongly associated with subsequent suicide, highlighting the difference between those that commit active suicide and populations that withdraw from treatment.[21] Although depression should be ruled out, it should not be assumed to be the underlying cause when a patient makes a request to withdraw from treatment.[19] Estimates indicate that approximately 20% of United States (US) dialysis patients voluntarily choose to discontinue ESRD therapy.[20–24] Age, medical complications, and failure to thrive are commonly associated with the decision to withdraw from ESRD therapy. (See Chapter 12 for a full discussion of withdrawing from dialysis.)

9.3.1.3 Treatment

Effective interventions will support individuals through the period of depression, helping them to regain a sense of well-being and optimism as well as giving them the ability to address the rigours of treatment and the life changes entailed by the condition. Treatment for depression may take the form of psychotherapy, antidepressive medication, or a combination of both. Although there have yet to be randomized clinical trials supporting the role of psychotherapeutic intervention,[25] preliminary evidence on this topic is encouraging.[26]

Although there is limited evidence for the effectiveness of psychotropic medications in ESRD populations, early evidence of antidepressant therapy shows both selective serotonin-re-uptake inhibitors (SSRIs) and tricyclic antidepressants (TCAs) to be beneficial.[27,28] Although the greatest body of experience is on the TCAs, these have largely been supplanted by the newer generation of antidepressants. Tricyclic antidepressants ought to be reserved for CKD patients with treatment-resistant depression, or for other indications, such as painful peripheral neuropathy. The hydroxylated metabolites of TCAs contribute to both therapeutic and toxic effects in ESRD. In psychiatric populations, imipramine and amitriptyline continue to be used for analgesia in neuropathic pain, while trazodone is commonly used in low doses as a sedative–hypnotic for patients with insomnia.

SSRIs are often used in ESRD, but have not been systematically or adequately studied. Fluoxetine is the best-studied medication in this class, and appears to be both non-toxic and efficacious.[29] The kinetic profile of single doses of fluoxetine is unchanged even in anephric patients. A study of multiple doses concluded that renal function does not significantly alter either fluoxetine or norfluoxetine serum levels.[28] Sertraline has not been as intensively studied in this population, but it is also widely prescribed. Like fluoxetine, it is metabolized in the liver, and excretion of the unchanged drug in urine is an insignificant route of elimination. Pharmacokinetic investigations in people with mild to severe renal impairment and matched controls show no significant differences.[30] Sertraline has been used to ameliorate sudden haemodialysis-related hypotension.[31] Like sertraline and fluoxetine, venlafaxine kinetics are minimally changed in patients with ESRD and dose-adjustment is probably not necessary.[32] Interestingly, plasma concentrations of paroxetine hydrochloride are increased in people with renal impairment, and the recommended initial dose for patients with severe renal insufficiency is one-half to one-third that of normal adults. A general guideline for treatment of depression in CKD patients is 'start low and go slow'.[33] The careful nephrologist may start with less than the recommended starting dose of an SSRI, and advance dose increases over a prolonged test period.

There are several non-SSRI antidepressant medications that should be used with caution or avoided.[27] For example, little is known about the pharmacokinetics of nefazodone hydrochloride in patients who have chronically impaired renal function. Careful dose-adjustment is also necessary with venlafaxine, which is chiefly eliminated in urine along with its metabolites.[27] Its elimination half-life is prolonged and clearance is reduced in people who have chronic renal insufficiency or ESRD. Regular monitoring of blood pressure is recommended for those taking this drug. Bupropion hydrochloride has active metabolites, which are almost completely excreted by the kidney. These metabolites may accumulate in dialysis patients and predispose to seizures. Care must be taken with patients receiving concurrent drugs metabolized by the cytochrome P-450 3A4 system (e.g. tacrolimus, cyclosporin, sildenafil) when using antidepressants which are inhibitors of this isoenzyme. These inhibitors include nefazodone, fluoxetine/norfluoxetine, fluvoxamine, paroxetine (a weak inhibitor), sertraline, and valproic acid (a weak inhibitor).

For many years, lithium has been the primary pharmacological treatment of bipolar affective disorder. It has efficacy in acute episodes and in prevention of relapses. It is being replaced by classic anticonvulsant medications, such as depakote, carbamazepine, and gabapentin, which also significantly help patients with bipolar depression. There are a small number of bipolar patients with ESRD who require lithium (and do not respond to the anticonvulsants). In these cases, treatment involves administration of a single dose (usually 600 mg) after each dialysis treatment. Because it is a small molecule, lithium is readily cleared by dialysis. A single dose given over time will result in a steady serum level.[34] Monitoring lithium levels is essential when treating patients with bipolar disorder and CKD or ESRD. Serum lithium levels obtained before and after dialysis sessions are used to establish the therapeutic dose. Ideally, these levels should be obtained immediately before dialysis and 2 h after its completion. The level obtained immediately after dialysis will often be lower than that observed later due to a post-dialysis redistribution effect. A smaller dose may be given to augment its therapeutic effect in patients with treatment-resistant unipolar depression. Lithium can be nephrotoxic, especially when taken over a period of years. Efforts should be made to substitute other drugs in patients with renal insufficiency. A long-term follow-up study has found that when the drug is discontinued, renal function may sometimes improve.[35]

9.3.2 Anxiety Disorders

9.3.2.1 Definition

Anxiety is probably the most common and pervasive emotion of people who receive hospital treatment. Renal patients are concerned about the severity and variation in their symptoms, and the restrictions the condition imposes on their lives and plans for their future. They worry about what the treatment will be like, the degree to which it will be successful, and their ability to manage its complexities. ESRD patients worry about untimely or approaching death and such concerns can pervade all aspects of their life. Excessive anxiety, like depression, often goes unrecognized and often requires treatment. In current psychiatric nosology, there are a variety of disorders that are characterized by overarching anxiety and stress, including generalized anxiety disorder, panic disorder, phobias, social anxiety, obsessive compulsive disorder, and post-traumatic stress disorder.[2] Anxiety disorders can be diagnosed by the same measures used to diagnose depression. Self-reported anxiety can be measured by the Beck Anxiety Inventory,[36] the Hamilton Anxiety Scale,[37] the Hospital Anxiety and Depression Scale,[38] and the Spielberger State Trait Anxiety Inventory.[39]

9.3.2.2 Prevalence/incidence

It is likely that the majority of dialysis patients experience episodes of anxiety and stress at some stage in their treatment and that some patients will experience these conditions throughout their life. Some studies[40] report that about one-third of patients experience episodes of moderate anxiety in their first year of treatment. One recent study[41] assessed psychiatric diagnoses in a sample of 70 predominately black ESRD patients and found that about 45% had at least one anxiety disorder. The most common diagnoses identified were phobias and panic disorder. The prevalence of panic disorder was much higher than community samples and may be related to hypervigilance to the bodily sensations associated with haemodialysis.

9.3.2.3 Treatment

There is a sizable shortage of literature relating to the psychological treatment of anxiety in patients with ESRD, with many of the reported studies being descriptive in nature. This reflects the general lack of psychological care in renal units and the statistically insignificant numbers that have been recorded in individual studies.

Optimum interventions should aim to reduce the stress associated with ESRD and increase patients' coping abilities. System-wide intervention should include provision of training at pre-dialysis clinics, facilitated interaction with other patients, and the inclusion of a partner/significant other in training and/or treatment sessions. An open relationship with the nephrologist and the dialysis clinic social worker is essential in allaying the patients' concerns. There are no clinical trials of psychotherapeutic intervention in ESRD samples, but there is a substantial literature highlighting the efficacy of cognitive behavioural interventions in treating the full gamut of anxiety disorders in other populations.[42] Aerobic exercise training, mental imagery, and social support enrichment are also thought to be useful techniques for managing the anxiety/stress experience.

Pharmacological management is typically either directed at acute episodes of anxiety and panic, or at more generalized nervousness.[27] Since benzodiazepines are metabolized in the liver, dosage-reduction is generally not necessary in ESRD, but it is prudent to use the lowest effective doses in such patients to minimize adverse effects. Exceptions include midazolam and chlordiazepoxide. SSRIs are being used increasingly to treat anxiety disorders.[43]

9.3.3 Cognitive ability

Research over the last 30 years relating to the effects of uraemia on the central nervous system has shown deficits in concentration, alertness, flexibility in thinking, and decreased speed of mental processing.[44,45] Patients with CKD frequently manifest neurological symptoms even when they are considered adequately dialysed. For patients aged over 65 years who are maintained with dialysis, organic brain syndromes are a leading cause of hospitalization.[46] As renal function worsens, it is increasingly likely that subtle or overt neurological symptoms will occur. Overall, there is evidence that cognitive dysfunction is prevalent in CKD patients[47] and that stage of disease may be an important predictor of the stage of cognitive decline. However, the course of the cognitive impairment[48] and the specific cognitive domains that are affected by CKD are less clear. The causes of the cognitive impairment may be multifaceted, as various consequences of renal disease can contribute to cognitive decline. Haemodialysis patients are often older, and are therefore at greater risk for cognitive difficulties. Uraemia itself has been associated with a reduction in concentration, memory impairment, and intellectual functioning.[49–51] Another risk factor for compromised cognitive functioning in renal patients is the occurrence of anaemia. [44] Reduced oxygen availability may result in decreased cognitive function, especially in patients with other forms of neurological or cerebrovascular diseases.[52]

9.4 **Social support**

Social support plays an integral role in health outcomes for ESRD patients, potentially impacting access to healthcare, treatment compliance, and psychological symptoms. Social support refers to a social network's provision of psychological and material resources intended to augment an individual's ability to cope with stress.[20,53–55] ESRD patients can receive social support from family, friends, and individuals on the dialysis unit (e.g. physicians, social workers, nurses, other patients). Increased levels of social support may positively impact outcomes by different mechanisms, including decreased levels of depressive affect, increased patient perception of quality of life, increased access to healthcare, increased patient compliance with prescribed therapies, and physiological effects on the immune system.[56]

Higher levels of perceived social support are thought to have a positive influence on health outcomes, utilization of healthcare services, and compliance. Previous research has demonstrated that social support is related to improved health outcomes and lower mortality for ESRD patients.[56–60] Social support, measured by quality of life[58] and family cohesion[61] has predicted survival in haemodialysis patients. In addition, level of social support experienced by an ESRD patient may play a role in utilizing healthcare services.[53,57,62] Previous research on ESRD patients indicates that social support may influence compliance with haemodialysis treatment.[57,61,62]

Patients receiving haemodialysis treatment spend a substantial amount of time every week at their dialysis units. The patient may form relationships with staff members, physicians, and haemodialysis patients. Research has suggested patients' increased satisfaction with the staff was related to better dietary compliance and increased satisfaction with physicians was associated with attendance and compliance.[63] It is possible that the culture and relationships of the dialysis unit may mediate outcomes in treatment outcomes. However, there are little data on the relationships between social support and these outcomes.

Social support has also been shown to improve psychological symptoms. Previous research has found a relationship of indices of social support and level of depressive symptoms, perception of illness effects, and satisfaction with life.[57,60,64–67] A recent study found that social support may alleviate psychological stressors caused by ESRD in peritoneal dialysis patients, such as worry about health.[68] Social support may act as a buffer for psychological symptoms for ESRD patients: psychological symptoms (e.g. depressive symptoms) may impact health or treatment outcomes; however, social support may mediate this relationship.

Marital and family relationships may influence levels of social support in ESRD patients. Perceptions of marital strain and psychological distress have been found to be related for dialysis patients and their spouses.[69] Previous research has found a relationship of spousal perceptions and social support,[69] as well as an association of spousal levels of depression and level of depression for patients receiving haemodialysis treatment.[70] When considering familial support beyond a marital dyad, family structures that include relatives and non-relatives living together were associated with increased risk of mortality.[71] It is important to consider the relationships of the source of social support and ESRD patient outcomes, particularly since social support may be seen as a modifiable risk factor.

9.5 **Sexual dysfunction**

Despite claims that the majority of patients on dialysis experience diminished frequency of or interest in sex, and the number of references to it in the renal literature suggesting that this is a major concern for most patients, the issue of sexual activity is oft not widely discussed between patients and care staff. Levy, e.g. observed that approximately 70% of men in the first generation of patients to receive dialysis had partial or total impotence, and the majority of women were amenorrhoeic or infertile.[72] More recently, Abdel-Kader and associates reported that 43% of a sample of patients with ESRD endorsed having a decreased interest in sex and 47% complained of trouble getting aroused.[73] Palmer noted similarly high rates of sexual dysfunction in men and women with ESRD.[74] There appears to be growing evidence that sildenafil can be used safely in ESRD patients.[74,75] One study found that about 85% of haemodialysis patients benefited from sildenafil, with only mild side effects reported.[76] The subject of sexual performance is complex with cultural, age, gender, racial, religious, and emotional factors to consider before including the impact of any physical disability.

9.6 Health disparities

There are racial, ethnic, and socioeconomic disparities for ESRD patients in disease incidence, access to healthcare, treatment, and survival.[77] Socioeconomic factors, such as low income, low levels of educational achievement, residence in low-income areas, and limitations in access to healthcare have been found to be strong predictors of the development of ESRD.[77] Socioeconomic status has been shown to have a significant impact on the incidence and treatment of ESRD.[78,79] Furthermore, there are racial disparities amongst which ESRD patients receive kidney transplantation, the optimal treatment method. According to recent data, of transplant waiting-list patients, 67% of patients who received living donor transplants were white, compared to 13% black patients and 13.6% Hispanic patients in July 2007 to July 2008 (Scientific Registry of Transplant Recipients, updated 1/13/09). For deceased donor transplants, 47% of patients who received transplants were white, compared to 31% black patients and 15% Hispanic patients (Scientific Registry of Transplant Recipients, updated 1/13/09). A possible explanation for the transplant disparity is the relatively lower organ-donation rates amongst minority communities. The relationships amongst race, socioeconomic status, and ESRD outcomes are complex and may result from synergistic combinations.[66,77]

There is some indication that there is an association between survival and socioeconomic status in ESRD populations, as higher socioeconomic status was associated with improved survival irrespective of race.[80] In addition, higher mortality rates and lower rates of transplantation were found amongst white and black dialysis patients living in communities that were predominately composed of blacks.[81] The reasons for this are unclear, but it is possible that cultural factors play a role in perception of illness, attitudes towards organ donation, and course of treatment for ESRD patients, as has been found in other populations.[82] Culture may also impact lifestyle factors that influence incidence and health outcomes, such as diet or exercise. The web of relationships amongst psychosocial functioning, culture, and socioeconomic status may explain their connection to health outcomes in the ESRD population.[83]

9.7 Adherence

It is also important for patients receiving renal replacement therapies to adhere to prescribed treatment. There are different types of adherence and measurement strategies, that examine medications, diet regimen, fluid intake, exercise, medical appointments, and behaviour (e.g. shortening time receiving dialysis or missing appointments). Previous research has reported that measures of behavioural compliance are clinically meaningful and partially related to more traditional measures of compliance.[57,84] A recent study examined medication adherence in ESRD and found that 37% of the haemodialysis patients reported less than perfect adherence to medication regimen.[85] Another study found that the median daily pill burden of an ESRD cohort was 19, and in one-quarter of the subjects it exceeded 25 pills per day. Phosphate binders accounted for about one-half of the daily pill burden, and 62% of the participants were noncompliant with the prescribed phosphate binder therapy.[86]

Lack of adherence to prescribed immunosuppressive medication leads to higher rates of graft failure and possible kidney rejection.[87] However, the minimum threshold of immunosuppressive medication adherence required to prevent increased risk of rejections has not been defined. Additionally, there is a lack of a standard assessment strategy for measuring medication adherence. Previous studies have used different measures such as blood chemistry, pharmacy and medical records, electronic monitoring (e.g. Medication Event Monitoring System), self-report, and in-office pill counts to assess compliance. Each of these assessment strategies has limitations and a summary measure incorporating a variety of different types of measurement might be best used to approximate true medication adherence.[88]

Non-adherence is related to a lower belief in needing immunosuppressant medication and having a transplant from a live donor for renal transplant recipients.[89] A recent study has also found that depression plays an important role in medication adherence in ESRD patients.[85] The issue of non-adherence among ESRD patients is another reason why it is important to identify patients suffering from depression.

9.8 Conclusion

The effort and psychological stamina required of an ESRD patient are considerable and sometimes little appreciated. The importance of a working partnership between care staff and patient is acknowledged but not always practised. There is an assumption that if patients have the details of their condition and the treatment required they will be able to conform to the medical model of care espoused by most renal teams. Their failure to match this expectation at all times creates difficulties in addition to those they already experience because of the illness. Greater tolerance and flexibility in the treatment may follow from increased understanding of the psychological and psychiatric factors in advanced renal disease.

This was highlighted in the case presentation of Mr. James. The sensitivity of the entire staff to Mr. James' circumstances led to referrals and the implementation of a psychosocially oriented, integrated treatment plan. If medical, nursing, and technical staff are given the encouragement and opportunity to become more familiar with the psychological and psychiatric considerations of their patients then there is every hope that their partnership with patients can become more meaningful and effective.

Ethical case analysis

The case of Mr. James illustrates how sensitive, knowledgeable clinicians working with dialysis patients can markedly improve quality of life. The nephrologist, nurse, and nutritionist all noted the changes in Mr. James's behaviour and appropriately arranged for a psychological evaluation. Well-grounded in the behavioural problems common among dialysis patients, the psychologist proposed an accurate biopsychosocial formulation of Mr. James's situation and a corresponding, effective treatment plan. The net effect of the team intervention is that Mr. James felt better emotionally and physically. What is ethically required of dialysis staff is knowledge of the common psychological problems of dialysis patients and training on how to detect them. As dialysis units become increasingly familiar with providing palliative care, screening of patients for psychosocial and cognitive disorders should become a standard part of orientation and continuing education for dialysis personnel. By including these topics in their educational programme for employees, dialysis units can help to achieve the goal of palliative care which is the best possible quality of life for patients and their families.

References

1 Cukor D, Peterson RA, Cohen SD, et al. (2006). Depression in end-stage renal disease hemodialysis patients. *Nat Clin Pract Nephrol.* Dec, **2**(12), 678–87.

2 Diagnostic and Statistical Manual of Mental Disorders (2000).

3 Cohen LM, Steinberg MD, Hails KC, et al. (2000). Psychiatric evaluation of death-hastening requests. Lessons from dialysis discontinuation. *Psychosomatics.* May–Jun, **41**(3), 195–203.

4 Beck AT, Steer R (1987). *Manual for the Beck Depression Inventory.* San Antonio, TX: The Psychological Corporation.

5 Kimmel PL, Peterson RA (2005). Depression in end-stage renal disease patients treated with hemodialysis: tools, correlates, outcomes, and needs. *Semin Dial,* Mar–Apr, **18**(2), 91–7.

6 Hamilton M (1960). A rating scale for depression. *J Neurol Neurosurg Psychiatry,* Feb, **23**, 56–62.

7 Zung WWK (1965). A self-rating depression scale. *Arch Gen Psychiatry,* **12**, 63–70.

8 Ware JE, Jr., Sherbourne CD (1992). The MOS 36-item short-form health survey (SF-36). I. Conceptual framework and item selection. *Med Care,* Jun, **30**(6), 473–83.

9 Radloff LS (1977). The CES-D scale: A self report depression scale for research in the general population. *App Psychol Measurement,* **1**, 385–401.

10 Hays RD, Kallich JD, Mapes DL, et al. (1997). *Kidney Disease Quality of Life Short Form (KDQOL-SF™), Version 1.3: A manual for use and scoring.* Santa Monica, CA: RAND.

11 Robins LN, Helzer JE, Croughan J, et al. (1981). National Institute of Mental Health Diagnostic Interview Schedule. Its history, characteristics, and validity. *Arch Gen Psychiatry,* Apr, **38**(4), 381–9.

12 First MB, Spitzer RL, Gibbon M, et al. (1996). *Structured clinical interview for DSM-IV Axis I Disorders, Clinician Version.* Washington, DC: American Psychiatric Press.

13 Spitzer RL, Kroenke K, Williams JB (1999). Validation and utility of a self-report version of PRIME-MD: the PHQ primary care study. Primary Care Evaluation of Mental Disorders. Patient Health Questionnaire. *JAMA,* Nov 10, **282**(18), 1737–44.

14 Hedayati SS, Bosworth HB, Kuchibhatla M, et al. (2006). The predictive value of self-report scales compared with physician diagnosis of depression in hemodialysis patients. *Kidney Int,* May, **69**(9),1662–8.

15 Watnick S, Wang PL, Demadura T, et al. (2005). Validation of 2 depression screening tools in dialysis patients. *Am J Kidney Dis,* Nov, **46**(5), 919–24.

16 Craven JL, Rodin GM, Littlefield C (1988). The Beck Depression Inventory as a screening device for major depression in renal dialysis patients. *Int J Psychiatry Med,* **18**(4), 365–74.

17 Kimmel PL, Peterson RA, Weihs KL, et al. (2000). Multiple measurements of depression predict mortality in a longitudinal study of chronic hemodialysis outpatients. *Kidney Int,* May, **57**(5), 2093–8.

18 Cukor D, Coplan J, Brown C, et al. (2008). Course of depression and anxiety diagnosis in patients treated with hemodialysis: a 16-month follow-up. *Clin J Am Soc Nephrol,* Nov, **3**(6), 1752–8.

19 Bostwick JM, Cohen LM (2009). Differentiating suicide from life-ending acts and end-of-life decisions: a model based on chronic kidney disease and dialysis. *Psychosomatics,* Jan–Feb, **50**(1), 1–7.

20 Kimmel PL (2001). Psychosocial factors in dialysis patients. *Kidney Int,* Apr, **59**(4), 1599–613.

21 Kurella M, Kimmel PL, Young BS, et al. (2005). Suicide in the United States end-stage renal disease program. *J Am Soc Nephrol,* Mar, **16**(3), 774–81.

22 Cohen LM, Germain MJ (2005). The psychiatric landscape of withdrawal. *Semin Dial,* Mar–Apr, **18**(2), 147–53.

23 Cohen LM, Germain MJ, Poppel DM (2003). Practical considerations in dialysis withdrawal: "to have that option is a blessing". *JAMA*, Apr 23–30, **289**(16), 2113–19.

24 Murtagh F, Cohen LM, Germain MJ (2007). Dialysis discontinuation: quo vadis? *Adv Chronic Kidney Dis*, Oct, **14**(4), 379–401.

25 Rabindranath KS, Daly C, Butler JA, et al. (2005). Psychosocial interventions for depression in dialysis patients. *Cochrane Database Syst Rev.* (3), CD004542.

26 Cukor D (2007). The hemodialysis center: a model for psychosocial intervention. *Psych Services*, **58**, 711–12.

27 Cohen LM, Tessier EG, Germain MJ, et al. (2004). Update on psychotropic medication use in renal disease. *Psychosomatics*, Jan–Feb, **45**(1), 34–48.

28 Finkelstein FO, Finkelstein SH (2000). Depression in chronic dialysis patients: assessment and treatment. *Nephrol Dial Transplant*, Dec, **15**(12), 1911–13.

29 Blumenfield M, Levy NB, Spinowitz B, et al. (1997). Fluoxetine in depressed patients on dialysis. *Int J Psychiatry Med*, **27**(1), 71–80.

30 Joffe P, Larsen FS, Pedersen V, et al. (1998). Single-dose pharmacokinetics of citalopram in patients with moderate renal insufficiency or hepatic cirrhosis compared with healthy subjects. *Eur J Clin Pharmacol*, May, **54**(3), 237–42.

31 Dheenan S, Venkatesan J, Grubb BP, et al. (1998). Effect of sertraline hydrochloride on dialysis hypotension. *Am J Kidney Dis*, Apr, **31**(4), 624–30.

32 Troy SM, Schultz RW, Parker VD, et al. (1994). The effect of renal disease on the disposition of venlafaxine. *Clin Pharmacol Ther*, Jul, **56**(1), 14–21.

33 Cohen SD, Norris L, Acquaviva K, et al. (2007). Screening, diagnosis, and treatment of depression in patients with end-stage renal disease. *Clin J Am Soc Nephrol*, Nov, **2**(6), 1332–42.

34 Port FK, Kroll PD, Rosenzweig J (1979). Lithium therapy during maintenance hemodialysis. *Psychosomatics*, Feb, **20**(2), 130–2.

35 Braden GL (ed) (2001). *Lithium-induced renal disease*. San Diego,CA: Academic Press.

36 Beck AT, Steer RA (1993). *Beck Anxiety Inventory manual*. San Antonio, TX: Psychological Corporation.

37 Hamilton M (1959). The assessment of anxiety states by rating. *Brit J Med Psychol*, **32**, 50–5.

38 Zigmond AS, Snaith RP (1983). The hospital anxiety and depression scale. *Acta Psychiatr Scand*, Jun, **67**(6), 361–70.

39 Speilberger CD, Gorsuch RL, Lushene RE (1970). *Manual for the State-Trait Anxiety Inventory*. Palo Alto, CA: Consulting Psychologists Press.

40 Nichols KA, Springford V (1984). The psycho-social stressors associated with survival by dialysis. *Behav Res Ther*, **22**(5), 563–74.

41 Cukor D, Coplan J, Brown C, et al. (2008). Anxiety disorders in adults treated by hemodialysis: a single-center study. *Am J Kidney Dis*, Jul, **52**(1), 128–36.

42 Rachman S (2008). Psychological treatment of anxiety: the evolution of behavior therapy and cognitive-behavior therapy. *Ann Rev Clin Psychol*, 97–119.

43 Vaswani M, Linda FK, Ramesh S (2003). Role of selective serotonin reuptake inhibitors in psychiatric disorders: a comprehensive review. *Prog Neuropsychopharmacol Biol Psychiatry*, Feb, **27**(1), 85–102.

44 Pereira AA, Weiner DE, Scott T, et al. (2005). Cognitive function in dialysis patients. *Am J Kidney Dis*, Mar, **45**(3), 448–62.

45 Murray AM (2008). Cognitive impairment in the aging dialysis and chronic kidney disease populations: an occult burden. *Adv Chronic Kidney Dis*, Apr, **15**(2), 123–32.

46 Kimmel PL, Thamer M, Richard CM, et al. (1998). Psychiatric illness in patients with end-stage renal disease. *Am J Med*, Sep, **105**(3), 214–21.

47 Murray AM, Tupper DE, Knopman DS, et al. (2006). Cognitive impairment in hemodialysis patients is common. *Neurology*, Jul 25, **67**(2), 216–23.

48 Murray AM, Pederson SL, Tupper DE, et al. (2007). Acute variation in cognitive function in hemodialysis patients: a cohort study with repeated measures. *Am J Kidney Dis*, Aug, **50**(2), 270–8.

49 Williams MA, Sklar AH, Burright RG, et al. (2004). Temporal effects of dialysis on cognitive functioning in patients with ESRD. *Am J Kidney Dis*, Apr, **43**(4), 705–11.

50 Pliskin NH, Yurk HM, Ho LT, et al. (1996). Neurocognitive function in chronic hemodialysis patients. *Kidney Int*, May, **49**(5), 1435–40.

51 Bae JS, Park SS (2008). Contingent negative variation before and after hemodialysis among patients with end-stage renal disease. *J Neurol Sci*, Apr 15, **267**(1–2), 70–5.

52 Johnson WJ, McCarthy JT, Yanagihara T, et al. (1990). Effects of recombinant human erythropoietin on cerebral and cutaneous blood flow and on blood coagulability. *Kidney Int*, Nov, **38**(5), 919–24.

53 House JS, Landis KR, Umberson D (1988). Social relationships and health. *Science*, Jul 29, **241**(4865), 540–5.

54 House JS (2002). Understanding social factors and inequalities in health: 20th century progress and 21st century prospects. *J Health Soc Behav*, Jun, **43**(2), 125–42.

55 Brissette I, Cohen S, Seeman TE (2000). *Measuring social integration and social networks*. New York: Oxford University Press.

56 Cohen SD, Sharma T, Acquaviva K, et al. (2007). Social support and chronic kidney disease: an update. *Adv Chr Kidney Dis*, Oct, **14**(4), 335–44.

57 Kimmel PL, Peterson RA, Weihs KL, et al. (1998). Psychosocial factors, behavioral compliance and survival in urban hemodialysis patients. *Kidney Int*, Jul, **54**(1), 245–54.

58 Christensen AJ, Wiebe JS, Smith TW, et al. (1994). Predictors of survival among hemodialysis patients: effect of perceived family support. *Health Psychol*, Nov, **13**(6), 521–5.

59 McClellan WM, Anson C, Birkeli K, et al. (1991). Functional status and quality of life: predictors of early mortality among patients entering treatment for end stage renal disease. *J Clin Epidemiol*, **44**(1), 83–9.

60 McClellan WM, Stanwyck DJ, Anson CA (1993). Social support and subsequent mortality among patients with end-stage renal disease. *J Am Soc Nephrol*, Oct, **4**(4), 1028–34.

61 Christensen AJ, Smith TW, Turner CW, et al. (1992). Family support, physical impairment, and adherence in hemodialysis: an investigation of main and buffering effects. *J Behav Med*, Aug, **15**(4), 313–25.

62 Patel SS, Peterson RA, Kimmel PL (2005). The impact of social support on end-stage renal disease. *Semin Dial*, Mar–Apr, **18**(2), 98–102.

63 Kovac JA, Patel SS, Peterson RA, et al. (2002). Patient satisfaction with care and behavioral compliance in end-stage renal disease patients treated with hemodialysis. *Am J Kidney Dis*, Jun, **39**(6), 1236–44.

64 Kimmel PL, Peterson RA, Weihs KL, et al. (1996). Psychologic functioning, quality of life, and behavioral compliance in patients beginning hemodialysis. *J Am Soc Nephrol*, Oct, **7**(10), 2152–9.

65 Kimmel PL, Patel SS (2006). Quality of life in patients with chronic kidney disease: focus on end-stage renal disease treated with hemodialysis. *Semin Nephrol*, Jan, **26**(1), 68–79.

66 Kimmel PL, Emont SL, Newmann JM, et al. (2003). ESRD patient quality of life: symptoms, spiritual beliefs, psychosocial factors, and ethnicity. *Am J Kidney Dis*, Oct, **42**(4), 713–21.

67 Patel SS, Shah VS, Peterson RA, et al. (2002). Psychosocial variables, quality of life, and religious beliefs in ESRD patients treated with hemodialysis. *Am J Kidney Dis*, Nov, **40**(5), 1013–22.

68 Ye XQ, Chen WQ, Lin JX, et al. (2008). Effect of social support on psychological-stress-induced anxiety and depressive symptoms in patients receiving peritoneal dialysis. *J Psychosom Res*, Aug, **65**(2), 157–64.

69 Chowanec GD, Binik YM (1989). End stage renal disease and the marital dyad: an empirical investigation. *Soc Sci Med*, **28**(9), 971–83.

70 Daneker B, Kimmel PL, Ranich T, et al. (2001). Depression and marital dissatisfaction in patients with end-stage renal disease and in their spouses. *Am J Kidney Dis*, Oct, **38**(4), 839–46.

71 Turner-Musa J, Leidner D, Simmens S, et al. (1999). Family structure and patient survival in an African-American end-stage renal disease population: a preliminary investigation. *Soc Sci Med*, May, **48**(10), 1333–40.

72 Levy NB (1985). Psychological problems of patients on dialysis. In Stevens PM (ed.). *Proceedings of the European Dialysis and Transplant Nurses Association–European Renal Care Association*. pp. 177–84. London: Baillière Tindall.

73 Abdel-Kader K, Unruh ML, Weisbord SD (2009). Symptom burden, depression, and quality of life in chronic and end-stage kidney disease. *Clin J Am Soc Nephrol*, Jun, **4**(6), 1057–64.

74 Palmer BF (2003). Sexual dysfunction in men and women with chronic kidney disease and end-stage kidney disease. *Adv Ren Replace Ther*, Jan, **10**(1), 48–60.

75 Zarifian A (1999). The role of Viagra in the treatment of male impotence in ESRD. *ANNA J*, Apr, **26**(2), 242.

76 Seibel I, Poli De Figueiredo CE, Teloken C, et al. (2002). Efficacy of oral sildenafil in hemodialysis patients with erectile dysfunction. *J Am Soc Nephrol*, Nov, **13**(11), 2770–5.

77 Norris KC, Agodoa LY (2005). Unraveling the racial disparities associated with kidney disease. *Kidney Int*, Sep, **68**(3), 914–24.

78 Powe NR (2003). To have and have not: Health and health care disparities in chronic kidney disease. *Kidney Int*, Aug, **64**(2), 763–72.

79 Agodoa L (2003). Lessons from chronic renal diseases in African Americans: treatment implications. *Ethn Dis*, Summer, **13**(2 Suppl 2), S118–24.

80 Robinson BM, Joffe MM, Pisoni RL, et al. (2006). Revisiting survival differences by race and ethnicity among hemodialysis patients: the Dialysis Outcomes and Practice Patterns Study. *J Am Soc Nephrol*, Oct, **17**(10), 2910–18.

81 Rodriguez RA, Sen S, Mehta K, et al. (2007). Geography matters: relationships among urban residential segregation, dialysis facilities, and patient outcomes. *Ann Intern Med*, Apr 3, **146**(7), 493–501.

82 Sue S, Dhindsa MK (2006). Ethnic and racial health disparities research: issues and problems. *Health Educ Behav*, Aug, **33**(4), 459–69.

83 Adler NE, Boyce T, Chesney MA, et al. (1994). Socioeconomic status and health. The challenge of the gradient. *Am Psychol*, Jan, **49**(1), 15–24.

84 Kimmel PL, Peterson RA, Weihs KL, et al. (1995). Behavioral compliance with dialysis prescription in hemodialysis patients. *J Am Soc Nephrol*, Apr, **5**(10), 1826–34.

85 Cukor D, Rosenthal DS, Jindal RM, et al. (2009). Depression is an important contributor to low medication adherence in hemodialyzed patients and transplant recipients. *Kidney Int*, Jun, **75**(11), 1223–9.

86 Chiu YW, Teitelbaum I, Misra M, et al. (2009). Pill burden, adherence, hyperphosphatemia, and quality of life in maintenance dialysis patients. *Clin J Am Soc Nephrol*, Jun, **4**(6), 1089–96.

87 Butler JA, Peveler RC, Roderick P, et al. (2004). Measuring compliance with drug regimens after renal transplantation: comparison of self-report and clinician rating with electronic monitoring. *Transplantation*, Mar 15, **77**(5), 786–9.

88 Fine RN, Becker Y, De Geest S, et al. (2009) Nonadherence consensus conference summary report. *Am J Transplant*, Jan, **9**(1), 35–41.

89 Butler JA, Peveler RC, Roderick P, et al. (2004). Modifiable risk factors for non-adherence to immunosuppressants in renal transplant recipients: a cross-sectional study. *Nephrol Dial Transplant*, Dec, **19**(12), 3144–9.

Chapter 10

Spiritual care of the renal patient

Chris Davies and Ira Byock

10.1 Introduction

The term 'spiritual' is one which can mean different things to different people. In 1992, the UK Department of Health produced a circular entitled 'Meeting the spiritual needs of patients and staff'.[1] This document, whilst clear, assumes that the reader will understand what spiritual needs actually are, yet little clarification is forthcoming within it. Despite the growing secularization of society on both sides of the Atlantic, healthcare professionals are still being asked to ensure that the spiritual and religious needs of their patients are fully taken into account at all times. This chapter aims to explore the terms 'spiritual' and 'religious' and to see how they may have bearing upon the supportive care of the renal patient.

Spirituality is an inherent characteristic of the human being. Although informed by evidence from anthropology, psychology, and medicine, spiritual care draws on philosophy, theology, and art as much as it does on science. Each human life is unique and precious. As a consequence, no single definition of spirituality or understanding of spiritual experience is likely to be satisfying to all; rather there are innumerable expressions of spirituality. It is indeed akin to an art class working on a portrait. Each student will create a painting that will be unique. So it is with spirituality. There may be a common theme, but the way an individual experiences that theme will depend upon their life's experience and system of beliefs. Attempts to describe and quantify spiritual care solely within a scientific model are destined to fail. Research is important to improving spiritual care giving, but clinicians seeking to meet their patient's spiritual and religious needs require a fuller understanding of spirituality that is informed by illness narratives, philosophy, theology, and art.

With this in mind, this chapter aims to address the subject in two distinct, yet complementary, ways. Ira Byock comes to it as an American physician and secular academic. Chris Davies explores it from the viewpoint of an Anglican priest steeped in theology and the culture of the UK. As with two people painting the portrait of someone sitting before them, there will not only some distinctive insights but also commonality.

It is to be hoped that readers will take from these authors insights and experiences that will help them develop clinical approaches to spiritual care for their patients that enhance their own integrity and well-being as clinicians and spiritual beings.

10.2 Portrait one: spiritual care from the perspective of a UK hospital chaplain

Modern best practice in healthcare demands that a patient is given the opportunity to exercise an 'informed choice' at every possible point in their treatment.

When speaking with nurses about such matters, I invariably begin by asking them to consider how they should ask a patient whether they might have any spiritual or religious needs whilst in hospital. The question ought to be routinely asked on admission but is often omitted. It is clear that how the question is asked is as important as asking it in the first place. A nurse who is an ardent member of a faith community may ask it in a way that can only elicit a 'yes response'; i.e. 'You would like to see the chaplain wouldn't you?' Whereas a nurse who is an atheist may ask in a way that will produce a 'no response'; i.e. 'You don't need to see the chaplain do you?' Both extremes are inconsistent with offering the patient balanced information in order for them to make an informed choice. As with the nurse who is admitting a patient, the doctor's views on spirituality and religion will also affect how comfortable a patient will feel about disclosing such needs. Unlike asking a phlebotomist to carry out a procedure, a doctor will not always be able to call in the chaplain or other spiritual care-giver to deal with matters raised at the bedside. I am not arguing for all clinicians to have a faith, far from it! I am, however, asking that clinicians, whatever their personal beliefs, take the spiritual needs of their patients seriously and allow for them to be addressed.

10.2.1 What is meant by spirituality?

In recent years, there has been an explosion of books addressing spirituality in the context of healthcare. It is clear from such written material that there is no single accepted definition of spirituality. If spirituality is seen as an aspect of human experience, one might expect that there will be as many definitions of spirituality as there are human beings! I understand spirituality to be about making sense of myself in relation to the world around me. It is about looking for meaning: who I am in relation to my past, my present, and my future and what the reference points are on my life journey. In the context of disease, I would add questions such as: 'Why is this happening to me?', 'What have I done to bring this upon myself?', 'So what has my life been all about and what has been the point of it all?', 'Who will be affected by my pain and death and why should they be?' Speck[2] notes that 'spiritual' relates to a concern with ultimate issues and is often seen as a search for meaning. This definition echoes Frankl[3] who has said, 'Man is not destroyed by suffering, he is destroyed by suffering without meaning'.

Religious needs, on the other hand, relate to how an individual seeks to find such meaning within a framework that gives expression to his or her life as a whole. This may be as one of an organized faith community or not. The essential aspect is that it is a framework that others are part of and share in whether they are physically present or not. There is, therefore, a significant difference between spiritual and religious needs.

Perhaps an analogy might help. I liken the difference between spiritual and religious needs to that of a four-stroke petrol engine. Such an engine powers a motor car and requires an electric spark in order to do so. This spark is produced by a spark plug. However, different makes of car have different types of spark plugs. The spark plugs perform an identical function but are usually brand specific. Humanity can be likened to such a car. Our spiritual nature is an integral part and can be compared with the engine. Our religious nature will depend upon our personal histories and will be different accordingly, as are the spark plugs in the various makes of cars. It is important that healthcare professionals, including chaplains, acknowledge such differences and seek to ensure that a patient's spiritual needs are addressed by appropriate means – be they religious in the traditional sense or otherwise. Chaplains are 'spiritual mechanics'. They carry a 'virtual tool bag' in which will be found the resources for a wide range of religious needs.

10.2.2 Assessing the spiritual and religious needs

'Am I going to die doctor?' is a question often asked by patients. This is a clear, straightforward question, or so it seems. Yet, what is being asked maybe something completely different.

The patient, rather than wishing to know the prognosis, may in fact want to be told that they are going to get better. Words convey a variety of meanings and it is only by 'listening to the whole person' that we communicate effectively. Listening is about using all our senses in harmony. Quietly asking for clarification of a patient's questions is essential to good care. Taking note of their countenance, their surroundings, and their network of relationships all play a part in seeking to help address their spiritual and religious needs.

10.2.2.1 Portrait one: spiritual care from the perspective of a UK hospital chaplain 193

It was 3 pm one Sunday afternoon, I had been busy with bedside prayers for most of the day and was very tired. The renal unit called me to attend one of their patients who had been missed off of my visiting list. The patient was a young blind woman with end-stage renal disease. I introduced myself and said that I had brought her Holy Communion to which she replied, "no thank you". I was perplexed by her reply and wondered why she had refused. She was sitting beside her bed and appeared quite agitated by my presence. I gently asked her if I had upset her in any way and she said, "no I hadn't".

As I sat with her and apologized for not coming during the morning, her agitation lessened. I said to her that I felt that she appeared upset by my arrival and wondered why. After a long pause she explained to me that ever since her childhood she would only go to church on a Sunday morning. She had expected me to come that morning and when I failed to arrive then she thought no more of it. However, to turn up unexpectedly on a Sunday afternoon had terrified her. She could not see my face but felt that I was rather anxious, which of course I was, for I had failed to see her earlier. Arriving as I did made her feel that there was some sort of emergency and that I was not just bringing her Holy Communion but had come because the staff had called me to attend as she was near to death. I had come, so she thought, to give her the 'last rites' and she did not want that at all. This was the starting point of a series of visits during which she began to talk of her fear of death.

(i) Case study

It may be that patients are unaware of some deep profound worry that has been thrown into focus by their disease. They may be unclear and unable to articulate what is troubling them. Listening to whole persons and not to just their words can enable the clinician to begin to help patients face what is upsetting them. Sometimes it is unwise to offer the services of a chaplain immediately. It may be that only after several difficult conversations does it become appropriate to suggest that perhaps someone like a chaplain might be able to help.

The most important factor in all of this is time and reflective listening. Assessing spiritual needs can be a slow process. This is not so when it comes to religious needs. Members of major faith communities will usually know what they need. It may be a place to pray, or the attendance of their minister for prayers and support. We all do well to remember that meeting the religious needs of a patient may not meet their spiritual needs at all. Assumptions can be made all too easily.

10.2.3 Questions, questions, and even more questions

When a patient is seeking to make sense of what is happening to them, they will ask themselves and may ask others a host of questions. Questions often begin seeking an adverbial answer such as 'how', 'where', or 'when'. The most powerful of them all is 'why'. It is all too easy for those working in a healthcare setting to proffer an immediate answer to a patient's questions. Yet for many of the 'why' questions, there is no ready answer. We may be able to answer why a patient's dialysis is no longer effective, i.e. vascular access is no longer possible and why it has come to this point.

But why with this particular patient at this particular point in their life is not a question that we can even begin to answer. It is here that we must be prepared to say that we just do not know. For some faith groups, sense is made of such an awful position by stating that it is the will of God. For many of our patients the struggle to make sense of what is happening to them is not satisfied by such a faith position. Their agony can only be helped by the listener staying with the patient's questioning and not running away from the pain that is engendered. Helping a patient by just being there as they seek to find words to articulate their innermost distress is fundamental to spiritual care at every level.

Many patients talk of their fear not of death but of dying. It is often a fear of a painful and undignified death. The great advances in palliative care over recent decades have gone a long way to ensure that no patient need die in physical pain any longer. However, it is not for us to decide for a patient that they should be pain free at the expense of all else.

On one occasion, a local minister called to commend one of his congregation to me. He was a recently retired professional man who was now actively involved in his church's outreach work. He had come in for tests and a tumour had been found in his kidney. He was awaiting its removal and further tests. I found him in a four-bedded unit with three other very talkative male patients. We sat on his bed and spoke for some considerable time about his new work with his church, of what was happening now, and how things might or might not go after surgery. As I drew our conversation to a close, I suggested that we pray together. He immediately withdrew from me saying, "no thank you I would rather not if you don't mind". I respected his wishes, shook hands, waved goodbye to the other three patients, and went on my way perplexed. Why did this committed Christian refuse to pray with me at such a difficult time in his life? Some weeks later, I met him after an out-patient appointment and asked how he was getting on. Before replying, he said how sorry he was for rejecting my invitation to pray with him. He went on to explain that it had been such a terrible shock to discover the tumour so soon after starting out on a ministry that he had really wanted from his youth. To have prayed openly with me in that unit would have meant that he would then have had to bring his message to the other three patients. At that moment his own inner turmoil was such that he just needed time to come to terms with what was going on in his life without having the pressure of wanting to tell others about his faith. In this instance, I had made wrong assumptions and this led me to focusing on what I perceived to be the patient's religious needs to the exclusion of his spiritual ones.

Care must be taken to ensure that both are addressed in a balanced and sensitive way. Hindsight is a wonderful gift; what would have been more helpful might well have been to have taken the patient into a quiet room off the ward where he could have shared both his spiritual and religious needs away from the ever watchful eyes and ears of other patients.

10.2.4 Peace and reconciliation

As a patient struggles with his disease and the prospect of death, it is often the case that part of his or her spiritual struggle is with events that have taken place in the past that have never been resolved. The patient may not know how to put things right, or believe that it is too late to make amends. Memories can come flooding back that feel unbearable. A patient's agitated state arises as much from the past as from their present circumstances and imminent death. Helping patients to talk through their painful past can be an important part of their spiritual care. It may be that they are torn apart by something they did, they said, or even thought which was hurtful to someone else. The person concerned may no longer be available for them to see and they are at a loss to know what to do. Feelings of guilt can become so great that the patient does not know how to cope.

In such cases, patients with a religious background may be helped by a recognized ritual such as sacramental confession. For those without such a framework, simply expressing what is troubling them to someone who is non-judgmental can in itself be all that is required. Similarly, a patient who has been wronged and has never come to terms with what took place may exhibit bitterness, anger, and depression that may be mistakenly attributed to the patient's disease pathway, rather than to past events. By telling their story slowly, and perhaps over and over again, the patient may begin to come to terms with all that had happened. The listener should be slow to reassure and to justify what took place; rather he or she needs to be present with the telling of the story, however painful and upsetting that might be. Acceptance and forgiveness can come about, but they may both be slow and painful processes.

Making present the past, in the presence of another and facing it head on can be a truly healing experience. To be at peace with oneself as death beckons has always been seen as most desirable. For some this will never be so, yet it is possible to facilitate it. Clinicians, as well as chaplains, may find opportunities with their patients to offer the support and encouragement needed for them to face the painful past in order that they may be more at peace with the present so as to accept the future with courage.

10.2.4.1 Case study

A 72-year-old widow dying slowly of end-stage renal disease had one son living in Australia at the time. She had not seen him for 26 years. He was flying across to see his mother but would not arrive until the following day. The staff felt that she would benefit from analgesia and sedation. However, her wish was to see and speak with her son. Care and expertise needed to be used in order that her wishes could be observed. It meant that until she and her son could have some time together her physical pain could not be as effectively controlled as the team would have wished. As a result of listening to her needs and respecting them she was able to be with her son in a way that meant so much to them both.

10.2.5 Meeting a patient's spiritual needs is a two-way process

Very often, renal patients have been associated with a renal unit for months or years. Their disease may have taken a long time to run its course. Doctors, nurses, and associated healthcare professionals will usually get to know much about such patient's families and friends and history. They can almost become part of the furniture! Staff may become very attached to such patients, which can be a positive experience but also a source of stress. Being with another person as they seek to come to terms with what is happening to them as a result of their disease has a cost to doctors and nurses. How we are with thoughts about our own mortality can help or hinder our involvement. The patient may remind us of a member of our own family who has gone through a similar illness. This may be extremely painful for us and we may avoid any references to death and dying because of this. The patient may also remind us of someone close to us now and this can be traumatic. 'It could be my wife or my child in that bed'. Again, such painful projections can lead the clinician to avoid any mention of issues relating to the patient's spiritual needs. My own father died after many months of illness in an intensive care unit (ICU). Treatment was withdrawn as my mother and I sat by his bed. He died peacefully and with dignity. However, when I was next called to an ICU to be with a family in a similar situation I found it extremely painful and difficult to be there with them fully. The emotional and spiritual cost to clinicians can be large.

It is vital, therefore, that appropriate support networks – including the provision of spiritual care to the team – and a system of clinical supervision are readily available. This is not only necessary for the well-being of the clinician but will also ensure that a patient's spiritual needs are not overlooked because of any unresolved issues that were raised for team members. It is also important to note that any supportive care of the patient will also include their closest family members and carers. They too will be struggling to make sense of what is happening to their loved one. It may well be that clinicians spend as much if not more time with family and friends than with the patient grappling with issues related to spiritual needs. Again, it is here that referral to a spiritual care-giver may be the most appropriate form of action. To care for and support the patient will always include support of their family and friends. All in all, the support of a renal patient as they move towards the end of their life is a complex web – involving staff, relatives, and friends. It is support that will take many forms and will vary from patient to patient.

10.2.6 **Final brush strokes**

I have tried to 'paint' my picture of the spiritual and religious needs of a renal patient that should be part and parcel of the supportive care offered by clinicians. As with all portraits it will be clear which of those aspects are particularly important to me as a hospital chaplain. It would be presumptuous of me to tell patients what to believe and how to address their spiritual agonies. However, it is a great privilege to be invited into a patient's life at such a personal and deep level. By actively listening to their searching questions, I hope, that should they ask me how I make sense of my life in relation to God and the universe, I might be able to share with them a sense of hope and peace that gives them courage to face all that lies before them.

10.3 **Portrait two: spiritual and religious issues from the perspective of a US clinician**

10.3.1 Case study

KF is a 79-year-old man with long-standing insulin-dependent diabetes, renal insufficiency, and peripheral vascular disease. He has been maintained on haemodialysis for the past 3 years and has needed bilateral below-knee amputations. Bouts of severe depression in the past have usually responded to antidepressant medication. Vascular access has become progressively more difficult and within the past 4 months, two vascular grafts have become unusable, despite multiple procedures.

He recently moved into the home of his daughter and her family as, 3 months previously, his wife of 27 years died suddenly of a stroke, plunging him into grief and depression. He now feels he is an increasing burden on his daughter and her family. He has a strong Christian faith, but has been unable to attend church regularly because his health problems have led to difficulties in access. During a routine visit with the dialysis social worker, KF asked about the option of discontinuing dialysis. He asked her whether it was allowed, and how it was different from suicide. Following a consultation with his nephrologist, the social worker and a peer counsellor[4] began meeting him over a period of weeks and listened to his concerns. He had many questions concerning what would happen and how he would be cared for if he were to stop dialysis. He was particularly concerned about his daughter and her family.

Hospice referral was made to respond to his questions. The hospice medical director spoke to his doctor and recommended a modest adjustment in his dose of antidepressant medication. The hospice chaplain contacted his congregation and encouraged the minister to visit. The minister visited the very next day and was apologetic that he had not known of KF's recent misfortunes. They prayed together. This visit affirmed his sense of worth and the minister arranged for him to be visited by members of the congregation's caring committee. Transportation was arranged and he was able again to attend services each Sunday.

On a follow-up visit, the hospice chaplain asked KF, "What is most important to you in your life now?" He readily responded that God, his children, and his grandchildren are what give his life meaning. Working with the chaplain, he was able to identify specific tasks he wanted to accomplish. He had in mind gifts of memorabilia and a photo album of his and their grandmother's early life he wanted to assemble for his family, especially his grandchildren. The church's caring-committee members helped and he found the projects enjoyable and meaningful. Through informal life review, KF developed a sense of how much he had contributed to others – his family, friends, and the community – and gradually came to accept their love and support. His depression lifted and he again engaged in life, exhibiting a renewed sense of self-worth. He assumed the responsibility of after-school childcare for his two grandchildren.

Through this process he came to feel that nothing was left unsaid, and to accept his new life, with all its difficulties. Although discontinuation of dialysis remains a consideration and may become necessary if vascular access is lost, KF now has a sense of worth and value in his current life.

10.3.1 Interior realms: responding to mystery, seeking meaning, and connection

Spirituality is an inherent aspect of the human condition. Our ability to reflect upon ourselves, our lives, and our relationships to others and to the world embeds human experience with spiritual dimensions. This is not a philosophical assertion as much as it is an anthropological fact. In the devoutly secular culture of American medicine, the existence of spirituality as a fundamental feature of humankind cannot be emphasized too strongly. A person may choose to characterize himself or herself as 'religious' or 'spiritual'. An individual's cultural heritage and upbringing, as well as his or her unique preferences and perspectives, influence his or her beliefs and the level of interest and intensity of feeling the person invests in spiritual aspects of life. Labels such as 'religious', 'spiritual', 'non-religious', 'atheist', or 'existentialist' may convey information about the individual's interest and particular beliefs, which at times proves clinically useful. However, any person with the capacity for self-awareness and reflection must be assumed to have aspects of his or her life experience that can properly be termed, spiritual.

The realms of the interior and transcendent commonly swell in proportion to other aspects of life for persons living with progressive illness, and they can be sources of solace or suffering. It is, therefore, especially important for clinicians who care for patients with life-limiting conditions to develop a vocabulary and some familiarity with spiritual domains of patients' experiences. Definitions and terms are critical to discussing spirituality. Often, the words spirituality and religion are used interchangeably. I use the term spirituality to refer to experiences, thoughts, and emotions that arise in response to the mystery of life and pertain to a source of meaning or to a sense of connection to something larger than oneself which extends into an open-ended future. The drive to seek meaning and a connection is a response to the awe-inspiring and, at times, terrifying mystery of life and is rooted in the depths of the human psyche. There is value in considering meaning and connection to be distinct; however, these constructs are frequently intertwined. A person's connection to God or to country, for instance, may also provide him or her with a predominant source of meaning.

Religion refers to a combination of beliefs, values, eschatology, knowledge, techniques, rituals, customs, and practices which foster a sense of connection and meaning and a way of dealing with the mystery of existence. Religion may be thought of as a primary vehicle through which human beings have reached out to one another, in community and across generations, in confronting primal issues of life and death. Particular religions often involve specific beliefs related to a supreme being. However, some religions – including Taoism, Shintosim, and Buddhism – do not include a belief in a deity. Therefore, someone may describe himself or herself as religious, yet not believe in God.

People who have a deep religious faith often find it affords a well of strength and source of comfort in dealing with injury, illness, disability, care giving, death, and grief. In some circumstances, however, religion can be at the root of a person's suffering. Such situations arise when people feel that their illnesses or misfortunes are caused by some moral failing or the lack of sufficient faith. Any such dilemmas need to be addressed with a patient with due care and sensitivity.

10.3.2 Spiritual care is integral to supportive and palliative care

Spiritual care is an integral part of whole-person supportive and palliative care for patients with end-stage renal disease. When a person is confronted with the new diagnosis of a life-limiting illness or when a serious complication of long-standing illness raises the possibility of death, questions of spiritual content often acquire special relevance and urgency. 'Why is this happening to me? Why now? What caused this illness or injury? Is there some deeper meaning to this misfortune? What is my life worth now that I cannot do the things I used to? What has my life meant to myself, to others? Will I be remembered, and if so, how will I be remembered? What will happen after I die? Does 'life' – my existence and self-awareness – really end, or will I awake in an afterlife? How does God view my life and me? What does God want from me in this situation?'

Some of these questions carry obvious religious assumptions and invite further inquiry and response within the context of a person's religious orientation. Others may sound distinctly philosophical. However, for a person living with the symptoms, functional limitations, and emotional and social consequences of renal disease, these questions accrue practical signifi-cance by arising from the physical reality and mundane events of life with illness.

10.3.3 Meaning

Although the concept of meaning is central to the definition of spirituality offered here, and has profound importance for clinicians engaged in spiritual assessment and care, the word 'meaning' may never be uttered by an individual who is ill. People universally have a sense of meaning, or suffer from the lack of meaning, but they may not think or speak in such terms. Many people do ponder meaning of and in their lives; however, meaning or its absence is predominantly felt. Far from being a merely philosophical construct, a person facing the end of life may have a visceral sense of meaning that is related to tangible entities, events, and people in his or her life. A father of three grown children, who are all successful with young children of their own, need only look around the room at a family gathering to feel a sense of meaning about his life. That sense of satisfaction may be eroded when he considers past failures in business, the loss of his children's inheritance in bad investments, or perhaps through gambling.

The myriad of influences that shape an individual's life and sense of meaning are diverse and unique. Yet this uniqueness does not exclude elemental commonalties. Cassell's construct of personhood encompasses an individual's physical body and emotional temperament, as well as his or her past, cultural heritage, habits and aversions, family, hopes and fears, and sense of the transcendent.[5] This multidimensional concept of personhood suggests predictable aspects of life in which both contributors to and detractors from meaning may reside. Accomplishments, failures, the people we have loved and lost, as well as those we have hated, all have roles in shaping a person's sense of themselves and their sense of meaning.

10.3.4 Therapeutic implications of the drive to make meaning

An inventory of contributions and barriers to meaning suggests a basic therapeutic strategy. If meaning is central to spiritual well-being, it follows that helping people to identify meaning in their lives is essential to achieving that process. A meaning-based interview can identify sources of satisfaction and pride as well as areas of regret and shame. Most often, this takes the form of life review.

The word meaning may or may not be used at all. The most direct question, 'What gives your life meaning?' may evoke a long and cogent reflection on life from one person and shrugged shoulders from another. 'What is most important to you in life?' may be more likely to yield a response.

Many people will readily identify the things in their lives they are most proud of and, along the way, mention things they wish they had done differently. In providing spiritual care to patients with life-threatening conditions, it is important to listen sensitively and avoid probing to uncover old wounds that have not been mentioned. Life review is not insight therapy. People need not sift through an inventory of failures to reach some predetermined spiritual goal. Within a developmental approach, our therapeutic goal is to help people to achieve a sense of meaning and sense of personal integrity. People can be helped to grieve, forgive, and let go of the sad, tragic, painful, and shameful regrets of the past.

I often reflect to patients that none of us is perfect. We are just human. When feelings of regret or shame or lack of worth are contributing to a person's suffering, I may ask the person to have some mercy. 'If you were reading this story as a biographical novel, how would you feel toward the main character? Can you please bring yourself a little mercy?'

10.3.5 Listening: the principal skill of spiritual care

Listening is the fundamental skill necessary for effective spiritual care. As a physician, I inevitably bring my own taxonomy and conceptual way of thinking about spiritual experience to the clinical encounter. However, it is important for me to learn how the patient thinks and talks about issues of mystery, meaning, and connection so that I may discuss these matters in his or her own terms. Familiarity with the worldview, beliefs, and traditions of majority denominations is valuable. However, it is prudent to assume that not every self-described Anglican, Catholic, Jew, or Buddhist thinks like every other, or has adopted the world view of his or her religious heritage. It is wise to explore how each patient's religion or philosophical stance is uniquely experienced and understood by them.

10.3.6 Connection

Humans share an inherent drive to feel connected. While relatively few people believe in immortality *per se*, it is nearly universal to seek a connection to something or to people who will remember us after we have gone. The sense of connection to something larger than oneself that will endure into an open-ended future is the basis for transcendence. For many people the sense of connection to God is vibrant and, in itself, is a response to the mystery.

This sense of connection to a supreme being has been described as a feeling that, 'mother is at home'. It is a confident sense of being loved, of being cared for.

It is not necessary to have a belief in God to have a passionate sense of connection. Dr Ned Cassem (personal communication, 2002) asks, 'Is there anyone or anything you would be willing to die for?' An individual's answer to this question may point towards a secular source of felt connection that transcends the boundaries of the person's finite life.

For many people, their family and the community of their friends and acquaintances provide a sense of connection that will endure beyond their life and death. When someone tells stories from her past, the process contributes to a sense of meaning about her life. In recording or otherwise preserving her life stories, she is creating an heirloom for her children, grandchildren, and generations yet to come. For people who are physically debilitated and feeling themselves a burden to others, the preserving and conveying of their personal history can be a tangible way of continuing to contribute to their family and community. In this way the connection to others is strengthened in a manner that not even death can destroy.

Not uncommonly, patients tell me that they are comforted by knowing that they will be buried on a plot of earth that has been in their family for generations; or that their ashes will be scattered from a peak or at a high mountain lake that has special importance for them. This sense of connection to nature and the understanding that their physical self will go back into the earth has value, dare I say meaning, for them.

The fundamental way in which clinicians can contribute to a patient's sense of connection is to remain involved. Many times in the past, when cure is no longer possible, patients have described feeling abandoned by their doctors. An often quoted American phrase is one that holds that 'ninety-five percent of life is "showing up".' It is certainly true in the realm of care for patients nearing the end of life. As clinicians, being present at the bedside or at the home of an ill and possibly dying person provides tangible evidence that we care; that the person still matters to us.

10.3.7 The developmental approach to spiritual experience with progressive, incurable illness

The uniqueness and individuality of each person is not diminished by recognizing that there are elemental commonalties within the human experience of living with the knowledge of the approach of death. By building on the methodologies and knowledge base of childhood development and developmental psychology, the conceptual framework and terminology of human development can be used as a valuable clinical tool for approaching the personal experience of life-threatening illness and injury. The developmental approach encompasses spiritual dimensions of experience and offers a robust framework for assessment and individualized, patient-centred intervention, and a well-established foundation for clinical research. Since the concept of life-long human development is commonly taught in primary and secondary schools, it also provides a familiar vocabulary for clinical training.

If human development is life-long, it follows that people may grow, or suffer developmental delays, during the latter stages of life, just as they might at its beginning. A schema of relevant developmental landmarks and task-work enables practical and clinically meaningful assessment of individual patients in a manner that informs therapeutic intervention (Box 10.1).[6]

An important advantage of a developmental approach is that it is not confined to recognizing and responding to suffering, as is the problem-based approach to medical care. Although all too common, suffering is not the human experience associated with nearness to death. Personal experience associated with illness and dying extends from suffering on one pole to a heightened sense of well-being on the other. Suffering in the context of end-stage illness may involve pain and other physical distress, but often extends to the realms of spirit. Suffering has been described as a sense of impending disintegration[5] based on a felt loss of meaning and purpose in life. In the resulting isolation that accompanies the gradual destruction of one's sense of value and purpose and in the resulting isolation that follows its loss, all suffering is spiritual. Pain is just pain if one knows it will end and if it does not threaten the integrity of one's self and one's place in family and community. Recognizing the myriad potential sources of suffering experienced by our patients, and encountering so much suffering in the course of our busy clinical practices, can at times make it seem that suffering is inevitable, and the best we can do is make it a little less intolerable. Sometimes that is true; however, our clinical models of human experience are challenged to accommodate the empiric evidence that some individuals experience preserved or even heightened quality of life in the face of death.

Box 10.1 Developmental landmarks and task-work for life closure

Sense of completion with worldly affairs
_ Transfer of fiscal, legal, and formal social responsibilities.

Sense of completion of relationships with community
_ Closure of multiple social relationships (employment, commerce, organizational, congregational, etc.).
_ Components include: expressions of regret, expressions of forgiveness, acceptance of gratitude, and appreciation.
_ Leave taking; the saying of goodbyes.

Sense of meaning about one's individual life
_ Life review.
_ The telling of 'one's stories'.
_ Transmission of knowledge and wisdom.

Experienced love of self
_ Self-acknowledgement.
_ Self-forgiveness.

Experienced love of others
_ Acceptance of worthiness

Sense of completion in relationships with family and friends
_ Reconciliation, fullness of communication and closure in each of one's important relationships.
_ Component tasks include: expressions of regret, expressions of forgiveness and acceptance, expressions of gratitude and appreciation, acceptance of gratitude and appreciation, and expressions of affection.
_ Leave taking: the saying of goodbyes.

Acceptance of the finality of life – of one's existence as an individual
_ Acknowledgement of the totality of personal loss represented by one's dying and experience of personal pain of existential loss.
_ Expression of the depth of personal tragedy that dying represents.
_ Decathexis (emotional withdrawal) from worldly affairs and cathexis (emotional connection) with an enduring construct.
_ Acceptance of dependency.

Sense of a new self (person hood) beyond personal loss
_ Developing self-awareness in the present.

Sense of meaning about life in general
_ Achieving a sense of awe.
_ Recognition of a transcendent realm.
_ Developing/achieving a sense of comfort with chaos.

Surrender to the transcendent, to the unknown – 'letting go'
_ In accomplishing this last landmark, the doer and 'task-work' are one. Ultimately, little remains of the ego except the volition to surrender.

We may be helped to understand our patient's experiences through the words of others such as Dr Roger Bone – an eminent American pulmonologist – who wrote during the months in which he was living with progressive, incurable renal cancer:[8]

> Death has opened my eyes to life—literally. Since learning that I have a terminal illness, I believe that my mind has expanded and its appetite has become insatiable. I want to know and experience everything.
> ... No life is without gift, even when it may seem giftless to others. Contemplation and introspection in the context of nature have brought me to a point of enlightenment I would probably not have had under other circumstances. Cancer has allowed me a measure of insight.

Marie de Hennezel observed:[9]

> Life has taught me three things: The first is that I cannot escape my own death or the deaths of the people I love. The second is that no human being can be reduced to what we see, or think we see. Any person is infinitely larger, and deeper, than our narrow judgements can discern. And third: he or she can never be considered to have uttered the final word on anything, is always developing, always has the power of self-fulfillment, and a capacity for self-transformation through all the crises and trials of life.

Understanding how some individuals who are approaching death are able to transition from experiencing a sense of meaninglessness and impending annihilation to a sense of wholeness and 'well-ness' has profound practical implications for psychosocial and spiritual assessments and interventions. If a sense of impending disintegration and the loss of meaning underlie suffering, it is not surprising that a sense of well-being involves the preserved or enhanced sense of integrity and meaning. We can aid people in developing a sense of meaning about their life and life in general. For instance, clinicians and trained volunteers can work with patients on life review and the recording of stories. We can help people explore things that they feel would be left undone if they were to die suddenly. It is often important to people to complete relationships with others who have been important to them in the past. At times, this involves resolving past differences. Care-providers can help patients make contact with significant others and assist with correspondence, phone calls, or travel arrangements.

As spheres of a person's life become less relevant to their changed situations, they can be completed and released. We can assist people to complete these tasks. In this manner, a person need not disintegrate, but may instead be thought of as becoming less 'corporeal' and progressively more 'ethereal' over time. The metaphor of a person dissolving out of life well describes the peaceful, transcendent deaths palliative care professionals and others sometimes witness.

Families suffering the recent or impending loss of a loved one also have needs and opportunities in spiritual realms. In approaching the death of a beloved friend or relative, people may struggle amidst sadness to find some meaning in the tragedy. Belief systems may help people cope with tragedy and death and religious teachings often provide guidance to those who grieve. People naturally look for ways to develop a lasting sense of connection to the person. Religious traditions offer prayers, holidays, and memorial customs as ways of establishing and maintaining a sense of connection. Common informal customs include collecting photos, stories, heirlooms, and ashes of the deceased.

In each age and culture, our innate human drive to make meaning and seek connection finds relevant expression. One strategy is in some way to deliberately invest the tragedy with meaning. An example of a secular practice that has become fairly common for making meaning from a seemingly senseless death is for the family and friends to establish a scholarship fund or annual event to benefit others in a manner that reflects the deceased's values. In modern America, I have observed in my own practice several family members thoughtfully design and undergo tattoos that memorialize loved ones they have lost. And finally, in a typically American fashion, one company has recently begun offering to manufacture individual cubic zirconium, or manmade diamonds, from carbon of the person's ashes. Those who wish, and can afford to, can wear a bit of their loved one on their finger, from a pendant or as earrings.

10.3.8 **Final brush strokes**

The specific work that a person feels a need for, or interest in doing, as they confront life's end will vary from one individual to another. The end-of-life developmental landmarks and the task-work that underlies them are intended to describe predictable personal challenges as well as important opportunities for people as they die. The general developmental approach can provide a valuable map to clinicians through the inherently difficult landscape of the dying experience and end-of-life care.

Importantly, within this model one need not sanitize nor glorify the experience of life's end to think of a person as having achieved a degree of wellness in their dying. Personal development is rarely easy. The touchstone of dying well is that the experience has value and is meaningful for the person and their family.

10.4 **Conclusion**

Two distinct, yet complementary, portraits of the spiritual care of the renal patient have been offered in this chapter. Much of what has been written will apply to patients whatever their illness or disease. It is to be hoped that readers will be encouraged to develop their own portrait of spirituality and religion that will enable them to address the needs of their patients and patients' families as carefully as possible.

The two portraits both highlight the search for meaning as central to any understanding of a person's spirituality. Equally significant is the need to assess a patient's spiritual needs in the context of their home environment, culture, and religious faith (if they have one). The importance of significant others to the patient will also be crucial to the support offered by healthcare professionals.

It is important to note that at times, however hard we try to meet such needs, a patient may die without resolving some, if not all, of the issues encompassed by the terms 'spiritual' and 'religious'. That fact does not detract from the importance of making sure that we are aware that, for many people, spiritual and religious experience is a fundamental part of their daily life. It is essential that, as healthcare professionals, we seek to care for the whole person and not just the disease; that we find ways of asking and then assessing a patient's spiritual and religious needs and opportunities, and that we use the services of spiritual care-givers such as chaplains who are a vital part of the multidisciplinary team to assist in this aspect of care.

As a patient travels along the renal disease trajectory from diagnosis to death clinicians can monitor their spiritual needs and experience at every point. Careful listening to what is going on at that moment for the patient, both what is said and what is not said, will enable the clinician to make an assessment of the appropriate support that should be offered. Whether that support is received and utilized will, in the last analysis, be up to the patient. That is only right and fitting.

Similar to all aspects of palliative care, and indeed all of medicine, those involved need the support of others. This is especially true when it comes to being with patients who are grappling with the deep and painful questions encompassed by the terms 'spiritual' and 'religious'. It is important that whatever one's own orientation to such matters there should be no hesitation in calling on the services of chaplains and spiritual care-givers to support not only the patient and their relatives and friends but also the professional care-giver.

Ethical analysis

Recent research has also revealed that physicians' spiritual and religious beliefs have an influence on their practices. In any ethical analysis, attention to the patient's values and preferences is central. The recent medical literature documents that patients' spiritual values are more important to them than previously appreciated.

In the United States, research shows that 95% of patients believe in God. Focus-group research of patients and families indicates that at the end of life, patients and families have broader – psychosocial and spiritual – concerns than physicians' often narrow tendency to focus on physical matters. The authors of this chapter emphasize that physicians should take the spiritual needs of their patients seriously and ensure that they are addressed. In this regard, the case of the 72-year-old widow whose son was flying in from Australia is instructive. The physicians were concerned about treating the widow's pain, but the widow was more concerned about being mentally alert for the visit from her son, whom she had not seen in 26 years. Physicians need to understand that patients' values may differ from physicians', and physicians should not underestimate the significance of achieving a patient's spiritual goals in providing treatment to them.

Similarly, the case of KF demonstrates how important having meaning in one's life is to one's overall well-being. KF was on the verge of discontinuing dialysis when interventions by the hospice chaplain and KF's minister helped him to see how continuing to live after his wife's sudden death could have meaning and value for himself and his family. Asking questions is key to helping patients understand the meaning of their lives. The hospice chaplain asked, 'What is most important to you in your life now?' Other helpful questions include 'What might be left undone if you were to die today?' and 'What legacy do you want to leave to your family?'[10] As was accomplished in the case of KF, the goal of a spiritual intervention is to see the patient as a person and help the patient appreciate his/her worth. The 'Patient as person history' presented in the Introduction is also helpful towards this end.

References

1 NHS Management Executive (1992). *Meeting the spiritual needs of patients and staff: Good practice guide.* London, Department of Health.
2 Speck P (1998). *Being there.* London, SPCK Publishers.
3 Frankl VE (1987 edition). *Man's search for meaning.* London, Hodder and Stoughton.
4 Kapron K, Perry E, Bowman T, Swartz RD (1997). Peer resource consulting: redesigning a new future. *Adv Renal Replacement Ther*, **4**(3), 267–74.
5 Cassell EJ (1982). The nature of suffering and the goals of medicine. *N Engl J Med*, **306**(11), 639–45.
6 Byock IR (1997). *Dying well: the prospect for growth at the end of life.* New York: Riverhead.
7 Byock IR (1996). The nature of suffering and the nature of opportunity at the end of life. *Clin Geriatric Med*, **12**(2), 237–52.
8 Bone RC (1996). A piece of my mind: Maumee: My Walden Pond. *J Am Med Assoc*, **276**(24), 1931.
9 de Hennezel M (1997). *Intimate death: how the dying teach us how to live.* New York, Knopf.
10 Lo B, Quill T, Tulsky J (1999). Discussing palliative care with patients. *Ann Intern Med*, **14**, 27–34.
11 Curlin FA, Lantos JD, Roach CJ, Sellergren SA, Chin MH (2005). Religious characteristics of U.S. physicians: a national survey. *J Gen Intern Med* 20: 629–34.
12 Curlin FA, Nwodim C, Vance JL, Chin MH, Lantos JD (2008). To die, to sleep: US physicians' religious and other objections to physician-assisted suicide, terminal sedation, and withdrawal of life support. *Am J Hosp Palliat Care* 25: 112–20.

Chapter 11

Support of the home-dialysis patient

Alastair Hutchison and Helen Hurst

11.1 Introduction

The development of the Scribner dialysis shunt in the early 1960s made intermittent haemodialysis (HD) treatment possible for people who would otherwise have died, both in North America and Europe. Despite specifically identified funding, dialysis was only available in a few centres, so that only people who were considered 'socially worthy' by hospital select committees were given this scarce and expensive treatment.[1] Consequently during the 1960s, the haemodialysis population consisted mainly of white, married, well-educated men who were <50 years of age.[2–5] However, as the spaces within dialysis centres were filled, it became common for patients and their spouses (or other family members) to be trained to perform haemodialysis at home, thereby allowing many more patients access to treatment.[6] The number of dialysis patients in the United States of America (USA) increased from around 300, in 1965, to nearly 3000 by 1969, of whom over a 1000 were dialysing at home.[7]

Even in these early years, it rapidly became apparent that patients and their carers experienced a variety of psychological stresses associated with home haemodialysis, and that it demanded a degree of technical expertise and psychological resilience beyond that of any other treatment available then or now. Some patients were reported to resist all efforts to train them, and others took many more months than expected.[1] Once a patient was established at home it became clear that carer-assistants experienced as much, or possibly more anxiety, in particular relating to the possibility of their spouse dying during dialysis.[8] The investigating psychiatrists highlighted the fact that home haemodialysis necessitated a spouse carrying out a treatment that is both life-saving and potentially lethal on their partner. During the 1970s, there was a dramatic decrease in home-haemodialysis patients with an increasing number of female patients whose employed husbands were not available as carer-assistants. Furthermore, in the US, Medicare legislation included some economic disincentives to home treatment and, consequently, the percentage of patients on home dialysis declined from 40% in 1972 to 13% in 1979. In response, health professionals – most notably nurses, social workers, and psychologists – began to design studies to examine the impact of home dialysis on patients and their families using conceptualizations derived from systems theory.[9] In turn, clinicians described interventions that focused on helping family assistants adapt to their situations through support groups and improved communication with their spouse. Gradually, an understanding of the support required by a home-dialysis patient and his or her family began to evolve.

The development of continuous ambulatory peritoneal dialysis (CAPD) in the late 1970s radically altered the nature of home dialysis and made it available to many patients who would previously not have been considered, including a greater proportion of women. CAPD had minimal capital costs compared to home haemodialysis and the training period of 1–2 weeks was vastly shorter than the 3–4 months required for haemodialysis. In addition, no carer-assistant was thought to be required if the patient was otherwise able-bodied. However, in time it became evident that older patients and those with significant additional co-morbidity did require the help of a carer, and that generally this was a female member of the family – wives, daughters, and even adult sisters.

Full rehabilitation of home-dialysis patients (return to gainful employment, full-time studies or homemaking, etc.) has been shown to be difficult, but equally possible amongst haemodialysis and CAPD patients. Rubin et al.[10] found no significant differences between dialysis modalities in this respect, whilst acknowledging that the majority of patients were not rehabilitated.

In order to understand the support required for a home-dialysis patient – whether on CAPD or haemodialysis – healthcare professionals require a significant understanding of the family relationships involved, as well as an awareness of stereotypical role expectations which can vary from one family to another and are influenced by a variety of cultural and ethnic factors. Anderson and Elfert[11] emphasized that the belief that women are responsible for family care giving is reinforced by many health professionals so that a wife may be expected to take on the role of dialysis assistant where a husband would not. Similarly, it was noted that a husband assisting his wife to dialyse was invariably offered in-home cleaning services, care services, and community resources, whereas a wife assisting her husband often did not receive or ask for such help.

The collective findings of a variety of studies leave no doubt that home dialysis has always been a complex and stressful experience for patients and their families.[1] Over the past 25 years, the dialysis population has become increasingly elderly and suffers from multiple complex and debilitating medical problems as outlined in the case study within this chapter. Long term survival is not a serious consideration for many patients taken on to home-dialysis programmes despite selection of patients. Nevertheless, advance care planning in patients with chronic kidney disease remains woefully inadequate considering that the average annual mortality for all dialysis patients is around 20%.[12] Indeed, recent figures from the UK Renal Registry show that the average 5-year survival rate for a 60-year-old patient commencing dialysis, who does not receive a kidney transplant, is around 46% – only slightly better than that expected for ovarian carcinoma (44%). The modification of the 'Sheffield model' for renal palliative care implicitly acknowledges that life expectancy is significantly shortened by end-stage renal disease (ESRD), and that increasing support therapies will be required in time, for all patients (Fig. 2.1 and Table 11.1). This model emphasizes the importance of advance planning and provides a useful template for healthcare

Table 11.1 Comprehensive supportive care as described by the Sheffield Model

Primary care team
Physiotherapy and Occupational therapy
Psychology
Rehabilitation
Dietetics
Social Work
Chaplaincy
Pain Clinic
Complementary Therapies
Information services
Palliative Care

professionals to be applied to home-dialysis patients, accepting that dialysis is not a curative treatment and that the nature of the required support changes with time. Although certain features of supporting a home-dialysis patient are unique to the home environment, many of the other chapters within this book will be of direct relevance. For example, the symptoms of renal disease, sexual problems, psychological and psychiatric considerations, and the use of advance directives are no different for the home patient than for the 'in-centre' patient.

11.2 **Selection of home-dialysis patients** (Table 11.2)

It is self-evident that not all patients are suitable for home dialysis, either because they are unable or unwilling to dialyse themselves, or because their home circumstances are unsuitable. However, in the UK, the National Institute for Clinical Excellence (NICE; on behalf of the government) has published guidance for healthcare professionals on the location in which haemodialysis is carried out.[13] Although use of home haemodialysis has declined compared to its peak in the early 1970s, NICE recommends that "all suitable patients should be offered the choice between home haemodialysis or haemodialysis in a hospital". The guidance alludes to selection of suitable patients, stating that patients suitable for home haemodialysis will be those who:

1 have the ability and motivation to learn to carry out the process and the commitment to maintain treatment

2 are stable on dialysis

3 are free of complications and significant concomitant disease that would render home haemodialysis unsuitable or unsafe

4 have good functioning vascular access

5 have a carer who has (or carers who have) also made an informed decision to assist with the haemodialysis unless the individual is able to manage on his or her own

6 have suitable space and facilities or an area that could be adapted within their home environment (NICE 2002).

The guidance also states that patients and their carers "will require initial training and an accessible and responsive support service". It does not identify how to assess ability, motivation, commitment, stability on dialysis, ability to make an informed decision, or what constitutes an accessible and responsive support service. Nevertheless, it is clear that support and training for the patient and their family should ideally begin in this 'pre-dialysis' phase in order that a firm bond of trust and support is built. Conversely, failure to address a patient's perceived problems at this stage, or for example failure to plan and create dialysis access appropriately will result in a loss of confidence

Table 11.2 Process of establishing home dialysis

Pre-dialysis education programme
Training for patient and helper
Input from nursing staff, dietician, social worker, clinician, and dialysis technician
Conversion of suitable area in home for dialysis and storage
Transition to home dialysis with community renal nurse (CRN) assistance
Independent home dialysis with visits from CRN

that may not be recoverable later. Under such circumstances, establishing a patient on home dialysis may become almost impossible.

11.3 **Pre-dialysis education**

A prospective home-dialysis patient needs to have sufficient knowledge, skill, and ability to carry out their treatment regimen without direct supervision from healthcare personnel. Therefore, patient education is an important component in the management of ESRD.[14] The suitability or otherwise of a patient for home dialysis may first become apparent during the process of pre-dialysis education.

A review of the literature shows that a number of different models has been used for patient education[15–18] but most include information on dialysis techniques and modalities, the impact on patients' and families' lives, plus information about the local renal unit and available resources. Commonly cited goals include informed choice of treatment options, decreased anxiety for patients and their families, and enhanced self-care strategies. Klang et al.[19] evaluated the effects of a pre-dialysis patient-education programme on functioning and well-being in 28 uraemic patients and compared them to an age- and sex-matched group of patients who had not been through the programme. She found participating patients to have better mood, less mobility problems, fewer functional disabilities, and lower levels of anxiety compared to controls. These differences disappeared after 6 months on dialysis, but it is not clear whether this was because the control group improved or the 'educated' group slipped back. However, the initial 6 months of home dialysis are perhaps the most important, as the patient and carers learn to adapt to a radically new home environment, so that the benefits listed above could only be helpful.

11.3.1 **Training for home dialysis and the patient's role in treatment**

Although technological advances have simplified many aspects of dialysis over the past 30 years, the statement of Lancaster in 1979 concerning home dialysis remains true in the twenty-first century; "No other chronic illness in today's society requires as many diet restrictions, as many medications, or as large a volume of technical knowledge as is required for the patient with end-stage renal disease".[20] However, self-care moves the patient away from traditional medical paternalism, fostering of dependence and the sick role, and offers a positive approach to adaptation to a chronic illness. It involves patient control over treatment and a choice of therapies.[21] Its medium and long-term aim is to place the patient back in their own environment and to make them independent, to the fullest extent possible, of the hospital environment and the sick role. In doing so, it makes the patient and their carer the 'experts' and equips them to prevent, or deal with, the majority of likely complications. The restoration of confidence to a previously devastated life can be almost miraculous to witness, but it requires a highly organized and skilful team to do so.

Methods employed in training patients for home dialysis are out of the scope of this chapter, but it is vital to realize the importance of the bond of trust and friendship that should develop between trainer and trainee. All of us remember our teachers, both good and bad, from our past education and realize the impact that the relationship can have on eventual 'grades'. So it is with the home-dialysis trainee. A good trainer will inspire confidence and trust, and the trainee's perception of the entire support structure of the renal unit will be influenced by this early experience. In this way, the process of involving the patient and carer in the multi-disciplinary 'renal team' will begin and, perhaps for the first time, they will start to feel that they are gaining control of the illness rather than vice versa.

The length of the training period varies according to the chosen mode of dialysis, the patient's aptitude and the frequency of training sessions and will include continued teaching on diet and fluid management. A predetermined expectation of length of training is unhelpful since it encourages both trainer and trainee to think in terms of 'slow' and 'fast' learners. If the selection process is essentially sound, and the trainer is good, very few patients should fail to 'graduate'. Nevertheless, a significant integration of manual dexterity and cognition is required by the patient and carer for home dialysis to be feasible.[21]

Once the initial training period is completed, further training will be required in the patient's home, initially under the close supervision of the Community Renal Nurse (CRN). He or she will continue the training process and lead the patient to real independence as a home-dialyser.

11.4 An accessible and responsive support service

'Accessible' and 'responsive' are key aspects of a home-dialysis support service. It is essential that from the first day at home, the patient feels secure in the knowledge that if a complication arises, the full resources of the local renal unit are readily available, and can deal with it promptly and efficiently. If at any stage (but particularly in the first few weeks and months) this appears not to be the case, the patient's confidence will rapidly diminish and home dialysis will become progressively more problematic.

The two most immediate sources of support for the newly established home-dialysis patient are the community renal nurse (CRN) and the telephone 'help-line' to the local Renal Unit (Table 11.3). Ideally the CRN will have already been involved with the patient at earlier stages of education and training, and must have several years of dialysis nursing behind them to exude an air of calmness, confidence, and 'seen it all before'! In the US, Medicare regulations require follow-up visits to home-dialysis patients, yet they consume a large amount of personnel time. Theoretically, the cost of these visits in both time and money may be offset, at least in part, by the savings from complications and in-patient episodes avoided as a result of recommendations made, and changes implemented during a home visit.[22] Many dialysis patients refer to 'their' CRN as their 'lifeline', and mean it quite literally. The CRN will usually act as a focal point

Table 11.3 Renal Unit support for the home-dialysis patient

Planned home visits from CRN
Telephone help-line giving 24/7 access to technical, nursing, and medical advice
Planned hospital clinic visits and blood testing
Drop-in clinic for unplanned medical examination and assessment
Monitoring of water quality for haemodialysis patients
Appropriate ease of access to;

- Renal medical and nursing staff
- Dietician
- Social worker
- Psychologist/counsellor
- Home-dialysis administrator
- Physiotherapist and Occupational therapist
- Chaplaincy and spiritual care
- In-patient bed and medical or surgical management of complications

for the majority of the patient and carers problems, and is ideally placed to refer on to other members of the multi-disciplinary support team such as the dietician, social worker, counsellor or physiotherapist (Table 11.3).

Obviously the CRN cannot be available 24/7, and therefore a telephone help-line is required for problems that arise at other times. Many home-haemodialysis patients will choose to dialyse at times outside the usual working day, and therefore adequate back-up must always be available. This is not as easy as it might seem at first thought. The telephone number must be invariable – an anxious patient in the middle of a dialysis does not want to have to consult a rota to decide which number to call. This means that for most renal units the phone line will be to ward area which is always open, rather than to a dialysis area which may close down overnight. When the phone rings it must be immediately obvious to the staff that the call is from a home patient, so that it is not left to ring for several minutes as can often happen on a busy ward. Whoever answers the phone must be capable of dealing swiftly with a distressed patient or carer in the midst of a dialysis crisis – the last thing the caller wants to hear is "could you hold on for a moment, all the nurses are busy just now", even though this may be true!

The outcome of a phone call may be that the patient needs to come up to the renal unit for a medical assessment, and therefore an 'open access' or 'drop-in' clinic facility is required. Peritoneal dialysis (PD) patients should be encouraged to utilize this facility immediately they develop 'cloudy bags' or think they may have peritonitis for any other reason. Patients will often use this facility for all manner of minor ailments rather than going to their general practitioner or primary care physician, but it provides an ideal setting for on-going education about dialysis and chronic kidney disease. It requires appropriate nurse staffing and ready access to patient notes, a renal physician, and the possibility of surgical review if required.

11.5 Psychosocial and social support

The availability of a psychologist or counsellor with experience of chronic disease is imperative, and can be useful to both patients and staff. The counsellor perhaps straddles the boundary between the multi-disciplinary renal team and the other sources of support that patients may utilize outside the renal unit's physical provisions.

The demands and coping skills required of people with chronic kidney disease and their families are enormous.[23] The home-dialysis patient must overcome, or at least cope with, a large number of internal and external stressors if the process of dialysis itself is to be acceptable within the home environment. Various coping strategies will manifest themselves initially and may be helpful or otherwise. Reactions such as fear, anxiety, depression, denial, anger, and emotional dependency must be recognized and carefully worked on in a partnership between the patient and carer, with the healthcare team with the psychologist/counsellor taking a lead role. The psychologist also has an important role in educating other members of the renal multi-disciplinary team whose reactions to patient denial or anger may otherwise be unhelpful.

'Crisis points' in chronic kidney disease have been identified by Steffen[24] and it is important that these are recognized in all dialysis patients, but particularly those dialysing at home (Table 11.4). A crisis occurs when the patient's state of equilibrium is disrupted and usual coping mechanisms are ineffective. The patient adopts new strategies in an attempt to restore equilibrium and these result in either healthy or unhealthy adaptation. The crisis may, therefore, eventually be a very positive experience for the patient who finds that they can adapt, but an awareness of the crisis points amongst the healthcare team allows unhealthy adaptation to be picked up as early as possible and appropriate support to be provided (Table 11.5).

Table 11.4 Crisis points in chronic kidney disease

First diagnosis of chronic kidney disease
Hospitalization
Access surgery
Initiation of dialysis
6 months after initiation of dialysis
Changes in restrictions or dialysis schedules
Modality change
Complications
Significant change in health status

11.5.1 **Patient peer support**

National and local peer support groups, such as the Kidney Patients' Association, provide invaluable aid to many home-dialysis patients, who may otherwise be relatively isolated from fellow sufferers. Information on peer support groups should be made available during the training period, but it should be recognized that some patients would rather have nothing to do with them because it 'places' them within a life-style group from which they are striving to escape. Nevertheless, for many home patients, communication with someone who has 'been there' provides enormous encouragement, and also an opportunity to help others. Meeting patients with successful renal transplants can also provide significant hope for the future and a sense of purpose. Purvis quotes a patient as saying "Having been on treatment for a long time, the group has helped me remove the isolation attached to life on home dialysis".[25]

In many renal units, formal peer support groups exist and meet together regularly, some coordinated by a psychologist.[26] Many units, such as our own, have a tradition of an annual holiday for PD patients organized by two or more CRNs. The favourite destination for these groups from Manchester is Majorca in the Mediterranean. For some patients this can be a very bonding time, and it is sometimes the first international holiday they have ever had. Travel abroad produces a great sense of achievement in both patient and carer and gives them a feeling of freedom, or of having broken the shackles that were clamped on them when they started dialysis. Many then go on to successfully organize their own family holidays in subsequent years. Another approach to

Table 11.5 Other sources of support for the home-dialysis patient

Family and friends
Primary care physician/General practitioner
Spiritual care
Palliative care teams
Patient organizations
Internet advice
Nursing homes and rehabilitation facilities
Employer

peer support is to pair experienced, coping patients with new dialysis patients to assist adjustment during the early months.[27]

11.5.2 **Family support**

The importance of a supportive family environment cannot be overestimated, and may be particularly important for the more elderly patient. Carey et al.[28] used the Beavers–Timberlawn Family Evaluation Scale to rate the supportive nature of families of 294 CAPD patients, with ratings from 1 (representing a chaotic family structure) to 9 (representing an orderly 'egalitarian' structure). Patients over the age of 60 years in families with low scores were 4 times more likely to transfer to in-centre haemodialysis as a result of peritonitis or psychosocial factors than were patients from families with high scores. As a result, almost 70% of patients greater than 60 years of age with low scores transferred within 1 year of starting home dialysis. The authors emphasize the importance of considering psychosocial factors in selection of patients suitable for home dialysis, and in particular those at the older end of the age spectrum.

Family members often assist with haemodialysis and may assume the total burden associated with dialysis therapy.[29] Since the 1960s, both clinicians and researchers have reported that home haemodialysis is as stressful, if not more stressful for the carer than for the patient.[1] Family involvement in home care significantly influences the outcome of home-haemodialysis patients, just as the patient's health and functioning influence the family. Haemodialysis patients assisted by paid care-workers experienced significantly greater morbidity and greater financial burden than patients cared for by family members.[30]

Family carers of PD patients are similarly affected, and often assume some, if not all, of the responsibility for providing care.[31] This is particularly common in certain patient groups such as infants, children, frail elders, and otherwise disabled patients such as those who have undergone lower-limb amputation.

11.5.3 **Financial support**

In most Western countries, financial support for dialysis patients is provided in varying ways by the state. Private health insurance usually ceases in whole or in part to contribute to the costs associated with home dialysis at around the time the patient first commences dialysis. In the UK, the National Health Service pays all the bills, although dialysis facilities overall do not match demand. This has resulted in greater dependence on home dialysis, and in particular peritoneal dialysis. All associated costs are paid by the local renal unit, to the dialysis-equipment manufacturer.

In the US, a dialysis patient may voluntarily choose to become a home patient, but the final decision is based on whether the patient meets Medicare guidelines. Medicare will pay 80% of the cost of home dialysis for all patients who are eligible for Medicare. The remaining 20% is usually paid either by the patient's private insurance company or by Medicaid and in many states other programmes will assist patients who have neither insurance nor Medicaid eligibility. The cost of home dialysis for each approved dialysis centre is determined by Medicare. Home-dialysis patients can choose between two payment options: method I and method II. Under method I, the patient's dialysis unit provides all the facilities required for home dialysis either directly or under arrangements with other providers, and Medicare pays the unit directly. Under method II, the patient chooses to deal directly with a single supplier to obtain all dialysis equipment and supplies, but a local dialysis unit must agree to provide backup dialysis and support services in the event of problems arising.

11.5.4 Support for the elderly dialysis patient

The average age at start of dialysis in the UK was 64 years by the end of 2007.[32] In the USA, the fastest-growing dialysis cohort is in the age group of 65–74 years,[33] and significant increases are being seen in patients ≥75 years. However, life expectancy in this elderly age group is on average only around 2 years.[32] It is clear that there are many barriers to the elderly starting peritoneal dialysis, and the de Nederlandse Coöperatieve Studie naar de Adequaatheid van Dialyse (NECOSAD) study demonstrated that people over the age of 75 years were 6 times more likely to choose in-centre haemodialysis.[34] The reasons for this have been explored by several authors,[34–36] who note that outcomes in terms of technique survival are no different for peritoneal dialysis than haemodialysis. Yet there are many advantages of a home-based therapy for the elderly, where it avoids issues such as lengthy transport to and from a dialysis unit, vascular access problems, and offers advantages relating to quality of life. However, the elderly may have other barriers to home dialysis such as frailty, living alone, additional co-morbidity, and poor manual dexterity. Assisted peritoneal dialysis (aPD) is an approach whereby healthcare assistants go into the patient's home and take on the task of setting up the peritoneal dialysis exchange.[35] In France, non-disconnect CAPD with UV-flash is the predominant method used, as this greatly shortens the time needed for the nurse visit – the nurse phones the patient, or a relative, to start the drain procedure so that when she arrives she only has to remove the old bag and connect the new one, leaving the fluid to drain in, and the patient to fold up the bag after her departure. In other countries, automated peritoneal dialysis (APD) is used as the modality for assisted patients, with two visits from the nurse – a longer visit in the morning when the patient is disconnected from the machine, the old bags removed, and new ones placed on the machine, then a shorter evening visit when the patient is re-connected to the machine. Alternatively the patient performs the connection and disconnection with the assistant only managing the machine set-up and take-down at single visit. In these ways, the assistant removes the majority of the dialysis-technique burden.[35]

Assisted peritoneal dialysis offers a useful alternative to in-centre haemodialysis for those patients not able to access peritoneal dialysis otherwise, and in whom life expectancy is poor. For such patients time spent at home is often particularly valuable.

11.6 Monitoring and audit of home-dialysis support

Regular monitoring or audit of home dialysis can provide early signs that support is not as good as it should be, and may point to inadequacies in the service. A monthly or quarterly review of parameters such as the number of in-centre haemodialysis sessions, in-patient days, drop-in clinic visits, telephone help-line calls, peritonitis, and catheter-exit-site infections in peritoneal dialysis patients, or unplanned home visits by CRNs or technical staff can quickly identify deficiencies in support to home patients. An increase in in-centre haemodialysis sessions may suggest inadequate home support, whereas an increase in unplanned home visits or peritonitis may suggest inadequate training.

11.7 The long-term home-dialysis patient

A patient who has managed their own dialysis for a number of years can present particular challenges for the healthcare team. In our own programme, we have a number of home-haemodialysis patients who have looked after themselves for over 20 years, and who therefore have more experience of their treatment than many quite senior staff members. Such patients will immediately recognize a junior nurse or doctor's inexperience, whilst the nurse or doctor may frequently fail to recognize the patient's vast wealth of experience! Under these circumstances conflicts may occur, particularly when the staff member's instinct is to be cautious and perhaps recommend admission when the patient was simply seeking advice or reassurance. They may specifically avoid junior members of the team at clinic visits, because they recognize that they themselves know more about dialysis and its complications than a recently qualified nurse or doctor. It is important that home patients of this type have access to the most senior staff available on a given day, and that all staff recognize that enquiries from them are unlikely to be frivolous or clinically unimportant.

Inevitably, long-term patients eventually enter a phase of decline, and will – by this stage – have seen many of their dialysis colleagues fall victim to complications of one sort or another. They will therefore be well aware of their own limitations and mortality so that managing the transition to greater dependency requires enormous skill and sensitivity. Although the multi-disciplinary team remains essential to provide the range of care required at this time as much as any other, it is likely that the patient and their carer will look to one or two particularly trusted members to advise and guide them through this period.

11.8 End-of-life care for the home-dialysis patient

Patients who have maintained the independence afforded by home dialysis rarely wish to relinquish it as they near the end of their life. Ninety percent of the respondents to a Gallup survey commissioned in the US by the National Hospice Organisation, in 1996,[32] expressed a desire to die at home. In contrast to this, as modern medicine developed advanced technology to treat illness, death moved out of the home and into institutions, so that now less than 20% of people in the US die within their own homes.[33] The majority of deaths are predictable and could be managed at home, as is the case for many dialysis patients – not just those utilizing home treatments. However, formal education in 'end-of-life care' is lacking in many medical schools but other organizations have taken a lead. The American Medical Association conceived the EPEC Project – 'Education for Physicians on End-of-life Care'. EPEC is intended to help physicians take care of their portion of the responsibility to develop good end-of-life care, and is particularly appropriate to any physician looking after home-dialysis patients. Topics include:

◆ negotiating goals of care and treatment priorities,

◆ advance care planning,

◆ medical futility,

◆ requests for physician-assisted suicide, and

◆ requests to withhold or withdraw life-sustaining therapy.

If the Sheffield Model is applied to care of the home-dialysis patient, then appropriate supportive care will have been deployed from the earliest signs of kidney disease, so that when a patient enters the end-of-life period described by the EPEC Project there should be no difficulty in initiating the change in the nature and intensity of support required to enable the home-dialysis patient to die peacefully at home. Planning end-of-life care for a home-based patient should in fact be easier than planning similar care for a hospital-based patient who may be less likely to have the network of support services already in place.

Planning the end-of-life care of a home-dialysis patient incorporates all the aspects discussed in Chapter 4 – Advance care planning; Chapter 10 – Spiritual care; Chapter 12 – Initiation, withdrawal, and withholding of dialysis: communicating with patients and family; and Chapter 15 – End of life. However, the role of the CRN in the end-of-life care of a home-dialysis patient cannot be over-emphasized. He or she will probably be the member of the multi-disciplinary team who will know the patient, the carer, and the home circumstances best.

It will probably be the CRN with whom the question of discontinuation of dialysis will first be discussed, and of whom questions about mode of death will be asked. If the patient becomes frail, visits to the hospital clinic, and repeated measurement of laboratory parameters, become unnecessary. The emphasis on dialysis as a life-prolonging treatment shifts towards it being a means of controlling symptoms. If the patient has acquired a life-threatening condition in addition to chronic kidney failure, such as an incurable cancer, then the dialysis patient may be in the 'fortunate' position of being able to decide at what point to discontinue dialysis and plan the timing of their death. Many questions arise in the patient's and carer's mind at this time and may require a home visit by the dialysis physician. EPEC-type training at this stage is invaluable to both the patient and physician.

Case study	Mary – 69-year-old female
Primary Diagnosis:	Type II diabetes mellitus from age 51
Co-morbidities:	Hypertension, retinopathy, neuropathy, and depression
Dialysis history:	Required temporary haemodialysis while on holiday in USA at age 68
	Commenced CAPD 7 months later
	System adjusted to needs, including assisted peritoneal dialysis
	Died 2.5 years later at home
Social:	Lived with husband
	One son died on honeymoon due to diabetic coma
	One son alive with two grandchildren
Mobility:	Poor and limited

Mary was referred to the renal team by her diabetes consultant at a local district hospital. In view of the known poor prognosis for patients with diabetic nephropathy and extensive co-morbidity, palliative care was discussed along with dialysis options. The patient decided that she wanted dialysis treatment, but, because she did not like hospitals, wanted a treatment that would reduce hospital admissions or attendances. CAPD was discussed and Mary felt that with help from her husband she would be able to do it.

For the first 18 months at home on CAPD, Mary managed reasonably well, though she and her husband experienced many emotions and difficulties and it became clear that she was having difficulty coping with her other disabilities rather than the dialysis.

Mary (now age 72) started becoming less communicative and displayed evidence of depression. She was reviewed by her nephrologist and commenced on an antidepressant. The community renal nurse (CRN) visited more frequently to provide support for both Mary and her husband. It became evident that Mary's husband was doing increasingly more as her level of independence deteriorated, and he required increased support from the Social Worker to organize various aspects of Mary's care, including carers to sit in the house whilst he was able to get out for short periods. Mary's general practitioner (GP) also became involved at this stage and a 1-week hospital admission was organized to allow Mary's husband a respite, and to reassess Mary's condition.

There was little evidence of any new medical issues but Mary was unable to carry out most of her daily living needs and required a lot of help from nurses. Her dialysis modality was switched to assisted APD on discharge. Once at home again Mary's condition stabilized initially for a few weeks but then continued to deteriorate. The CRN arranged a home visit by the nephrologist to discuss with Mary and her husband how best to manage her from this point. Her bed was now downstairs and her assistant was doing all her dialysis with help from her husband as well.

She had become increasingly immobile and had significant pain from her arthritis. Mary expressed clearly that her quality of life was now so poor that she could no longer battle against all her difficulties. A referral was made to the palliative care team who liaised closely with the GP, district nurses, and CRN. Although dialysis was not stopped the volume of APD exchanges was reduced. Mary's husband needed a lot of support and the family were at the bedside constantly. Mary died peacefully at home, approximately 30 months after starting dialysis.

Ethical case analysis

High quality care has been described as the right care for the right patient at the right time. Quality should be the goal of all medical care including renal supportive care. This case highlights such quality. Mary's wish to engage in home dialysis was honoured, and when she started to fail, she and her husband received support from the CRN, her GP, the hospital who provided respite care for the husband, the home-dialysis team who switched her to assisted APD, the palliative care team, and their family. Such coordinated, compassionate care should be the goal of all who seek to develop renal supportive care teams.

References

1 Brunier GM, Mckeever PT (1993) The impact of home dialysis on the family: literature review. *ANNA J*, Dec, **20**(6), 653–9.

2 Brunner FP, Gurland HJ, Harlen H, et al. (1972). Combined report on regular dialysis and transplantation in Europe, II, 1971. *Proceedings of the European Dialysis and Transplant Association*, **9**, 3–34.

3 Katz AM (1970). Patients in chronic haemodialysis in the United States: A preliminary survey. *Social Science & Medicine*, **3**, 669–77.

4 Morrin PAF (1966). A survey of chronic renal failure in Southeastern Ontario. *Can Med Assoc J*, **94**,1353–6.

5 Price JDE, Ashby KM, Reeve CE (1978). Results of 12 years treatment of chronic renal failure by dialysis and transplantation. *Can Med Assoc J*, **118**, 263–6.

6 Shambaugh PW, Kanter SS (1969).Spouses under stress: Group meetings with spouses of patients on haemodialysis. *Am J Psychiatry*, **125**(7), 928–36.

7 Evans RW, Blagg CR, Bryan FA (1981). Implications for healthcare policy: A social and demographic profile of haemodialysis patients in the United States. *J Am Med Assoc*, **245**(5), 487–91.

8 Shambaugh PW, Hampers CL, Bailey GL, et al. (1967). Hemodialysis in the home: Emotional impact on the spouse. Transactions American Soc Artificial Internal Organs, **13**, 41–5.

9 Osmond MW (1987). Radical-critical theories. In Sussman MB and Steinmetz SK (eds) *Handbook of marriage and the family*, pp. 103–24. New York. Longman.

10 Rubin J, Case G, Bower J (1990). Comparison of rehabilitation in patients undergoing home dialysis. Continuous ambulatory or cyclic peritoneal dialysis vs home haemodialysis. *Arch Intern Med*, **150**(7), 1429–31.

11 Anderson JM, Elfert H (1989). Managing chronic illness in the family: Women as caretakers. *J Adv Nursing*, **14**, 735–43.

12 Annual Data Report 2000. United States Renal Data Service http://www.usrds.org/2008.htm

13 Adam J, Akehurst RL, Angris S, et al. for the National Institute for Clinical Excellence (2002). Guidance on home compared with hospital haemodialysis for patients with end-stage renal failure. National Institute for Clinical Excellence. London.

14 Goovaerts T, Jadoul M, Goffin E (2005). Influence of a pre-dialysis education programme (PDEP) on the mode of renal replacement therapy. *Nephrol Dial Transplant*, Sep, **20**(9), 1842–7.

15 Motiwala SS, McFarlane PA (2008). Standardized preplanned patient education to encourage transfer from hospital hemodialysis to home dialysis. *Perit Dial Int,* Jul-Aug, **28**(4), 403–7.

16 Ahlmen J, Carlsson L, Schonborg C (1993). Well-informed patients with end-stage renal disease prefer peritoneal dialysis to hemodialysis. *Perit Dial Int*, **13** Suppl 2, S196–8.

17 Binik YM, Devins GM, Barre PE, et al. (1993). Live and learn: patient education delays the need to initiate renal replacement therapy in end-stage renal disease. *J Nerv Ment Dis*, **181**(6), 371–6.

18 Hayslip DM, Suttle CD (1995). Pre-ESRD patient education: a review of the literature. *Adv Ren Replace Ther*, **2**(3), 217–26.

19 Klang B, Bjorvell H, Berglund J, et al. (1998). Predialysis patient education: effects on functioning and well-being in uraemic patients. *J Adv Nursing*, **28**(1), 36–44.

20 Lancaster LE (1984). The patient with end-stage renal disease. 2nd ed. John Wiley & Sons, Inc.

21 Pagels AA, Wǎng M, Wengström Y (2008). The impact of a nurse-led clinic on self-care ability, disease-specific knowledge, and home dialysis modality. *Nephrol Nurs J*, May–Jun, **35**(3), 242–8.

22 Farina J (2001). Peritoneal dialysis: a case for home visits. *Nephrol Nurs J*, Aug, **28**(4), 423–8.

23 Gathercole WK (1987). Psychosocial aspects of end stage renal disease. *Nursing*, **17**, 633–6.

24 Steffen C (1989). Psychosocial issues at critical times in the course of dialysis. *9th Annual Conference on Peritoneal Dialysis (presentation)*. University of Missouri, Columbia.

25 Purvis PJ (1991). A support group for patients with renal insufficiency on maintenance dialysis. *EDTNA-ERCA J*, **17**(3), 25–7.

26 Cerruti G, Cotto M, Rivetti M, et al. (1993). Patients' group experiences. *Periton Dialy Int*, **13**(Suppl 2), s199–201.

27 Prater J (1985). An exploration of coping behaviors within a dialysis caseload. Dialy Transplant, **14**(9), 504–10.

28 Carey H, Finkelstein S, Santacroce S, et al. (1990). The impact of psychosocial factors and age on CAPD dropout. In Nissenson AR (ed.) *Peritoneal dialysis in the geriatric patient. A supplement to advances in peritoneal dialysis*. 6, 26–8.

29 Wicks MN, Milstead EJ, Hathaway DK, et al. (1997). Subjective burden and quality of life in family caregivers of patients with end stage renal disease. *ANNA J*, Dec, **24**(5), 527–38.

30 Walker PJ, Diaz-Buxo JA, Chandler JT, et al. (1981). Home care: Paid home dialysis aides: The experience of a single program. *Contemp Dialy*, **2**(4), 50–4.

31 Srivastava RH (1988). Coping strategies used by spouses of CAPD patients. *ANNA J*, **15**, 174–9.

32 Ansell D, Feehally J, Feest TG, et al. (2007). UK Renal Registry Report 2007. UK Renal Registry, Bristol, UK.

33 Afolalu B, Finkelstein SH, Finkelstein FO (2009). CKD education and treatment choice. *Semin Dial*, 22, 25–7.

34 Jager KJ, Korevaar JC, Dekker FW, et al. for Netherlands Cooperative Study on the Adequacy of Dialysis (NECOSAD) Study Group (2004). The effect of contraindications and patient preference on dialysis modality selection in ESRD patients in The Netherlands. *Am J Kidney Dis*, May, **43**(5), 891–9.

35 Brown EA (2008). Peritoneal dialysis for older people: overcoming the barriers. *Kidney Int*, **108**, s68–71.

36 Oliver MJ, Quinn RR (2008). Is the decline of peritoneal dialysis in the elderly a breakdown in the process of care? *Perit Dial Int*, Sep–Oct, **28**(5), 452–6.

37 The Gallup Organisation (1996). Knowledge and attitudes related to hospice care. Survey conducted for the National Hospice Organisation. Princeton, NJ: The Gallup Organisation; September 1996.

38 Emanuel LL, von Gunten CF, Ferris FD (1999). The Education for Physicians on End-of-life care (EPEC) curriculum. The Robert Wood Johnson Foundation.

Initiation, withdrawal, and withholding of dialysis: Clinical

Lionel U Mailloux

12.1 Introduction

As patients and their families realize they can use their 'rights' in the medical decision-making process, more numbers are becoming involved in decision-making about all aspects of their care, e.g. dialysis, cancer chemotherapy, surgical procedures. This has a direct impact on practising nephrologists as many patients consider never initiating renal replacement therapy (RRT) as their renal function deteriorates. There has been limited literature on patients not starting dialysis, but of late more information has been published (see Chapter 13). However, there is more information with regard to patients who withdraw from dialysis. Based upon national, Canadian, and regional data, about 20–25% of end-stage renal disease (ESRD) patients receiving RRT later withdraw from dialysis; this withdrawal from dialysis is the second most common cause of death in Canada (after cardiovascular disease) among patients with ESRD and the third most common cause in the United States (after cardiovascular and infectious diseases).[1–3] With the ready availability of dialysis in the USA, nephrologists may feel 'forced'/'obligated' to offer RRT to all patients with clinical indications for dialysis.

Many patients and more nephrologists are willing to discuss advanced directives and end-of-life (EoL) decisions; this has become a national objective in most hospitals and out-patient practices. In addition, the Renal Physicians Association/American Society of Nephrology (RPA/ASN) workgroup to formulate guidelines concerning initiation and withdrawal of treatment has stimulated much discussion in this area; the guideline is currently being revised.[4] The group involved multiple disciplines, including physicians, ethicists, nurses, social workers, and clergy. They recommended the following: shared decision-making, informed consent or refusal, estimating prognosis, conflict resolution, advance directives, withholding or withdrawing dialysis, special patient groups, time-limited trials, and palliative care. For complete guidelines see "Introduction to Ethical Case Analysis" in this volume.

Although there are few available data, withholding dialysis probably occurs more frequently than commonly thought. In a survey of American nephrologists over 10 years ago, nearly 90% reported withholding dialysis at least once during the preceding year and over 30% reported withholding it at least 6 times [5]. By comparison, a prospective Canadian study reported that about one-quarter of patients referred for initiation of haemodialysis were not offered dialysis following due consideration.[6] These patients had very poor functional capacity, severe cardiovascular disease (50% with diffuse atherosclerosis and renovascular disease), diabetes mellitus, or neurological disease. Only two of the 23 patients survived for 6 months, confirming the diagnosis of ESRD in 91% of the patients. Primary care physicians may play a more important role in withholding dialysis by not referring patients to nephrologists for evaluation. One study from West Virginia found that 20 of 76 primary care providers (26%) had effectively withheld dialysis for at least one patient because of nonreferral to a nephrologist.[7] The most common reasons cited by the physician were end-stage heart, liver, or lung disease, old age, and patient refusal. In a report from Feehally of visits to UK renal units, he acknowledged the challenge of providing bias-free information and expressed concern at the confidence of some staff that the decisions made by patients they had counselled were independent and free from professional or family influence.[8] Noble, who has done considerable clinical research in this area, recently published an article about reasons patients give for not initiating dialysis.[9] These include: the need for patients to make an autonomous decision, the arduous nature of dialysis, difficulties in getting to the dialysis center 3 times weekly, previous experience with friends or family members on dialysis, age, the fact that for them dialysis equated to a death sentence, dialysis venepunctures, and the inability to make a decision.[9] In fact, many patients and nephrologists feel uraemia is a "good death".[10]

Patient decision-making process for dialysis: whether to start or to withdraw later

Clinical scenarios to highlight pertinent points

12.2 Annotated clinical cases

Mr. N.

A 77.25-year-old gentleman with known progressive (10–12-year course) advanced chronic kidney disease (diabetic nephropathy) who is practically ready to initiate RRT, has estimated glomerular filtration rate (eGFR) of 14 cc/min. He has had a prior nephrectomy for renal cell cancer, has active metastatic prostate cancer, and peripheral vascular disease with several bouts of dehydration causing acute renal failure superimposed on his chronic kidney disease. He had an arterio-venous fistula placed several months previously, but it did not mature appropriately because of the many venepunctures and intravenous therapies required in the previous 4 years. He had a fall at home and broke his left femur leading to surgical repair of the fracture; it was not possible to confirm a pathological fracture. He became more catabolic post-operatively and was eventually discharged to subacute rehabilitation. While there, he developed sepsis and had to be transferred back to the hospital. Subsequently, he became oliguric, uraemic, and developed early encephalopathy. His arterio-venous fistula malfunctioned, so he eventually required a tunnelled dialysis catheter. Although the patient was comfortable with the possibility of not undergoing dialysis, his children could not come to grips with that decision and he and his family were not sure of which course to take. His advance directive did not mention withholding RRT, although he had stated some ambivalence towards RRT on a few occasions and it was noted that he felt that just going to the oncologists was burdensome and a detriment to the quality of his life. A palliative care consult was called to assist the nephrologists with the on-going care and support its team was providing. He and his family agreed to a 'trial of dialysis' for 3 weeks. The dialysis treatments were very difficult and arduous with frequent hypotension, severe cramping, tachycardias, disequilibrium, and an overall lack of improvement. After six treatments, although mentally improved slightly, he agreed to palliative care only. He was transferred to an 'in-patient' hospice facility a few days later. His wife called to inform the team that he was at the most peaceful and communicative that she had seen him in 4–6 months following the transfer. He was not in pain. He expired 4 days later.

Case comment

The patient felt initially ambivalent about dialysis but did not refuse an attempt at arterio-venous fistula placement. He did not want not want to burden his family. The wife and children were more positive towards RRT than the patient. Neither the healthcare proxy nor the advance directive addressed dialysis but did mention parenteral nutrition, chest compressions, etc. Because of the acuteness of the situation with sepsis, the nephrologists concurred with the decision-making process for a trial of dialysis to correct the encephalopathy and clinical uraemia, but the dialysis treatments were very difficult no matter how the prescription was modified. The patient eventually made the decision that the 'trial' was a failure. He passed away peacefully at hospice in peace with his wife at the bedside. There was considerable relief in the family with closure of the whole situation.

This case demonstrates several of the principles outlined above, i.e. shared decision-making, conflict resolution, time limited trial, palliative care, incomplete advance directive and informed decision to withdraw from an extraordinary therapy. The patient, with the support of children, consciously decided to withdraw from dialysis and go to hospice. He was capable of making decisions. The family supported his decision-making process.

Mrs. L.

A 90-year-old lady with known very slowly progressive renal insufficiency for several years superimposed upon peripheral vascular disease, degenerative joint disease, hypertension, recent trauma with dislocated right shoulder, and poor urinary bladder control, who then required dialysis. Although she lived semi-independently, she required assistance for activities of daily living. She felt quite tired and lethargic and more recently fell on a staircase and fractured her right hip, which required surgical fixation. She then went to a geriatric-rehabilitation facility from which she was discharged to her daughter's home where she required more assistance to ambulate. She often expressed her feelings that she had now become a 'real burden' to her family. One of her neighbours was on dialysis and tried to convince her to think positively about it. She is on numerous cardiac medications. Physical examination revealed a frail, chronically ill lady ambulating with difficulty with one assistant and a walker. She had obvious wasting but was alert, oriented, and fully responsive. Pertinent laboratory data revealed a depressed serum albumin.

Case comment

This lady felt unable to perform peritoneal dialysis and did not want to burden her family; she was also extremely negative about the possibility of initiating haemodialysis, therefore no planning was made for either, including no provision for vascular access. In addition, she showed clinical evidence of protein calorie malnutrition. Her children were in full agreement with her decision, because she was competent. She had no healthcare proxy or advance directive but had clearly expressed her views which were supported by her family. Her grandchildren were quite upset that she was not willing to start dialysis; however, they respected her wishes. The nephrologists concurred with the decision-making process, made over a period of months as she deteriorated. She passed away peacefully at home in her own bed 3 weeks later. There was considerable relief in the family with the closure of the clinical situation.

This case demonstrates several of the principles noted above, i.e. shared decision-making, conflict resolution, and informed refusal to initiate an extraordinary therapy. The patient, with the support of children, consciously decided to forego dialysis – a decision which was accepted despite the fact that she did not have an advanced directive. She was uraemic, but competent to make her own decisions and her family supported her.

Case study 3: Patient HA

Mr HA was 76-years old at the time of his death. He had been on dialysis for more than 6 years when he elected to withdraw. His ESRD was caused by adult polycystic kidney disease with significant underlying coronary artery disease, hypertension, peripheral vascular disease (S/P bilateral lower extremity amputations), and severe pulmonary hypertension with right-heart failure. One of his children had begun dialysis in 2001 and another child had advanced chronic kidney disease awaiting a renal transplant. The patient himself had chronic pain requiring narcotic analgesia. In mid-2001, he began to express concern about his inability to care for himself. He used expressions such as 'my son has to carry me', 'I can't breathe', 'I need oxygen at all times', and 'my wife doesn't have a single free minute except when I'm in the hospital'. He needed six hospitalizations in 2001 and five in 2002. He was, however, well dialysed, often receiving additional ultrafiltration or dialysis. At this time, because of his increasing dependence and his need for constant oxygen therapy, he started to talk about his wish to stop dialysis.

Initially, his family had great difficulty discussing the idea of withdrawal from dialysis, feeling that one did everything medically until death occurred. They were referred to their pastor for a discussion in which the nephrologists participated. His wife and daughter had been appointed healthcare proxies and were aware of his concerns. Six months after opening the conversation about withdrawal, a decision to withdraw was made. It was accomplished after a quick trip to their summer home for a last visit (the journey 250 miles away nearly killed the patient). The daughter on dialysis also had to arrange for a trip east from California; she stayed for 3 months receiving dialysis in the same ambulatory unit as her father. He died in the hospital within 18 h of admission when he developed agonal breathing, 5 days following withdrawal. His family was at his bedside.

Case comment

This patient was absolutely miserable on dialysis as his peripheral vascular disease and pulmonary hypertension progressed further. He did have an advance directive, in which he had expressed his wish not to be a 'total burden', but his entire family needed to be involved in the decision-making process. They eventually 'bought into' the process and everyone was at peace with the decision. This case also illustrates some of the above principles: shared decision-making, informed consent or refusal, estimating prognosis, conflict resolution, and having advance directives in place.

Case study 4: Patient GA

Mrs GA was 68-years old, legally blind with Type 2 diabetes mellitus, hypertension, underlying coronary artery disease, and had undergone a two-vessel coronary artery bypass graft years earlier (S/P myocardial infarction, angina pectoris, and arrhythmias). During the previous 6 months, she had been hospitalized twice for a myocardial infarction and cerebrovascular accident with minimal residual weakness on the left side. It was noted that she had chronic kidney disease. Three months later, a full evaluation for anaemia revealed the presence of multiple myeloma with bony lesions. The patient was hospitalized on several occasions for pain control, congestive heart failure, and eventual initiation of chemotherapy after developing severe hypercalcaemia. Her renal function deteriorated and she developed progressive uraemia. She had expressed the wish to withhold dialysis. Despite an advance directive, her two children felt that she should initiate dialysis in the hope of controlling the myeloma. She therefore consented to a 'trial' of dialysis. Additional therapy included thalidomide, narcotics, oral hypoglycaemic agents, antianginal medication, antihypertensive medication, and erythropoietin. At that time, she had generalized pain and discomfort throughout her body, she had experienced episodes of bleeding, and examination revealed a debilitated lady with markers of chronic ill-health and numerous bruises, and ecchymoses. In addition, she had decompensated congestive heart failure. She remained significantly anaemic and thrombocytopaenic (haemaglobin always <8.8 g/dl) despite escalating doses of erythropoietin with appropriate iron replacement. Dialysis was initiated with her as an in-patient. There was no recovery of renal function; bone pain persisted, and she developed gastrointestinal symptoms which became worse. By week 9, the patient met her whole family, held private discussions with the oncologists and nephrologists, and decided to withdraw from dialysis at the end of week 10. She died at home with her children and grandchildren 16 days later.

Case comment

This lady's advanced directive had clearly stated that she wished no extraordinary measures undertaken should she be critically or terminally ill. She had also expressed the desire to withhold dialysis, but following full discussion with her oncologist, nephrologists, and family, she elected to set a time-trial on dialysis because her healthcare team had convinced her that there was a possibility of some recovery. A review was subsequently undertaken, as agreed, although following a longer time trial than usual, at which time her family acquiesced with her wishes.

12.2.1 Comments pertaining to the clinical scenarios

There has been more information published about the ethical issues of foregoing of dialysis and withdrawal from dialysis since the last edition of this textbook 6 years ago than in the previous

15 years.[2,8,9,11–20] Withdrawal from dialysis means the discontinuation of maintenance dialysis, while withholding of dialysis is defined as foregoing dialysis in a patient in whom dialysis has yet to be initiated. The terms may be used interchangeably in patients with acute or chronic renal failure. The expected outcome from choosing either one of these options is death within a variable period of time (usually 7–14 days following withdrawal, and up to 90 days when not initiating dialysis – though it can be much longer).

12.3 **Withholding dialysis** (also see Chapter 13 on conservative management)

Many nephrologists feel it is appropriate to withhold dialysis in the following specific clinical settings:[3,6,7,21,22]

- Patients with severe and irreversible dementia.
- Patients who are permanently unconscious (as in a persistent vegetative state).
- Patients with end-stage lung, liver, cancer, or heart disease, who are confined to bed or chair or in hospice and need assistance with activities of daily living.
- Patients with severe mental disability who are uncooperative with the procedure of dialysis itself, are unable to interact with the environment or other people, or are persistently combative with family or staff.
- Patients with severe, continued, and unrelenting pain in whom dialysis may prolong life for a short period of time but will also prolong suffering.
- Hospitalized patients (especially elderly) with multiple-organ-system failure that persists after 3 days of intensive therapy. The mortality rate of such patients is very high.

There usually is a proximate reason to consider foregoing dialysis; e.g. reasons for foregoing dialysis noted on the United States Renal Data System death-notification form in order of declining percentage in 1991 to 1992 were:[1]

- Failure to thrive (42%)
- Medical complications (35%)
- Access failure (4%)

12.4 **Withdrawal from dialysis**

Several factors are known to be associated with withdrawal from dialysis: advanced age, diabetes mellitus, extensive atherosclerotic disease, white race, low Karnofsky scores, female gender, higher physical discomfort index, and higher educational level.[23–26] The withdrawal rate rises with age, representing a significant part of the high mortality rate in the elderly ESRD patient population. For example, in one review of USRDS data, dialysis was discontinued in about 6% of patients under 65 years of age, but in 14% of those over 65 years of age.[26] In one of the original reports about discontinuation of dialysis, 56% of those over the age of 85 died because of withdrawal from chronic dialysis.[27]

Certain co-morbid conditions are also frequently present near the time of withdrawal, including diabetic gastropathy, neuropathy, the need for surgery, overall burden of dialysis, neoplastic disease, neurological deterioration, extremely poor or worsening quality of life, and increasing pain.[3,27–29] Dialysis is occasionally begun as a therapeutic trial in an attempt to improve an extremely poor quality of life; it is subsequently discontinued if no improvement occurs.

12.5 **Factors for consideration when withholding or withdrawing dialysis**

There has to be an appropriate sequential clinical approach to the withholding or withdrawing of dialysis, which involves some or all of the following important elements:

◆ Assessment of the patient's decision-making capacity
◆ Assessment of possible reversible factors
◆ Detailed and effective communication with the patient
◆ Full family involvement and appointment of a surrogate if so desired
◆ Interdisciplinary dialysis-team involvement
◆ The presence of an advance directive; either through a living will or healthcare proxy
◆ A trial period of dialysis (when felt to be appropriate)
◆ Commitment to support the patient's decision whether to forego, continue, or withdraw
◆ On-going support following withdrawal or withholding of dialysis.

12.5.1 **Assessment of patient's decision-making capacity**

The withholding of or withdrawal from dialysis may be suggested by the patient, the patient's family, the nephrologist, or other members of the healthcare team. Before proceeding with such a decision, the physician should satisfy himself that the patient (or appropriate surrogate) is competent and fully comprehends that the consequences of the decision include deaths, usually within 1–2 weeks in the case of withdrawal. See also Chapters 9, 12-Part 2, and 15).

12.5.2 **Assessment of possible reversible factors**

The healthcare team should explore why the patient requests withholding of, or withdrawing from, dialysis. Some patients may consider withdrawal because of irremediable factors (listed above), but reversible issues may precipitate contemplation of withdrawal. Potentially remediable factors may include painful needle insertions, frequent hypotensive episodes, intradialytic muscle cramps, uncontrolled pain, and depression. The nephrologist – with other members of the healthcare team – should address and modify these factors. (See also Chapters 7 and 9.)

12.5.3 **Detailed and effective communication with the patient**

Effective communication about foregoing dialysis or the possibility of withdrawal starts at the first nephrology consultation and should continue as appropriate throughout the patient's care. This will help the nephrologist determine the patient's true wishes. It is particularly important to ensure that requests for withdrawal are not either a reflection of untreated depression or a cry for help for unrecognized distress. Using the full resources of the multidisciplinary team will aid recognition of remediable family or communication issues. A full and open communication, maintained at all times, will contribute to the patient being able to reveal his or her true needs.

12.5.4 **Involvement of patient's family and appointment of a surrogate**

The nephrologist must ensure that the patient and his or her family or significant others are aware of a decision to forego or withdraw from dialysis and the consequences of such a decision; this includes the designated surrogate, if appointed. The patient, in most cases, is likely to be helped by the support of these people as he or she comes to a decision. Where there is conflict between the patient's wishes and those of his family, professionals from the nephrology team or separate from that team may be helpful for an individual to clarify his or her own wishes.

12.5.5 Interdisciplinary dialysis-team involvement

Since the decision to withdraw or withhold dialysis is complex, it is helpful to have other members of the healthcare team – i.e. the social worker, family members, physician, clergy, and dialysis nurses – complete the assessment. This team will be involved support and understanding of the patient and family.[9,11,13,28]

12.5.6 Importance of having an advance directive (living wills or healthcare proxies) (see Chapter 4)

If the patient has limited capacity, the presence of an advance directive detailing his or her desires concerning their future care in the event they become incompetent (or critically ill on life support) or has identified a surrogate agent (healthcare proxy) simplifies the entire matter. There are data suggesting that, in ESRD patients, advance directives may contribute to "good and peaceful deaths".[28]

12.5.7 Trial period of dialysis

A trial period of dialysis may be useful in a patient with depression, other psychological conditions, or when the fear over the dialysis technique is contributing to the decision to withhold dialysis. Many such patients often remain on dialysis once their trial period is over. The trial may last 30–60 days during which the patient is closely monitored. At the end of the trial, a discussion is held with the patient and family to assess the success or failure of the trial and a decision made to continue or withdraw treatment.

12.5.8 Commitment to support the patients and family's decision

Once the discussions are completed, the competent patient who desires to withdraw from long-term dialysis should be supported in this decision (even if the nephrologist does not agree). Likewise, this is similarly true for the occasional patient who the nephrologist feels is not a good dialysis candidate, but who nevertheless chooses to continue or initiate dialysis treatments. [11,13,30,31]

12.5.9 Support to patient and family following withdrawal of dialysis (see also Chapter 15)

Patients typically survive 1–2 weeks after discontinuing long-term dialysis. Most patients express great relief with the lifting of a heavy burden, become very comfortable, and are at peace with their decision. At this point, major healthcare attention should be directed towards the total comfort of the patient, including pain control if that was a precipitating factor. Care in the place of the patient's choice should be offered, if possible; this will include care within the hospital familiar to them, their own home, or hospice care. Palliative care can be provided in whatever setting. Comfort care includes the prevention, where possible, of foreseeable problems – so intravenous fluids, tube, or parenteral nutrition become inappropriate since they may precipitate fluid overload and pulmonary oedema which are most uncomfortable. Fluid and sodium intake should be limited to what is desired by the patient. As Kjellstrand has stated, if a patient has willingly begun dialysis with a fully open communications policy (atmosphere), then this same patient should be able to withdraw, exercising his or her own best judgement. The expertise of the nephrology team should remain available to the patient and family to guide the care of the dying patient by supporting the patient's priorities and discussing, in advance, the effects of the dying process with the patient and family. Non-palliative medications should be withdrawn and optimum pain control instituted. (See Chapter 15.)

12.6 **UK practice (by Edwina Brown)**

The different healthcare culture and patient expectations in the UK, as well as a different emphasis, means that the approach to the problems discussed are, at times, dissimilar. Referral patterns differ and very few patients will have advance directives. The sick elderly are often cared for in the community by primary care physicians and will initially be referred to physicians for the elderly. Historically, few such patients, especially if no longer independent, have been referred to nephrologists, although this is changing. Older, frailer patients are often referred or present late when someone notices the severe renal impairment, or when severe renal failure results from complications related to other co-morbidities. In such circumstances, patients do not have the opportunity to discuss treatment choices in terms of different dialysis modalities or opting for conservative care. The situation is further complicated as many patients in this situation are no longer competent to make their own decisions. The nephrologist then needs to make treatment decisions by determining the patients best interests (Mental Capacity Act 2005) (see Chapter 4). To be able to have appropriate discussions with the family, the physician needs to be honest about the prognosis. Unfortunately, this is often not the case and patients can be started on dialysis inappropriately. The various strategies and policy documents to improve EoL care in the UK are discussed elsewhere in this book (Chapters 2 and 4).

12.7 **Summary**

The dialysis population is increasingly represented by an elderly and frail group of patients with multiple co-morbidities (see Chapter 14). Many of these patients may not benefit from dialysis and/or may have an unacceptable quality of life with dialysis. Withholding and withdrawing dialysis is therefore appropriate for many. Appropriate counselling of the patient and family ideally results in shared decision-making and the establishing of goals of care. When initiation of dialysis can not be recommended, or the clinician feels it is no longer indicated, but the patient and or family requests dialysis, conflict resolution needs to take place.[4]

While all attempts should be made to accept the patient's/family's request in this situation, ultimately the clinician is responsible for ordering dialysis and must be comfortable with this decision.

12.8 **Conclusion and ethical analysis**

This chapter presents four cases – two involving time-limited trials of dialysis, and one each involving withholding dialysis and withdrawing dialysis. All four cases have, in common, that the patient did not want to start or continue dialysis, but at least some family members had difficulty accepting the patients' wishes. All four patients had poor prognoses because of multiple severe co-morbidities and decreased functional status. The RPA/ASN guideline recommends that, as part of the process of shared decision-making about starting, withholding, continuing, or stopping dialysis, the patient's prognosis should be estimated. In each of these four cases, the nephrologist should have not only estimated prognosis but taken a more active role in communicating the patients' poor prognoses and advocating for the patients to the families to honour the patients' wishes.

Because of the failure of the patients' nephrologists to more actively advocate for their patients, each patient experienced significant, **unnecessary** suffering. An underlying premise of this book is that nephrologists in conjunction with other clinicians can improve the care at the EoL of ESRD patients. As all four cases illustrate, nephrologists and renal care teams will need to improve their skills in communicating with and supporting families so that dialysis of those patients for whom the burdens substantially outweigh the benefits will not be undertaken.

References

1 United States Renal Data System (2008). USRDS 2008 Annual Data Report. U.S. Department of Health and Human Services. The National Institutes of Health, National Institute of Diabetes and Digestive and Kidney Diseases, Bethesda, MD.

2 Murtagh F, Cohen LM, Germain MJ (2007). Dialysis discontinuation: quo vadis? *Adv Chronic Kidney Dis*, **14**, 379–401.

3 Mailloux LU, Bellucci AG, Napolitano B, et al. (1993). Death by withdrawal from dialysis: A 20-year clinical experience. *J Am Soc Nephrol*, **3**, 1631–7.

4 Moss AH for the Renal Physicians Association and American Society of Nephrology Working Group (2001). A new clinical practice guideline to assist with dialysis-related ethics consultations. Shared Decision-Making in Dialysis: The New RPA/ASN Guideline on Appropriate Initiation and Withdrawal of Treatment. *Am J Kidney Dis*, **37**, 1081.

5 Singer PA (1992). Nephrologists experience with and attitudes towards decisions to forego dialysis. *J Am Soc Nephrol*, **2**, 1235.

6 Hirsch DJ, West ML, Cohen AD, et al. (1994). Experience with not offering dialysis to patients with a poor prognosis. *Am J Kidney Dis*, **23**, 463.

7 Sekkarie MA, Moss AH (1998). Withholding and withdrawing dialysis: The role of physician specialty and education and patient functional status. *Am J Kidney Dis*, **31**, 464.

8 Feehally J (2007). A View of UK Nephrology. Bristol, UK: Renal Registry.

9 Noble H, Meyer J, Bridges J, et al. (2009). Reasons Renal Patients Give for Deciding Not to Dialyze: A Prospective Qualitative Interview Study. *Dialy Transplant*, **38**, 82–90.

10 Cohen LM, McCue JD, Germain M, et al. (1995). Dialysis discontinuation: A 'good' death? *Arch Intern Med*, **155**, 42.

11 Noble H (2008). Supportive and palliative care for the patient with end-stage renal disease. *Br J Nurs*, Apr 24–May 7, **17**(8), 498–504.

12 Wong CF, McCarthy M, Howse ML, et al. (2007). Supportive and palliative care for the patient with end-stage renal disease. *Ren Fail*, **29**(6), 653–9.

13 Noble H, Meyer J, Bridges J, et al. (2008). Patient experience of dialysis refusal or withdrawal–a review of the literature. *J Ren Care*, Jun, **34**(2), 94–100.

14 White Y, Fitzpatrick G (2006). Dialysis: prolonging life or prolonging dying? Ethical, legal and professional considerations for end of life decision making. *EDTNA ERCA J*, Apr–Jun, **32**(2), 99–103.

15 Young S (2009). Rethinking and integrating nephrology palliative care: a nephrology nursing perspective. *CANNT J*, Jan–Mar, **19**(1), 36–44.

16 Patel SS, Holley JL (2008). Withholding and withdrawing dialysis in the intensive care unit: benefits derived from consulting the renal physicians association/american society of nephrology clinical practice guideline, shared decision-making in the appropriate initiation of and withdrawal from dialysis. *Clin J Am Soc Nephrol*, Mar, **3**(2), 587–93.

17 Holley JL, Davison SN, Moss AH (2007). Nephrologists' changing practices in reported end-of-life decision-making. *Clin J Am Soc Nephrol*, Jan, **2**(1), 107–11.

18 Davison SN, Jhangri GS, Holley JL, et al. (2006). Nephrologists' reported preparedness for end-of-life decision-making. *Clin J Am Soc Nephrol*, Nov, **1**(6), 1256–62.

19 Holley JL (2007). Palliative care in end-stage renal disease: illness trajectories, communication, and hospice use. *Adv Chronic Kidney Dis,* Oct, **14**(4), 402–8.

20 Davison SN, Holley JL (2008). Ethical issues in the care of vulnerable chronic kidney disease patients: the elderly, cognitively impaired, and those from different cultural backgrounds. *Adv Chronic Kidney Dis,* Apr, **15**(2), 177–85.

21 Moss AH (1995). To use dialysis appropriately: the emerging consensus on patient selection guidelines. *Adv Ren Replace Ther,* **2**, 175.

22 Moss AH, Stocking CB, Sachs GA, et al. (1993). Variation in attitudes of dialysis unit medical directors towards decisions to withhold. *J Am Soc Nephrol,* **4**, 229.

23 Eiser AR, Seiden DJ (1997). Discontinuing dialysis in persistent vegetative state: The roles of autonomy, community, and professional moral agency. *Am J Kidney Dis,* **30**, 291.

24 Leggat JE, Bloembergen WE, Levine G, et al. (1997). An analysis of risk factors for withdrawal from dialysis before death. *J Am Soc Nephrol,* **8**, 1755.

25 Bloembergen WE, Port FK, Mauger EA, et al. (1995). A comparison of mortality between patients treated with hemodialysis and peritoneal dialysis. *J Am Soc Nephrol,* **6**, 177.

26 Nelson CB, Port FK, Wolfe RA, et al. (1994). The association of diabetic status, age and race to withdrawal from dialysis. *J Am Soc Nephrol,* **4**, 1608.

27 Neu S, Kjellstrand CM (1986). Stopping long-term dialysis. An empirical study of withdrawal of life-supporting treatment. *N Engl J Med,* **314**, 14.

28 Cohen LM, McCue JD, Germain M, et al. (1995). Dialysis discontinuation: A 'good' death? *Arch Intern Med,* **155**, 42.

29 Tobe SW, Senn JS (1996). End-stage renal disease group. Foregoing renal dialysis: A case study and review of ethical issues. *Am J Kidney Dis,* **28**, 147.

30 Holley JL, Nespor S, Rault R (1993). Chronic in-center hemodialysis patients' attitudes, knowledge towards advance directives. *J Am Soc Nephrol,* **3**, 1405.

31 Holley JL, Nespor S, Rault R (1993). The effect of providing chronic hemodialysis patients written material on advance directives. *Am J Kidney Dis,* **22**, 413.

Initiation, withdrawal, and withholding of dialysis: Communicating with patients and family

Tom Sensky and Celia Eggeling

12.9 Introduction

This chapter begins by highlighting some general principles of communications between people with established renal failure and the professionals looking after them. The principles included relate to decision-making from the patient's[1] perspective, patients' reactions to information about their illness, and clinicians' reactions. Following this general overview, consideration is given to starting dialysis, withdrawing from dialysis, and withholding dialysis.

12.10 The patient's perspective

For patients, as for clinicians, knowledge of the likely outcomes of any decision is important – being able to weigh up the potential benefits and risks of different options. One might imagine that a necessary prerequisite would be to have sufficient knowledge and understanding in order to formulate the options available. While this is likely for most patients, some (particularly older patients) will put much more emphasis, in reaching their decision, on their trust in the clinician. Consistent with this, there is research evidence that the extent to which a person seeks information about the illness shows only a weak correlation with the extent to which he or she wishes to be involved in making decisions.[1] Some people prefer to have as much information as possible about their illness, while others show a strong preference towards having less information.[2] It is always helpful for the clinician to try to ascertain where an individual sits in the continuum between minimal and exhaustive information, because giving too much or too little information might not only make decision-making more difficult, but can also lead to the patient experiencing distress. Patients' preferences in this respect can usually be elicited by direct questioning. Sometimes, it may be helpful to negotiate how much information the person wants by starting off by regarding it as hypothetical. The clinician might say something like: "People differ in how much they want to know about their illness, and even about different aspects of their illness. I'm interested to know how much *you* would find helpful to know. For example, were I to consider that X might happen, how much would you want to know about that?" Clearly, such an approach must be used sensitively, but describing a particular clinical situation as hypothetical often allows the patient to see it as such if he or she wishes to.

---

[1] It would be preferable to avoid the use of "patient", and to refer throughout to "person with end stage renal failure", to acknowledge that dealing with the person is as important as managing the illness, and sometimes more so. "Patient" is chosen only because it is more concise.

Beyond knowledge and evidence, the patient's values are crucially important.[3] For example, someone who values personal independence particularly highly may prefer choices which support that independence – even to the extent that these choices go against the best available research evidence. A widely used textbook[4] defines evidence-based medicine as "the integration of best research evidence with clinical expertise and patient values". In this context, patient values are defined as "the unique preferences, concerns and expectations each patient brings to a clinical encounter and which must be integrated into clinical decisions if they are to serve the patient".

For each person, the values that he or she regards as particularly important are formed in a complex way, and developed as well as revised over time. They form an integral part of Personhood – how the person sees him or herself. Events during illness commonly threaten these important values, as well as other aspects of Personhood.[5] This is one important reason why people have strong reactions to aspects of their illness (see below). Both the development of Personhood and the means to modify this when it is threatened by illness depend on the person's story – his or her narrative. Events during illness disrupt this narrative, e.g. by jeopardizing a person's ambitions for the future, or by forcing the person to re-evaluate aspects of the past.[6] When this happens, the individual has to find a new narrative, or at the least modify the old one. This is usually done by telling and re-telling one's story. This offers the opportunity of rehearsing different narratives. None of these narratives is necessarily comprehensive or totally factually accurate, but this is not their main purpose.

While clinicians recognize the importance of individual patients' values in influencing their decisions, it is sometimes more difficult to see that these decisions have to be incorporated into a personal narrative. This can sometimes be a complex and lengthy process, involving not only patient and clinical team, but also family and others. Thus if – having been given as much information as possible relevant to a decision that needs to be taken – a person still appears reluctant to reach a decision, this may be because more work is required to modify the personal narrative, and the individual's Personhood, rather than merely because of obfuscation or denial. When this occurs, it would be helpful to consider how the person might be assisted in reaching the decision. Under such circumstances, it might be worth involving a counsellor, if the clinical team includes someone in this role.

12.11 Role of the family

Families commonly have an important influence on patients' decisions regarding any chronic illness. However, in people with end-stage renal failure (ESRD), there is sometimes an important additional dimension to this influence. In many instances, family members can potentially improve the course of the patient's illness by live donation of a kidney. Unless this possibility is raised by the clinical team, it may not be discussed within the family.[7] If the clinical team does raise the possibility, the ensuing discussions are probably best shared with the patient, even when a live donor is not forthcoming; otherwise, this can become "the elephant in the room", and can lead to longer term difficulties. For example, family members may feel guilty about deciding not to offer themselves as live donors – particularly when the patient experiences complications or deterioration. In some instances, family members may try to assuage this guilt by arguing for interventions which may be more active or even more "heroic" than the clinical situation justifies.

More generally, the family is a very important part of the individual's Personhood, and provides both material and psychological support. This is perhaps most striking where the person has dialysis at home, where the illness and its treatment often become part of the family's routine.

However, family influences can sometimes be complex and unexpected. The following clinical vignettes also illustrate the complex role of the family.

Case 1

Mrs GN – a woman in her 60s – had, prior to the diagnosis of ESRD, been acknowledged by the whole family as its matriarch. She effectively ran the family business, and even allocated the wages to her husband and other family members. As her overall physical state deteriorated while on dialysis, little by little, each of the important roles she held within the family was taken over by another family member. After some years, a successful cadaveric transplant led to a dramatic improvement in her physical health. However, her role within the family remained as it had done while she was on dialysis. She took to phoning her children several times each day, checking that they were safe and well. She herself remarked "All I can do now is worry".

In the case above, Mrs GN's family, although well intentioned, inadvertently removed key elements of her Personhood from her. In the following case, family dynamics became increasingly distressing because the family had to cope with illness and its treatment.

Case 2

Mr PC was a self-employed carpenter, married, and with four children. His wife had scleroderma and was currently in remission when, at the age of 44, he was diagnosed with renal failure. Financial commitments meant he needed to integrate hospital-based dialysis 3-times weekly into his lifestyle, and this could only be achieved by overnight dialysis. This put tremendous strain on his wife who complained she never saw him, that he no longer took his share of child-care responsibilities, or helped in the house when she was feeling unwell. Despite the symptoms and consequences of renal failure being explained to her, she remained in complete denial as to the severity of her husband's illness – possibly because of fear of facing such an uncertain future. When Mr C became too unwell to continue to work, the relationship began to break down. The impact on the children was catastrophic. One refused to attend school or leave her father's side fearing he was going to die and another exhibited antisocial behaviour which resulted in police involvement. The eldest child – feeling he had to take over his father's role – offered to forego his place at college and find employment. Meanwhile, Mrs C had taken a part-time job and angrily told her husband "Despite my illness, I can work". No longer able to communicate with each other and angry at their individual and joint losses, they became polarized. Mrs C coped by seeking support from friends to whom she could repeatedly tell her story and be 'heard', whereas Mr C became withdrawn and increasingly depressed. Feeling completely disempowered, undervalued, misunderstood, unsupported and a burden to his family, he said they would be 'better off' without him and requested to withdraw from dialysis.

12.12 **Shared decision-making**

Current guidance, regarding decisions concerning initiation of or withdrawal from dialysis, emphasizes the importance of shared decision-making.[8,9] Curiously though, the guidance does not elaborate on this. Shared decision-making has four key characteristics.[10] First, both clinician and patient are involved in the decision-making process. Secondly, both clinician and patient share information with each other. Thirdly, both clinician and patient take steps to participate in the decision-making process by expressing and sharing their preferences. Finally, both clinician and patient agree on the treatment to implement. Published research evidence provides some support for the benefits of shared decision-making, particularly in chronic illness.[11]

By the criteria above, it is clear that shared decision-making is not universally applied in this context. What might be described as rigorous shared decision-making is often more time consuming than other forms of decision-making. In addition, it can only work when both clinician and patient agree to undertake it; thus if the patient and/or the family are not ready to make a decision – or do not see the need to make a decision – then shared decision-making is impossible. Under such circumstances, the clinical team should work to assist the patient and family to reach the point where shared decision-making can begin. However, this can sometimes be extremely difficult to achieve.

Numerous other models of decision-making have been described in the clinical encounter. Two that are particularly relevant in this context are informed decision-making,[10] and what might best be described as postponed decision-making. As noted above, shared decision-making involves clinician and patient reaching a shared decision about treatment. In informed decision-making, the clinician provides the patient with all the necessary information to reach a decision, but the decision is then left to the patient to make. This is probably quite a common approach, but it is important to stress that this is not shared decision-making, and is not without its problems (see below). Postponed decision-making is not decision-making at all. Here, the patient is invited to reach a decision by the clinical team, but does not do so. This is commonly associated with applying the informed decision-making model – the clinical team gives the patient and family all the information that the team considers they need, then waits for the patient to reach a decision. Strictly speaking, this is not shared decision-making and goes against current guidance. However, when this occurs, the clinical team often faces a difficult dilemma. Postponing the decision can often make further treatment more difficult, and hence can have adverse consequences for the patient. On the other hand, working to motivate the patient to reach a decision, is either very time-consuming or can be perceived by those involved as pressurizing the patient. Striving to implement shared decision-making is perhaps the best approach to minimize the chances of such problems arising.

The following vignette illustrates some features of postponed decision-making, and highlights the difficulties patients might have in accepting the clinical team's view of how ill they are while they have few or no symptoms, or can continue to deny their severity.

Case 3

Mrs BD was a very active and youthful 75-year-old lady who enjoyed a good quality of life with her husband. She was referred to the pre-dialysis team several months before it was anticipated that renal replacement therapy would be required. As is standard practice among such teams, Mrs BD was offered a series of appointments with the team, to receive in-depth education relating to active treatment and conservative management, as well as offering time for reflection and clarification. Despite what she had learned, Mrs BD continued to deny feeling unwell – even while admitting to severe renal-related symptoms, such as fatigue, loss of appetite, itching, swollen ankles, and shortness of breath. She blocked and avoided any discussion about treatment modalities, other than to say she doubted she could tolerate the rigours of dialysis but she would 'wait and see' – eventually adding that she felt this was a decision her renal consultant should make as 'he knows best'. It was only when Mrs BD's symptoms were so severe as to precipitate emergency in-patient admission to the renal unit that she accepted she had to take responsibility and could not postpone decision-making any longer. Although she initially elected to have haemodialysis, she found it too arduous with no appreciable benefit to her quality of life, and then chose to withdraw and follow the conservative management pathway.

12.12.1 **Individual reactions and their management**

For the person with ESRD, management of their renal failure commonly involves threats to valued aspects of life, and uncertainty whether these threats can be overcome. Not surprisingly, such threats to the individual's Personhood can give rise to a wide range of emotions. Conversely, the presence of strong emotions should act as a cue to clinicians to explore whether the person perceives a threat to his or her Personhood.

Where it is necessary to make decisions about treatment in the context of worsening symptoms or developing complications, the patient is forced to acknowledge his or her state of health. In some instances, this can give rise to features of bereavement. If the person is able to make appropriate adjustments to his or her narrative and Personhood to begin to accommodate the changed state, such reactions are usually short lived. However, if a person is unable to find any way of accommodating the change in his or her physical state, including the changed prospects for the future, this can give rise to a depressive episode, which then warrants management in its own right.

In some instances, a person will react by remaining more optimistic than the circumstances warrant. This can be particularly difficult for clinicians to manage. On the one hand, if the patient is overly optimistic, clinicians have a harder task to engage him or her in decision-making. On the other hand, for some people, remaining optimistic is an important way of coping with their circumstances. Sometimes, it is possible to seek advice from family members about such reactions. Occasionally, it emerges that the individual has always been overly optimistic, or has perhaps avoided confronting difficulties, as in the following case.

Case 4

Mrs VF – a woman in her 40s who was married but had no children – found herself an in-patient after having been admitted via the Accident and Emergency Department. Prior to admission, she had been very unwell but ESRD was only diagnosed following admission. Her husband was a business executive, and Mrs VF used to spend most of her time entertaining him and his business colleagues at home, and going swimming with friends. Since her marriage, she had avoided taking important decisions, preferring to pass these to her husband – who appeared content to assume the role of decision-maker for her. She had always given the impression to friends that she was a "happy" person. However, following admission, she was not only confronted by the possible impact of her renal failure on the lifestyle she regarded as important, but also by the need to make decisions about treatment, which she found very threatening.

Another reaction – similar in some ways to over-optimism – is denial. In some instances, denial can be substantial – either of the seriousness of the person's circumstances, or of the decision needing to be taken. One similarity between this and over-optimism is that both of these reactions focus not on managing the situation (i.e. the decision needing to be taken) but rather on managing the person's emotions.[12] Such emotion-focused coping can create difficulties in reaching decisions. There is no easy formula to apply in managing such situations, although recognition by the clinical team that coping is predominantly emotion focused rather than problem focused is an important start.

12.12.2 Other factors that can support people in their decisions and decision-making

People strive to find meaning in everything that happens to them, including changes in their health, whatever their nature. For most individuals, meanings are a much stronger influence on decision-making than facts or evidence. Finding meaning (and reviewing this as necessary in the light of what happens to the person) is another feature of Personhood. Crucially, although meaning is multidimensional, the process of finding meaning is essentially cognitive and emotional, hence meanings can often be changed when they do not serve the individual well, and these changes can where necessary be facilitated by help from suitably experienced professionals.

Researchers have distinguished two major types of finding meaning – in the context of experiencing an illness, these are making sense of the illness or features of it, and finding benefit from the illness experience.[13] An important part of making sense of illness is to find explanations. These explanations do not have to be comprehensive, nor even necessarily accurate. The key point is that such explanations should fit adequately into the personal narrative. Making causal attributions is one element of making sense. The majority of people make causal attributions about the illness, and there is evidence that the failure to do so is associated with less favourable outcomes.[14] Related to this is the concept of sense of coherence.[15] This measures the extent to which the individual finds adversities in his or her life to be understandable and meaningful, and has confidence in having resources to deal with adversities. Sense of coherence is probably related to the personal narrative – someone with a low sense of coherence probably has difficulty integrating the experiences of illness into the personal narrative. There is substantial research evidence that a high sense of coherence is associated with a more satisfactory quality of life, and may even have an impact on mortality.[16]

The relationship between making sense of the illness experience, and finding benefit from it, remains unclear. Some have argued that the desire, or need, to find benefit from the illness experience is driven – at least in part – by a failure to make sense of the illness. However, not uncommonly, those who report having found benefit will also have made some sense of the illness experience. Patients report a variety of different types of benefit from the experience of illness, but these can be classified into two main groups.[13] Not uncommonly, patients report that they are able to appreciate aspects of life more (such as support from family or friends, appreciating nature, and so on) because their illness has forced them to go through a process of existential re-evaluation. The other main type of benefit might be described as finding strength through adversity. For example, patients sometimes report that their religious faith has been strengthened by their experience of illness.

For some people, their spirituality is very important in coping with the illness.[17] This is perhaps most easily recognized when it shows itself in "conventional" expressions of religious faith, but may involve other forms of transcendence beyond the person. The research literature has often failed to discriminate between experiential and ritual aspects of religion.[18] The former are largely private and include personal expressions of belief and faith, while the latter are mainly public and include, e.g. attendance at religious worship. Although these are conceptually very different, and might affect coping with illnesses in different ways, current evidence suggests that both types of spirituality can have substantial positive effects on health.

Hope is also crucial, both for the patient and for the clinical team.[19] Hope helps to keep relationships alive. It stops close family (and indeed also involved professionals) from treating the patient as though he or she has already died. The absence of hope also leads to demoralization. [20] Recent evidence suggests that, at least for family members, being given truthful information even when prognosis is poor does not undermine hope.[21]

How do the factors just described relate to decision-making? In essence, when someone has been unable to find meaning in important aspects of the illness experience, this may make it more difficult for the person to contribute to further decisions. If the personal narrative is fragmented, so too is the individual's Personhood. The importance of recognizing this is that it may contribute to explaining why someone is having difficulties in making a decision, and this might encourage the clinicians involved to review the time and other resources which might be helpful. This is not to say that clinicians should necessarily become directly involved in helping their patients find meaning, as the vignette below indicates.

Case 5

Mr JD was a devout Catholic, and also homosexual. He had been a successful piano teacher, and his success contributed substantially to his self-esteem, but his illness had forced him to give up most of his teaching. His relationship with his elderly parents was somewhat distant, because he had been unable to tell them about his homosexuality. He felt extremely guilty, because he considered that his illness represented a punishment from God for his homosexuality. He had sought guidance from his local priest, who reinforced this view, making him feel even more desperate.

In Mr JD's case, the clinical team sought help from the hospital chaplaincy. Mr JD was put in touch with another priest who had extensive experience of dealing with problems like his, who was able to provide reassurance and support.

12.12.3 Clinicians' reactions

Collaborating with patients and families in shared decision-making is seldom easy or straightforward. A number of particular difficulties have been described,[22] some of which have already been touched on above. These include initiating discussion about the future goals of care without considering the readiness of the patient and family to have this discussion. Sometimes, this is associated with an attempt to convince patient and family of the 'medical reality' of the patient's state. Both of these can be understood as attempts to apply the informed decision-making model – giving the patient the information necessary to reach a decision. The opposite approach – colluding with patient and family to postpone a necessary decision – can have equally unfortunate consequences.[23] If a patient has a poor prognosis, minimizing or ignoring the prognosis may prevent patient and family from managing the time before death as they might have wished. The same might result from the clinical team deciding to continue active treatment when this is difficult to justify clinically, although such a decision may sometimes ease the discomfort and distress of the clinical team. Information that is not exchanged between the patient and the clinical team may be as significant as information that has been shared, sometimes even more so.[24] Because of such considerable difficulties, it has been argued that clinicians involved in end-of-life decisions should have specific training to help to manage their own emotions.[25]

As noted above, hope is important for all concerned. When clinicians form the view that "nothing else can be done", this commonly leads them to distance themselves from the patient and family, and even to avoid contact, at exactly the time when the patient needs support and reassurance. The belief that there is nothing further than can be done is seldom justifiable, because there is always a place for palliative care. On the other hand, offering unrealistic or false hope is also likely to create difficulties for patient and family as well as for the clinical team.

For renal clinicians involved in the withdrawal of dialysis, there is likely to be an added difficulty. Terminally ill patients are commonly transferred to the care of the palliative care team. This transfer marks a transition for the patient, the family, and the patient's care. It can almost be seen as a ritual moving from one mode of treatment to another. For the clinicians involved, transferring the patient to the palliative care team commonly marks a clear change in the care plan, and in the priorities for care. Where the same team is involved first in 'curative or remedial' treatment and then moves to provide palliative care, this physical transition does not occur. Members of the clinical team have to shift their own mindset to the changed focus of care. Perhaps more importantly, this has to be negotiated with the patient and the family, without the benefit of the 'rituals' above. For clinicians who are accustomed to doing everything they can to keep their patients alive with the best quality of life possible, this shift can be extremely difficult. This is one argument for the clinical team having easy access to, and regular contact with, a palliative care physician.

12.13 Decisions with life-and-death consequences

The factors described above are relevant to all decisions facing people with ESRD, including those which have life-and-death consequences – such as withdrawing from dialysis, or deciding not to commence dialysis. It is helpful to consider the person's suffering in relation to the options available.[5,26] In fact, alleviation of suffering is relevant to all decisions about illness, but is introduced here because it is particularly pertinent in the context of decisions with serious consequences.

Suffering is best understood as "a state of severe distress associated with events that threaten the intactness of the person.... Suffering occurs when an impending destruction of the person is perceived; it continues until the threat of disintegration has passed or until the integrity of the person can be restored in some other manner".[27] In other words, suffering is a property of Personhood. From this definition, it follows that there are essentially three ways to alleviate suffering.[28] Attempts might be made to remove or change the "events that threaten the intactness of the person". In the context of illness, this is equivalent to curing the person and restoring him or her to health. In people with renal failure, having a successful transplant is the closest approximation to this, although this is not a cure in the strict sense, because the individual must continue on treatment indefinitely, and the prospect of failure of the transplant remains. Alternatively, suffering may be alleviated by reducing the severity of the perceived threat, or by the person revising his or her Personhood.

This conceptualization not only helps to gain a better understanding of the person's experience, but also makes it possible to consider treatment options in terms of the extent to which each can potentially alleviate that person's suffering. Although options for intervention may be constrained, e.g. by the patient's physical state, there are some instances in which intervention can be very effective, as in the following vignette.

Case 6

Mr BS was a married man in his 40s, with two young sons. Two failed transplants meant that his prospect of having a successful transplant was substantially reduced, and he had been on haemodialysis for some years. The clinical team caring for him saw him as a "model" patient, who bore his illness calmly and with dignity. He developed an arthropathy, which gradually lead to progressive limitation of his normal activities, to the extent that he had to start using a wheelchair. At this point, he decided that life was no longer worth living. He and his wife had agreed a long time ago that when he reached this point, he would end his life. However, they were unable to go through with this plan. At this point, he became profoundly depressed. Exploring with him why he had decided that life was no longer worthwhile, he focussed on his role as a father to his two young sons. Specifically, he thought that he could not be a good father unless he was able to remain physically active, e.g. being able to play football with his sons.

This vignette illustrates a number of important points. It is significant that Mr BS had approached his illness and circumstances with calm and dignity, to the extent that this was remarked on by members of the clinical team. This contrasted dramatically with what happened when he found that he could not go through with his long-standing plan to end his life at the time of his choice. Mr BS was clearly suffering, because the progressive consequences of his illness threatened a crucial aspect of his Personhood – namely how he saw himself as a father. Characteristically, the cause of Mr BS's suffering was highly personal, and even idiosyncratic. In some instances, as in Mr BS's case, people are able to tolerate considerable suffering if they perceive some mechanism of gaining control over the suffering. Suffering is exacerbated when its causes are intrusive and/or uncontrollable, and being able to exert some control over whatever causes of suffering is expected to reduce the extent of the suffering. Thus, e.g. suffering due to chronic pain may be alleviated if the person appreciates that the pain can be consistently reduced by analgesia. Mr BS was probably able to cope with his circumstances to the extent that others saw him as calm and dignified because he thought that if his circumstances became intolerable, he could end his suffering as he chose to do. His recognition that he could not go through with this plan caused considerable distress, and worsened his suffering.

Another crucial point about Mr BS's case was that, while he saw his worsening physical state as a serious threat to his Personhood, he could see no way of adjusting either the perceived severity of the threat, or his perception of his Personhood. However, exploring with him the events that led to his contemplating ending his life, it became clear that his view of himself as a father had focussed on his physical state to the exclusion of other qualities that good fathers have. Reviewing this allowed him to recognize that he was still able to be a good father to his sons even with his increasing reliance on the use of a wheelchair. In essence, Mr BS was able to revise his perception of his Personhood and, in doing so, he was able reduce the extent of his suffering. While this was successful for Mr BS, for some people the distressing perception of their Personhood and the threats to it are more difficult to shift, and may be intractable.

If consideration of treatment options is thought of in terms of alleviation of suffering then it involves reviewing how, and to what extent, a person can change his or her Personhood, or the extent to which the threat to that individual's Personhood from the illness might be reduced. All the factors reviewed above may be relevant. Reflecting on his experiences in a concentration camp, the psychotherapist Viktor Frankl noted that suffering ceases to be suffering when it takes on meaning.[29] While it is almost always helpful for members of the clinical team to form an understanding, in each individual case, of the person's suffering, factors contributing to it, and the scope for alleviating it, exploring in depth the individual's illness experience is a luxury in a busy clinical setting, and arguably less of a priority than focussing on clinical management of the symptoms and the disease. However, particularly where the patient appears "stuck", having great difficulty in making decisions either because of too much distress, or sometimes too little, this should raise the possibility of trying to identify other resources which might be helpful to the patient. This might include engaging the help of the family or others, such as religious or spiritual advisers. Fundamental to changes to the individual's Personhood is the need to revise the personal narrative, and this can be supported and facilitated by a renal counsellor.

12.14 Summary

The decision to withdraw dialysis, or to withhold it, is seldom straightforward. However, an appraisal of the extent to which other treatment options might alleviate the person's suffering can and should contribute to such decisions. It is also very important that such decisions cannot be isolated from their consequences. In many instances, a person is unable to reach a decision about withdrawing from dialysis until he or she understands adequately what is likely to happen after dialysis is stopped. Here, the general principles of palliative care apply, working with the patient to plan "a good death",[30] with attention to spirituality and dignity.[31,32]

Ethical case analysis

The six cases the authors present raise a number of issues including informed and postponed decision-making. As the authors note, when the prognosis is not good, physicians may tend to distance themselves from the patients and not communicate. The failure to communicate is unfortunate, because it deprives the patient and the family of three opportunities: (1) to participate in appropriate decision-making; (2) to express their preferences for end-of-life care and ensure that they are respected; and (3) to prepare for the patient's death. Families adjust better to a patient's poor prognosis and can be more supportive when they are realistic about the patient's likely outcome. Interestingly, the cancer literature provides evidence for physicians including pessimistic statements in their discussions with families of patients with advanced disease and shows that such families are more realistic.[33] Physicians may want to withhold prognostic information to maintain hope, but the vast majority of families (93% in one study) do not view withholding prognostic information as an acceptable way to maintain hope, largely because timely discussions of prognosis help families to prepare emotionally, existentially, and practically for the possibility that a patient will die.[21] The challenge for physicians is to provide accurate information in a sensitive manner so that patients are not allowed to be unrealistically optimistic to the detriment of themselves and their families.

In a couple of the cases the patients denied being unwell and used their denial to postpone needed decision-making regarding their subsequent care. In some semi-urgent situations in the care of ESRD, there is not the luxury of postponing decisions and allowing the patient to pretend that things are fine. If the patient chooses not to participate in shared decision-making, the urgency of the need for decision-making should be pointed out to the patient, and the patient should be asked to name a surrogate who can participate for the patient in decision-making. In a sense, the physician is forcing the issue for the good of the patient. In practice, patients often agree to participate once they realize that the physician is serious and will talk to another family member if the patient will not be involved in decision-making.

References

1 Ende J, Kazis L, Ash A, et al. (1989). Measuring patients' desire for autonomy: decision making and information-seeking preference among medical patients. *J Gen Intern Med*, **4**, 23–30.

2 Miller SM, Rodoletz M, Mangan CE, et al. (1996). Applications of the monitoring process model to coping with severe long-term medical threats. *Health Psychol*, **15**, 216–25.

3 Petrova M, Dale J, Fulford KWM (2006). Values-based practice in primary care: easing the tensions between individual values, ethical principles and best evidence. *Br J Gen Pract*, **56**, 703–9.

4 Sackett DL, Straus SE, Richardson WS, et al. (2000). *Evidence-based medicine: how to practice and teach EBM*. Churchill Livingstone, Edinburgh.

5 Cassell EJ (2004). *The nature of suffering and the goals of medicine*. Oxford University Press, Oxford.

6 Frank AW (1995). *The wounded storyteller*. University of Chicago Press, Chicago.

7 Sensky T, Mee AD (1989). Dilemmas faced by dialysis patients in search of a living-related kidney donor. *Dialy Transplant*, **18**, 243–9.

8 Renal Physicians Association and American Society of Nephrology (1999). *Clinical practice guideline on shared decision-making in the appropriate initiation of and withdrawal from dialysis*. Washington DC: Renal Physicians Association and American Society of Nephrology.

9 National Service Framework for Renal Services – Part Two: Chronic kidney disease acute renal failure and end of life care (2007). London: Department of Health.

10 Charles C, Gafni A, Whelan T (1999). Decision-making in the physician-patient encounter: revisiting the shared treatment decision-making model. *Soc Sci Med*, **49**, 651–61.

11 Joosten EA, Fuentes-Merillas L, de Weert GH, et al. (2008). Systematic review of the effects of shared decision-making on patient satisfaction, treatment adherence and health status. *Psychother Psychosom*, **77**, 219–26.

12 Folkman S, Lazarus RS (1988). The relationship between coping and emotion: Implications for theory and research. *Soc Sci Med*, **26**, 309–17.

13 Janoff-Bulman R, Yopyk DJ (2004). Random outcomes and valued commitments: existential dilemmas and the paradox of meaning, In Greenberg J, Koole SL, Pyszczynski T (eds) *Handbook of experimental existential psychology*, pp. 122–38. Guilford, New York.

14 Sensky T (1997). Causal attributions in physical illness. *J Psychosom Res*, **43**, 565–73.

15 Antonovsky A, Sagy S (1986). The development of a sense of coherence and its impact on responses to stress situations. *J Soc Psychol*, **126,** 213–25.

16 Eriksson M, Lindstrom B (2006). Antonovsky's sense of coherence scale and the relation with health: a systematic review. *J Epidemiol Community Health*, **60,** 376–81.

17 Miller WR, Thoresen CE (2003). Spirituality, religion, and health. An emerging research field. *Am Psychol*, **58,** 24–35.

18 Sinclair S, Pereira J, Raffin S (2006). A thematic review of the spirituality literature within palliative care. *J Palliat Med*, **9,** 464–79.

19 Johnson S (2007). Hope in terminal illness: an evolutionary concept analysis. *Int J Palliat Nurs*, **13,** 451–9.

20 Clarke DM, Kissane DW (2002). Demoralization: its phenomenology and importance. *Aust NZ J Psychiatry*, **36,** 733–42.

21 Apatira L, Boyd EA, Malvar G, et al. (2008). Hope, truth, and preparing for death: perspectives of surrogate decision makers. *Ann Int Med*, **149,** 861–8.

22 Weiner JS, Roth J (2006). Avoiding iatrogenic harm to patient and family while discussing goals of care near the end of life. *J Palliat Med*, **9,** 451–63.

23 Fallowfield LJ, Jenkins VA, Beveridge HA (2002). Truth may hurt but deceit hurts more: communication in palliative care. *Palliat Med*, **16,** 297–303.

24 Bugge C, Entwistle VA, Watt IS (2006). The significance for decision-making of information that is not exchanged by patients and health professionals during consultations. *Soc Sci Med*, **63,** 2065–78.

25 Weiner JS, Cole SA (2004). Three principles to improve clinician communication for advance care planning: overcoming emotional, cognitive, and skill barriers. *J Palliat Med*, **7,** 817–29.

26 Hutchinson TA (2005). Transitions in the lives of patients with End Stage Renal Disease: a cause of suffering and an opportunity for healing. *Palliat Med*, **19,** 270–7.

27 Cassell EJ (1982). The nature of suffering and the goals of medicine. *New Eng J Med*, **306,** 639–45.

28 Sensky T (2009). Suffering, In Mezzich JE, Snaedal J, van Weel C, et al. (eds), *Person-centered medicine: a conceptual exploration*, Proceedings of the 2008 Geneva Conference on Person-Centered Medicine [in press].

29 Frankl VE (1984). *Man's search for meaning: an introduction to logotherapy.* Pocket Books, New York.

30 Coyle N, Adelhardt J, Foley KM, et al. (1990). Character of terminal illness in the advanced cancer patient: Pain and other symptoms during the last four weeks of life. *J Pain Symptom Management*, **5,** 83–93.

31 Chochinov HM, Hack T, McClement S, et al. (2002). Dignity in the terminally ill: a developing empirical model. *Soc Sci Med*, **54,** 433–43.

32 Chochinov HM, Cann BJ (2005). Interventions to enhance the spiritual aspects of dying. *J Palliat Med*, **8, Suppl 1,** S103–S115.

33 Robinson TM, Alexander SC, Hays M, et al. (2008). Patient-oncologist communication in advanced cancer: Predictors of patient perception of prognosis. *Supportive Care Cancer*, **16,**1049–57.

Chapter 13

Conservative management of end-stage renal disease

Fliss Murtagh and Neil Sheerin

13.1 Overview

In common with failure of other organs, kidney failure leads to death. However, unique to renal disease, dialysis treatment, which is life-sustaining in patients with renal failure who do not have a kidney transplant, is available. This has been one of the major advances in modern medicine. Although attempts were made to dialyse patients in the early part of the twentieth century, the development of dialysis is largely confined to the last 50 years. In the early stages, dialysis was a short-term treatment for patients with acute renal failure, with no provision of maintenance dialysis for patients with chronic renal failure. The first maintenance dialysis programmes started in the 1960s and became increasingly numerous over the following 10–15 years. Despite this expansion, dialysis programmes were largely confined to major centres and the criteria for acceptance onto them were relatively strict. Therefore elderly patients or patients with multiple co-morbidities were usually excluded from renal replacement therapy (RRT) programmes.

Over the last 25 years, this situation has changed significantly. There are many more centres offering maintenance dialysis with a loosening of the criteria for acceptance onto renal replacement programmes. This has led to rapid growth in the number of patients receiving dialysis. For example, the number of patient receiving dialysis in the United Kingdom rose from 5000 in 1984 to 25 000 in 2006.[1] This increase reflects several factors, including an increase in the prevalence of renal disease, ethnic variations in renal disease, and an older population. However, dialysis treatment is now being offered to patients who previously would not have been considered.

Despite technical advances and changes in the way dialysis is delivered, e.g. assisted home dialysis, it still remains a challenging treatment for many patients. Dialysis delivered in its typical form requires invasive procedures prior to its initiation and then visits to a dialysis centre 3 times each week for 3–4 h of treatment. While some uraemic symptoms are relieved by dialysis, the overall symptom burden of those receiving dialysis remains high.[2] For some patients with severe co-morbidity and short life expectancy, dialysis is either not feasible or is unlikely to improve quality or quantity of life. Other patients – when they are informed about their treatment options – decide not to have dialysis, instead choosing supportive treatment of their renal disease. Renal management focusses on delaying progression of renal disease and controlling complications, alongside control of symptoms and psychosocial support as the disease progresses towards death. This chapter will discuss this important group of patients – who opt not to have dialysis – either through preference or necessity, and instead are managed conservatively.

13.2 **Epidemiology**

The classification of Chronic Kidney Disease (CKD) proposed by the National Kidney Foundation Kidney Disease Outcome Initiative in 2002[3] has allowed reproducible estimates of the prevalence of CKD. The New Opportunities for Early Renal Intervention by Computerised Assessment (NEOERICA) project estimated that the age-adjusted prevalence of Stage 3–5 CKD in the UK is 11% of women and 6% of men.[4] This is equivalent to approximately 4 million people in the UK. A similar prevalence of CKD has been reported by studies from other European countries, the United States of America, and Australia.[5,6]

Only a small proportion of these patients will progress to the point at which a decision between conservative or dialysis treatment is required, and older patients, in particular, may have greater likelihood of death from other causes or have non-progressive or slowly progressive renal disease. [7] Nevertheless, the prevalence of CKD is so high that even a small proportion progressing to end-stage renal disease (ESRD) translates into large numbers of patients reaching end stage, and this number is likely to increase further. Certainly, the number of patients on RRT is increasing steadily (see Fig. 1.8 in Chapter 1) and it is likely that this trend will continue for some years to come.[8] The United States Renal Data System reports 354 000 people on dialysis in 2006, with the prediction that this will increase to 533 000 by 2020.[9] By implication, as the number of patients reaching ESRD increases, so will the number of patients choosing conservative treatment. Data are not available to confirm this at the moment, but conservative treatment will increasingly feature as part of registry data collections, and national data on the numbers being managed conservatively will become available.

It is also evident from epidemiological studies in CKD and ESRD that their prevalence increases almost exponentially with advancing age. Stage 3–5 CKD is present in 40% of people older than 75, but in less than 1% of people younger than 35.[4] Initiation of dialysis is, therefore, much more frequent in the elderly (see Fig. 1.5 in Chapter 1); the proportion starting dialysis (per million population in that age band) increases sharply among those older than 65, peaks between 75 and 85 years, and only drops off in the >85-year age group.

The increasing proportion of older people in developed countries is therefore one of the main drivers behind the marked increase in the prevalent dialysis population. This change is also likely to increase the number of patients opting for conservative treatment. The exact number of patients who die of renal failure without receiving dialysis is very difficult to ascertain, partly because of the lack of routinely collected data, but also because few population-based, rather than service-based, studies are conducted. Some patients with severe co-morbidity – e.g. advanced cancer – may never be referred to renal services. In reported series of patients known to renal services and managed in specialist low-clearance clinics, approximately 15–20% will follow a conservative pathway.[10,11] In reality, this figure is likely to vary considerably between units, depending on the demographics of the catchment population and on how services are structured. However, these numbers provide only limited information concerning the numbers of patients whose death is directly attributable to their renal disease, because many deaths will be due to non-renal causes.

There have always been some patients managed conservatively, without dialysis, but practice has varied over time and between countries,[12] and between individual nephrologists.[13] The various national Renal Registries have collected data on those patients who are dialysed or transplanted, but not on those patients managed conservatively, so it is difficult to know accurately how many patients are being conservatively managed, and how trends are changing over time. It is only recently that there has been greater recognition of the conservatively managed group of patients, with systematic study beginning to be undertaken in order to address some of these very relevant questions.

13.3 **Survival**

For a variety of reasons, there is little evidence about the duration of survival of conservatively managed patients. First, although there have always been patients managed without dialysis, only recently has this group been recognized as a distinct population needing study. Second, it has been difficult to identify *from* what point survival should be measured – patients may not require dialysis until well into Stage 5, as they begin to experience worsening uraemic symptoms. In addition, even if dialysis is planned, some will die of co-morbid disease before dialysis can commence, and others experience only a very slow decline in renal function – such that dialysis is not actually needed for some time. Third, documented survival may well reflect the demographics, co-morbidity, and local practice at any one renal unit, rather than provide mortality data that is readily generalizable to other units.

There have been no prospective randomized trials which assess the benefit of dialysis versus conservative management in this population. The ethical challenges that this would raise are such that a randomized trial is unlikely to occur, and only a few observational studies are currently available to inform practice. Smith et al. report survival of 38 patients who, after multi-disciplinary assessment, were recommended palliative (conservative) treatment rather than dialysis.[11] In this cohort, 10 patients did not follow the recommendation and instead chose to have dialysis, while the remainder followed the conservative pathway as recommended. Statistically, survival was not significantly different between the two groups, although numbers were too small to be sure that there was not a Type II error. A second study considered all patients over 75 years with Stage 5 CKD managed in specialist nephrology care.[10] Notably, this study excluded those who were referred into nephrology care late, after estimated glomerular filtration rate (eGFR) reached <15 ml/min (late referrals are more likely to be managed conservatively,[14] and are known to have worse survival). A total of 77 patients (60%) were established on a conservative (non-dialytic) treatment pathway.[10] Patients managed without dialysis had a 1- and 2-year survival (measured from first reaching stage 5 CKD) of 68% and 47%, respectively. Those managed conservatively had a significantly worse survival than those on a dialysis pathway, suggesting some benefit from dialysis for older patients – at least in terms of survival. However, it was impossible to exclude a selection bias, with fitter patients choosing dialysis, and factors other than dialysis

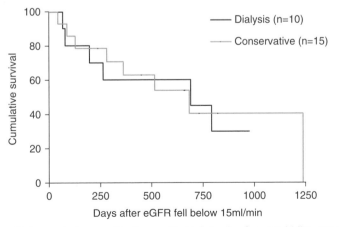

Fig. 13.1 Kaplan–Meier survival curves for those with high levels of co-morbidity, comparing dialysis and conservative groups[10].

were almost certainly contributing to the better survival in the dialysis group. In confirmation of this, 31% of the dialysis group had not actually started dialysis before the end of the study. More importantly in this study, if the patients with higher co-morbidity were considered in isolation, then the difference in survival between the two groups was much reduced (see Fig. 13.1) although the numbers in the study were small. This concurs with the experience of other renal units,[15] and with early evidence that conservative management is both feasible and provides comparable quality of life.[16] In addition to co-morbidity predicting survival,[17] functional capacity should also be assessed when considering whether a patient will benefit from dialysis, as this is also a good indicator of survival in stage 5 CKD.[18] This is discussed further in the next section.

13.4 **Trajectories**

A trajectory is a pattern of change over time. Disease trajectories are usually described in terms of changes in the functional ability of the patient, or in the symptoms experienced, over time. Several authors have proposed that study of trajectory in advanced renal disease is needed to help inform care; Jablonski, for instance, has recommended that ESRD should be studied from the perspective of the trajectory of illness in order, comprehensively, to explore the different phases of trajectory and to help inform care and identify changing concerns of patients and their families. [19] Holley also proposes this approach to explore the wider and related issues of communication, advance planning, and related patient experiences.[20]

While there is no doubt that nephrologists need more evidence about survival times,[10] these alone are not sufficient to inform complex and challenging dialysis decisions. Patients themselves find statistical prediction or likelihoods difficult to make sense of in the context of their own illness; they want a more individualized and personal approach, with better understanding of how the illness might affect their day to day lives.[21] Delivering this demands better insights into the most likely course or trajectory of illness the patient might expect,[22] so as to best advise patients on what they might expect following the dialysis decision. Many patients want to know their prognosis.[23] Questions frequently asked by patients include 'how long do I have to live?' (which relates to prognosis and survival) but also 'what can I expect?', 'what symptoms will I get?', and 'what will happen near the end?' (all of which relate more specifically to functional and symptom trajectories). The answers to these questions will inform the patient's expectations for the future and may influence their dialysis choices and choices about place of care and death. Sensitive, yet honest, discussions about these issues – carefully matched to the patient's preferences for information – help patients maintain hope and realistic expectations, rather than removing hope as professionals often believe.[24] Unrealistic expectations – which can develop when issues relating to the advance and likely course of the illness are not discussed – may lead to anger and frustration as advancing illness robs patients and families of the quality and quantity of life they had hoped for. Evidence also shows that, alongside good symptom control, patients give high priority to the opportunity to prepare for death.[25,26] Without knowledge of trajectories, advance care planning, effective service delivery, and anticipating and preparing for end of life is much more difficult, if not impossible.

Thus, for the medical professionals who are planning and delivering care to patients with conservatively managed Stage 5 CKD and their families, it is important to understand functional and symptom trajectories. However, trajectories are also important for the patients themselves. There is, therefore, a considerable need for research into the trajectory of illness for those managed conservatively, without dialysis, as well as older dialysis patients.

The concept of distinct patterns of functional decline over time leading to death is well established in palliative care.[27] Four distinct trajectories in the last year of life have been described.[28,29] First, sudden death can occur at any stage without a prior diagnosis or symptoms of underlying disease. Second, following the diagnosis of a terminal illness such as cancer, there is a steady relentless decline over weeks or months. The third pattern is one of fluctuation, with acute episodes, frequently requiring hospital admission, and often without recovery to the previous level. Eventually, death occurs during one of these acute episodes. This pattern is typical of patients with organ failure, such as end-stage cardiac or respiratory disease. The final pattern is one of gradual decline from a baseline of already poor function and is typically seen in frail older patients or those with dementia (see Fig 15.2).

Patients with ESRD were not included in this original trajectory work, but there is some limited evidence about how these trajectories might apply to conservatively managed renal patients. Clinical experience indicates that conservatively managed patients can remain stable for long periods of time, and preliminary work from Williams and Burns suggests that they may have relatively rapid functional decline (with the last episode of illness lasting about 7–10 days) in the late stages of their disease.[30] This concurs with recent more detailed study of trajectories in conservatively managed Stage 5 CKD patients which confirmed that functional decline is maintained often at a low level until late in the illness, with rapid decline occurring over the last month of life.[31] Murtagh has documented the average functional trajectory over the last year of life in her recent longitudinal study of conservatively managed stage-5 CKD patients, and this average functional trajectory is presented in Fig. 13.2.

This trajectory is initially very stable, but with a steeper decline in the last 2 or 3 months than that seen in advanced cancer, although for individual patients with co-morbid cardiac or respiratory disease, the pattern may be more fluctuant than seen here in this mean trajectory for the whole study population.

The same study also evaluated symptom trajectories in conservative stage 5 CKD patients.[31] This showed that, although the average trajectory of symptoms in the last year life shows marked increase in symptoms in the last 2–3 months before death, individual patients showed considerable variation in their symptom trajectories. Three different patterns could be distinguished; steadily increasing symptoms over time, fluctuating symptoms over time (the unpredictability of which was highly distressing for patients), and a smaller group of patients with stable symptoms which did not change over time. This data indicates that services for conservatively managed patients

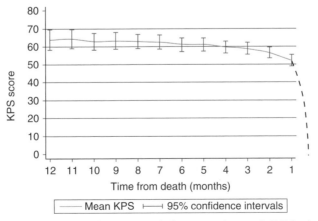

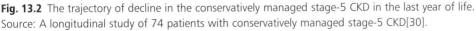

Fig. 13.2 The trajectory of decline in the conservatively managed stage-5 CKD in the last year of life. Source: A longitudinal study of 74 patients with conservatively managed stage-5 CKD[30].

need to be flexible and highly responsive to individual needs, and that those with a fluctuating pattern of symptoms may have the greatest need – not only in terms of symptom control, but also in terms of psychological and social support. The rapid functional decline towards the end of life also highlights the need for rapidly responsive services, particularly community services,[32] if home death (the place of preference for most to die) is to be facilitated.

13.5 **Symptoms**

There has been little study into the symptoms of those managed conservatively, without dialysis, although this may change as this population grows and there is greater recognition of their specific needs. Most of the work to date has been undertaken in the UK[31,33,34] but needs to be duplicated in other settings and countries. There is also little work on the patient experience of conservative management,[35] or the impact of it on families and caregivers.[36,37] The symptom work that has been done shows that patients with conservatively managed stage-5 CKD have a high prevalence of symptoms,[33] similar in terms of overall burden to patients with advanced cancer, although with differences in the patterns of symptoms and the level of distress caused.

Details of the actual prevalence of key symptoms in conservatively managed patients are provided in Chapter 7. Around the time that the decision for conservative management is made (late stage-4 or early stage-5 disease), a number of physical symptoms – fatigue, itch, drowsiness, dyspnoea, oedema, pain, loss of appetite, dry mouth, and poor concentration – are highly prevalent, occurring in 50–80% of all conservatively managed patients.[33,38] Certain symptoms are also disproportionately distressing to patients, including fatigue, pain, and dyspnoea. Renal-specific symptoms – such as restless legs and itch – are also unduly distressing.[31] Psychological symptoms are somewhat less common than physical symptoms, and severe levels of psychological symptoms are infrequent. The average symptom burden is moderate, with a mean number of symptoms of 15, but with a wide range (from 5 to 30).[31] Clearly, some individual patients experience very few symptoms, while others have a very high overall symptom burden. This has implications for services; a 'standard' approach for conservative patients is unlikely to be optimal, but instead a 'tailored' service, which is responsive to the level of symptoms and related distress, is more likely to be effective.

In early stage-5 disease, physical symptoms and physical functional impairment appear to contribute more to the overall burden of illness at this stage, while psychological functioning appears to be little impaired. Quality of life is mostly impaired across physical rather than psychological domains. The considerable psychological, practical, and social consequences of certain physical symptoms (e.g. fatigue and itch) also need to be recognized, and assessment/intervention for these needs to be extended beyond disease-orientated and pharmacological interventions to include appropriate psychological and practical assessment and support.[31] Renal professionals tend to under-recognize both pain[39] and other symptoms.[40] This needs to be addressed through training in symptoms assessment and management, and through the incorporation of symptom assessment into routine clinical practice.

Symptoms change as patients approach death. On average, symptoms increase steadily in the 2–3 months preceding death.[31] Professionals should be alert to increasing levels of symptom distress, and be aware that it may precede decline towards death. Although teams may wish to focus symptom-management resources into this last 2–3 months to provide maximum benefit, it is not yet clear whether targeting symptoms *before* they increase is more effective or not. It is likely that a combination of targeting of symptoms before they worsen, and increased proactive management in the last months when symptoms are more prevalent and severe will be needed. As death nears, the physical symptoms that were previously common become almost ubiquitous, and the associated levels of distress reported by patients are high. Dyspnoea is particularly dominant and distressing, especially for those with cardiac or respiratory co-morbidity, and needs to be actively managed. Psychological symptoms, although still less dominant than physical symptoms, become much more prevalent, with associated increase in severity. There continues to be – even close to death – considerable diversity among patients, ranging from relatively little symptom burden and related distress, up to very high levels of burden and distress from symptoms. Close to death, quality of life is impaired across both physical and mental domains, with physical aspects most affected, but psychological quality also notably impaired as well.[31]

In developing services for conservatively managed patients, these patterns of symptoms should be recognized and addressed. Detailed and skilled assessment and management of symptoms is important, and is addressed in Chapters 7 and 8. A further consideration for conservative patients is the frequency with which assessment of symptoms and concerns should be undertaken, especially if symptom assessment tools are being routinely administered to increase proactivity and improve identification of symptoms. The patterns of change over time suggest that such assessment should not be dictated by infrequent clinical attendance – e.g. if symptoms are assessed every 3 months, then the worsening symptoms and concerns in the 2 months prior to death may be missed. Symptom scores could be triggered by a patient's own concern that there is a notable change and/or by monitoring mild symptoms that may worsen, in addition to administering routine symptom assessment at follow-up clinic or home appointments. Appropriate tools are discussed in Chapter 7. A relatively small numbers of patients will follow a fluctuant symptom trajectory; these patients may need intermittent symptom interventions and fluctuating levels of involvement of services throughout their illness trajectory; again, a 'standard' approach is not ideal for accommodating the care of these patients.

Given the relatively short terminal decline, as described earlier, patients and families also need to be able to call on renal or palliative services for help at short notice, and find it helpful to have a single point of contact 24 h a day, 7 days a week, if feasible. This is especially useful in the last few weeks or months of life.

The use of clinical tools to assess symptoms is not, of itself, sufficient. Social and practical concerns may not always emerge from a symptom measure. Use of an assessment tool will help identification of symptom concerns, but cannot be a substitute for identification of symptoms and other concerns within the clinical consultation, where more complex or less easily elicited issues need to be identified. As symptoms increase and death approaches, the information concerns of these patients increase notably. Information that relates largely to the conservative-management decision is not enough – different information is needed as functional status falls and symptoms increase. This includes information about what to expect, where to seek help and support, when to call, and what might be feasible for place of care and death. Information is also important to support family and other informal caregivers. These increased information concerns need to be identified and addressed appropriately – through awareness of staff and appropriate advanced communications skills training. A recent national survey in the UK identified that only 39% of renal units employed nursing or non-medical professionals with a specific remit for the palliative and end-of-life care of renal patients.[41] Although the assumption cannot be made that staff without this specific remit do not assess symptoms and other concerns fully in clinical interviews, it is perhaps less likely that they will do so effectively – given the difficulty of prioritizing the care of these patients in busy renal units with increasing workloads. Staff with a dedicated remit, and specific training, need to be identified and supported within renal units to deliver improved symptom assessment and management, and to help identify and address other concerns.

A number of factors contribute to preventing patients expressing symptoms and other concerns.[31] Some perceptions, especially in these older patients, militate against the volunteering of symptoms or concerns. The belief that symptoms are an expected part of ageing, or due to conditions other than renal disease, plus uncertainty about their cause, and reduced expectations of relief may all play a part in reducing the likelihood of seeking help. Patients and families need proactive and skilled assessment, with the time and environment for them to be listened to. Advanced communication skills are important – not only in breaking bad news or addressing difficult issues in relation to approaching death, but also in eliciting and addressing the symptoms and other concerns of these patients.

The largely older age of the conservatively managed stage-5 CKD population also has major implications – both in practical terms and in modifying their experience of symptoms and other concerns. Consideration needs to be given to the place of delivery of care (home rather than clinic where possible), the amount of informal care available, the age of informal caregivers (who may be a spouse or partner of similar or older age), and the increasing isolation that often comes with ageing. The material and practical consequences are also different from those in a younger population, with less effect on work and finances, and more impact on social isolation and functioning.

Interventions, therefore, need to include social and practical components; evidence from other end-of-life populations, with similar breadth of symptoms and concerns, suggests that multi-disciplinary teams – including psychologist, social worker, physiotherapist, and occupational therapist – are likely to provide these best.[42] Given the level of concern for family anxiety expressed by patients, additional family support may also be necessary. With regard to psychological support, severe psychological symptoms were infrequent in the earlier course of illness, but increased notably in the weeks and months before death.[30] Identifying this change in individual patients may be difficult. This conservatively managed population also has different psychological symptoms. In contrast to the dialysis population, support is needed, not to come to terms with dialysis, but to deal with the negative emotions that may come with conservative management and related decline: guilt, hopelessness, or frustration with loss of independence and growing reliance on family and others. Teams need good liaison, a high degree of responsiveness to changing patient symptoms, and need to be aware of the higher levels of psychological symptoms in the last few months of life, and how these will present. Much of the symptom burden and other concerns identified in this population can readily be addressed by renal teams who have developed some of the skills needed, although further advanced communication and detailed symptom assessment and management skills are often needed. There may be some individual patients and families for whom specialist palliative care expertise is required or for whom specific palliative care services (such as hospice, day or in-patient care) are needed. It is also important to note that only a small proportion of these conservatively managed patients die a 'true' uraemic death – many will die of other causes before this stage arrives.

13.6 **Advance care planning**

There is some overlap between making the decision for conservative management and planning ahead for subsequent care, because the former will inevitably involve some exploration of the patient's preferences and priorities. However, there are other areas of advance care planning which need to be considered for the conservatively managed patient; such as what to expect at different stages, when and why hospitalization might be appropriate, what other active management is right for the individual, who is available to care for them at home, and where do they prefer to be cared for and to die, if practicable. This is a dynamic and evolving process, not one – or even a few – fixed episodes, and there needs to be good liaison to ensure it is effective.

Timing is critical; not all issues will be right to discuss at any one time, and there will need to be evolution in discussions as the disease itself advances. There is a fine balance between introducing issues for discussion too early, and leaving them too late, so that opportunities are missed, and 'default' care becomes inevitable.[43] Family and other caregivers need to be actively involved in discussions whenever possible,[44] to enable consistent responses at times of crisis or decline. There may be a number of professionals who also need to be aware of decisions, preferences, and priorities, including primary care professionals, who may have major responsibility if the patient is at home.

Unfortunately, little is known about the conservatively managed group of patients; why they make the decision for conservative management, what preferences they have for future care after the decision is made, the determinants of those preferences, and how preferences might change over time and towards death.[45] Advance care planning has been fairly widely studied in dialysis patients, and, together with the limited evidence in conservative patients, some conclusions can be drawn.

First, detailed discussions about the future and about preferences and priorities do not remove hope, as some professionals believe; rather, they sustain realistic hope and empower patients to work towards possibilities consistent with their own values.[24] They help patients and families to make the most of life, in the face of an advancing, life-threatening condition. Second, there are a variety of reasons why patients opt for conservative management.[46] These will influence how patients and families view the future, after the decision is made; a patient who views conservative management as a 'logical and affirming choice' will respond differently to one who is 'angry and believed they were somehow giving up on life'.[46] Subsequent advance care planning, therefore, needs to be responsive to the perspective patient and family bring to the process; it is about helping them towards greater empowerment, whatever the starting place, but some will have a very different psychological journey ahead, as compared with others. Third, advance care planning is not only about key medical decisions, such as decisions about dialysis or agreement to 'not for resuscitation' order when in hospital. When done well, it also involves enhancement of the final days, weeks and months with positive decisions about family relationships, resolution of conflict, and living well until the end of life[47] – all priorities which patients themselves rate highly. [48] This approach helps move away from isolated decisions about the utilization of medical supportive measures, which are sometimes influenced more by transient factors than by stable 'core' values,[49] and builds on a more integrated, person and family-centered care, consistent with the priorities of specialist palliative care.

There has been some study of the experience of illness among conservatively managed Stage-5 CKD patients,[31] and this work suggests that loss of control and related uncertainty are a particular feature for these patients. Advance care planning can help reduce this sense of loss of control.[50] This is important, since for a number of these patients, the prospect of death was not their main concern; uncertainty about the path of their illness before death troubled them more. Most understood – and expressed either explicitly or implicitly – the terminal nature of their illness, but responded to their illness in different ways. Achieving some kind of acceptance, and the related dignity that could be maintained, were important for many. Above all, participants expressed a wish not to be a burden to their family and others;[31] advance care planning helps to make explicit preferences and priorities about care, and identifies what can be provided to support families and reduce that burden (provided, of course, that appropriate services are available).

Advance care planning is discussed more fully in Chapter 4; much of the evidence on this area which is derived from dialysis populations applies also to patients managed conservatively, without dialysis.

13.7 **Implications**

This chapter has outlined the current evidence about patients who opt not to undergo dialysis and are managed conservatively. But what does this mean for nephrology and palliative care teams? Older patients with high levels of co-morbidity can perhaps be given choice whether or not to dialyse without a major adverse effect on survival. Evidence suggests that 15–20% of all Stage-5 CKD patients will choose not to dialysis.[11] This is a patient group with a high symptom burden equivalent or greater than that of patients with malignant disease,[33] and diverse disease trajectories. They, therefore, need significant medical, psychological, and social input.

The suggestion that older patients with significant co-morbidity gain only marginal benefit, if at all, from dialysis identifies a second group of patients that have significant palliative care needs, namely those that do start dialysis. These patients continue to have a large symptom burden because: dialysis will not alleviate all symptoms of renal failure; dialysis itself will add to the symptom burden and many symptoms may relate to other co-morbidities not affected by dialysis. [51] It is vital that we do not ignore palliative and supportive needs of this patient group because they are being actively treated, and remember that dialysis is itself a palliative treatment for renal failure and not a cure. If we consider all patients older than 75, irrespective of co-morbidity, 40–50% will die in the first year following commencement of dialysis.[52] With such a high mortality and no robust tool to predict which patients will die, a case could be made for considering the palliative needs, e.g. symptom control, resuscitation status, and preferred place of care, for all older incident dialysis patients. Generally, this is not done well by nephrologists with limited expertise and resources allocated to this important element of patient care.

No single model of care for conservatively managed patients can be defined as optimal for delivering services. There is, as yet, insufficient evidence available to inform this, although evidence is emerging as to the needs of these patients, and how the best practice might look. Over the next years, growing recognition of the conservatively managed patient group (and increase in their numbers) will undoubtedly lead to more research – including better understanding of trajectories of illness – and evaluations of specific interventions, so that care of patients and families can be improved.

13.8 **The roles of Renal and Palliative medicine**

The optimal management of conservatively treated patients is likely to be best achieved through the interaction of Renal and Palliative Care services, although much will be dependent on how local services are set up and coordinated – particularly the extent to which specialist palliative care services are available. The input required from each service will vary depending on the individual patient and the stage of disease, and it is clear that there is diversity of healthcare needs across this population. Therefore, provision of a service responsive to individual healthcare needs is critical; one size does not fit all.

13.8.1 **Renal medicine**

Most patients with CKD will only discover the implications of their renal disease when they meet a nephrologist. Usually there is time for their treatment choices, including conservative treatment, to be discussed and a plan formulated. It is vital that patients and their relatives are given time, an appropriate environment, and access to experienced staff who can provide the information required to inform the decision-making process. This will probably be provided by renal services. There is no fixed formula for this but a busy renal outpatient clinic is not the ideal environment. Use of nephrology staff with advanced communication and other palliative care training will be important, particularly when issues relating to end of life are discussed. It may be appropriate for specialist palliative care professionals to assist when particularly challenging issues arise, such as complex and ethically challenging decisions in the face of impaired capacity, or major family conflict.

One problem when considering informed decision-making in this context is the paucity of available data. There is very little comparative data on patient survival between conservative and dialysis treatment for the elderly, infirm patients increasingly being seen in nephrology clinics. The ethical issues are such that any form of randomized study comparing dialysis and conservative treatments is unlikely to occur, and use of Renal Registry data has the drawback that patients have already been selected. There is an urgent need for the renal (and palliative medicine) community to generate high-quality outcome data in this area to guide treatment choice. It is also vital to generate data as to the numbers of patients that choose conservative treatment and their treatment needs. Inclusion of this data in Renal Registry data collections will provide some insight into the number of patients being managed this way and, in time, data about survival. This, combined with descriptive studies of their symptoms and care needs, will allow an estimate of the resources required to treat this patient group.

Once the decision not to have dialysis has been made, most patients will still require input from renal medicine, jointly with primary care and palliative care professionals. Renal medicine will provide input in areas such as anaemia treatment, control of calcium and phosphate balance, and control of fluid status. As disease progresses care will increasingly be delivered away from the out-patient setting, with care moving to the community and perhaps hospice setting. Exactly how renal medicine inputs into this phase of patient care will vary depending on what is currently available, and how services are developed. Certainly there should not be complete withdrawal of renal input, and areas such as education and development of treatment guidelines should be considered even if direct patient contact is not maintained. Equally renal medicine should not duplicate services that are already provided by palliative medicine. Close liaison and collaborative working are essential.

13.8.2 **Palliative care**

In understanding the potential role of palliative care services in providing care for the conservatively managed population, it is important to understand the distinction between general and specialist palliative care. General palliative care is provided by the usual professional caregivers of patient and family, as an integral part of routine clinical practice.[53] Specialist palliative care is, on the other hand, provided by accredited palliative care specialists who work in multi-professional specialist teams; the difference is usually in the level of complexity of the palliative and end-of-life care needs of those patients seen.[53] Specialist palliative care services, therefore, have a role in supporting the development and provision of nephrology-based services to these patients and their families. How this evolves will often depend on local provision, because specialist palliative care services vary nationally, regionally, and locally, but the best way forward is through collaboration and liaison between nephrology and palliative professionals.

Specialist palliative care also brings a highly patient- and family-centred approach, distinctive in its holistic perspective and through the level of detail it brings to addressing the whole range of issues and concerns. This approach has already driven a number of research collaborations in the field of conservatively managed care for renal patients,[54] and is likely to bring more fruitful collaboration as this research area expands. Clinically, specialists in palliative care can bring advanced communication skills, expertise in symptom control, detailed awareness of psychological, social, and spiritual needs (including appropriate interventions), to improve care for individual patients and families, but they are perhaps best placed to help support nephrology services to develop general palliative and supportive care skills themselves. This may be through education, training, and collaborative research, as much as through patient and family care 'on the ground'.

Specialist palliative care professionals do not necessarily have the nephrology skills and experience to optimize management of the renal disease, delay disease progression, and minimize complications – all important priorities for conservatively managed patients, as for those on dialysis.[55] Questions arise as to how long such active disease management should be continued, and these can only be answered on an individual patient basis. However, it is important to maintain a broad, patient-centred perspective when deciding how long to continue renal interventions (such as anaemia treatment, control of calcium and phosphate balance, and control of fluid status), and not to revert to a narrower, disease-focussed approach.

Specific palliative services will perhaps always be available only through specialist palliative care, such as hospice or palliative in-patient care, hospice-based day care, hospital specialist palliative care teams, community-based specialist palliative care towards the end of life, and consultation/intervention for more complex healthcare needs. This may include difficult symptom-control issues, situations of family conflict, ethically challenging decision-making, or complex bereavement. The challenge for nephrology teams will be how best to develop general palliative and supportive skills, while coping with increasing demand for all nephrology services, and the challenge for both nephrology and palliative care specialists is how best to take forward effective, integrated services for conservatively managed patients and their families, which draw on the best in both specialties, and which develop the much-needed evidence base.

13.9 **The future of conservative care**

Life expectancy in developed countries continues to increase and with it the number of patients with CKD will also increase. Early identification and treatment of patients with Stage 1–3 CKD will reduce the proportion reaching Stage 5 CKD and the need to decide between conservative or dialysis treatment. Nevertheless, absolute numbers of patients are likely to increase. These patients may be more elderly than the patients currently seen, presenting logistical problems relating to the delivery of dialysis and with limited evidence for improved quality or quantity of life. Undoubtedly many challenges lie ahead.

One important implication of this change for renal and palliative services is that a patient's decision about dialysis or conservative care may become less important. When planning palliative and supportive services, there may be lessening need to distinguish between two patient groups, as their survival and symptom burden becomes more similar. Both groups will need significant input from palliative and supportive services. The study by Smith et al.[11] clearly illustrates the equivalent survival in a selected group of patients irrespective of whether they chose to dialyse or not. It is likely that both groups will require similar care. Therefore, nephrology teams will need to develop more general palliative care expertise and services will be required to deal with several groups: conservatively managed patients, patients with a limited life expectancy on (or withdrawing from) renal replacement therapy, and those with better life expectancy but with high symptom burden and need for palliation of those symptoms.

More patients will require more resources, and conservative treatment of patients should not be viewed as the cheap option. The number of patients on dialysis has increased and this has required a similar increase in funding. The model used in many countries bases funding on the number of patients dialysed. Therefore, conservative treatment of patients results in reduced income and increased expenditure. It is important that conservative treatment is recognized as an appropriate treatment choice for some patients and funded accordingly.

There is still much we do not know about conservative management of advanced kidney disease. Opportunities are available for both renal and palliative care professionals to develop research programmes in this important area, and collaborative research is likely to be most fruitful, drawing on the expertise of nephrologists in understanding renal disease, and the expertise within specialist palliative care in researching populations with advanced disease (where recruiting into studies is difficult, and levels of attrition from studies are high). Many questions remain to be answered. Can we more accurately identify which patients will most benefit from dialysis? What is a patient's life expectancy with or without dialysis? How do we best treat symptoms and improve quality of life? What trajectory of illness can a patient expect, with or without dialysis? Finally, above all, how can care best be delivered to ensure that the last months, weeks, or days of life for every patient are lived to the full, despite their advancing disease?

Case study

A 75-year-old gentleman with long-standing hypertension, diabetes mellitus, ischaemic heart disease, osteoarthritis, and diabetic nephropathy had been attending the nephrology clinic regularly for management of his progressive chronic kidney disease. It became apparent during discussions with his nephrology team that he was the main carer at home for his wife, who had moderately severe dementia. Following several discussions, and with the involvement of his only daughter, he decided that dialysis would prove too disruptive – both for himself and for the care of his wife – and that he would rather be managed conservatively, despite the potentially reduced survival.

As his renal function declined below an eGFR of 10 ml/min, he became increasing symptomatic, with reduced appetite, nausea, and gastric fullness suggestive of delayed gastric emptying, localized itch, and chronic pain from osteoarthritis. His symptoms were managed with metoclopramide orally, buprenorphine transdermally, plus skin care, emollients, and topical capsaicin cream for his pruritus.

He was reluctant to attend hospital, wanting to spend as much time as possible with his wife. Symptom review and psychological support was, therefore, provided for him at home by the community palliative care team. Advance planning as his renal function declined was especially important – both for himself and to consider his wife's care. Following family discussions, his daughter increased her support to them both, with the plan for his wife to move to the daughter's home after his death.

When he deteriorated quite rapidly 4 months later, he wanted to remain at home rather than be admitted. He quickly became less well, with cognitive impairment, restlessness, and joint and back pains. These symptoms were managed with low-dose alfentanil and midazolam subcutaneously via syringe driver. With support from his daughter, general practitioner, district nurses, and local community palliative care team, he died peacefully at home 2 days later.

Ethical analysis

This case illustrates the value of advance care planning (see Chapter 4), which is an expanded concept from the original recommendation #5 in the RPA/ASN guideline. It is now widely accepted that more important than the mere completion of a form, a written advance directive is a discussion with the patient and family about the patient's values, preferences, and goals for care in his present situation and in the future. The discussion about the future will be most useful if it is based on predictable contingencies of the patient's life-limiting illness. Such discussions help the patient to decide what treatment he does and does not want at the end of life, prepare the family emotionally and practically for what lies ahead, and identify for the healthcare team what interventions will and will not be appropriate as the patient's disease progresses. As the patient deteriorated, there was a coordinated escalation of palliative care treatments that was facilitated by the decisions reached in the advance care planning discussions. This approach was anticipated by the RPA/ASN guideline recommendation #9, "Palliative care. All patients who decide to forgo dialysis or for whom such a decision is made should be treated with continued palliative care. With the patient's consent, persons with expertise in such care, such as hospice healthcare professionals, should be involved in managing the medical, psychosocial, and spiritual aspects of end-of-life care for these patients. Patients should be offered the option of dying where they prefer including at home with hospice care. Bereavement support should be offered to patients' families." This book provides clinicians with the knowledge and skills to implement recommendation #9 in the care of their ESRD patients. This chapter assists clinicians to determine which patients might be more appropriate for a conservative approach to the treatment of their ESRD rather than one involving dialysis.

References

1 Ansell D, Feehally J, Feest T, et al. (2008). UK Renal Registry Report 2007. UK Renal Registry, Bristol, UK.

2 Murtagh FE, Addington-Hall J, Higginson IJ. (2007). The prevalence of symptoms in end-stage renal disease: a systematic review. *Adv Chr Kidney Dis,* **14**(1), 82–99.

3 CKD Work Group (2002). K/DOQI Clinical Practice Guidelines for Chronic Kidney Disease: Evaluation, Classification, and Stratification. *Am J Kidney Dis*, **39**(2 Suppl 1), S1–S266.

4 Stevens PE, O'Donoghue DJ, de LS, et al. (2007). Chronic kidney disease management in the United Kingdom: NEOERICA project results. *Kidney Int,* **72**(1), 92–9.

5 Coresh J, Astor BC, Greene T, et al. (2003). Prevalence of chronic kidney disease and decreased kidney function in the adult US population: Third National Health and Nutrition Examination Survey. *Am J Kidney Dis,* **41**(1), 1–12.

6 Chadban SJ, Briganti EM, Kerr PG, et al. (2003). Prevalence of kidney damage in Australian adults: The AusDiab kidney study. *J Am Soc Nephrol*, **14**(7 Suppl 2), S131–S138.

7 O'Hare AM, Choi AI, Bertenthal D, et al. (2007) Age affects outcomes in chronic kidney disease. *J Am Soc Nephrol*, **18**(10), 2758–65.

8 Roderick P, Davies R, Jones C, et al. (2004). Simulation model of renal replacement therapy: Predicting future demand in England. *Nephrol Dialy Transplant*, **19**(3), 692–701.

9 US Renal Data System (2008). USRDS 2008 Annual Data Report. Bethesda, MD.

10 Murtagh FEM, Marsh JE, Donohoe P, et al. (2007). Dialysis or not? A comparative survival study of patients over 75 years with chronic kidney disease stage 5. *Nephrol Dial Transplant*, **22**(7), 1955–62.

11 Smith C, Silva-Gane M, Chandna S, et al. (2003). Choosing not to dialyse: evaluation of planned non-dialytic management in a cohort of patients with end-stage renal failure. *Nephron Clinical Practice*, **95**(2), c40–c46.

12 Lambie M, Rayner HC, Bragg-Gresham JL, et al. (2006). Starting and withdrawing haemodialysis–associations between nephrologists' opinions, patient characteristics and practice patterns (data from the Dialysis Outcomes and Practice Patterns Study). *Nephrol Dialy Transplant*, **21**(10), 2814–20.

13 Kee F, Patterson CC, Wilson EA, et al. (2000). Stewardship or clinical freedom? variations in dialysis decision making. *Nephrol Dialy Transplant*, **15**(10), 1647–57.

14 Joly D, Anglicheau D, Alberti C, et al. (2003). Octogenarians reaching end-stage renal disease: cohort study of decision-making and clinical outcomes. *J Am Soc Nephrol*, **14**(4), 1012–21.

15 Dasgupta I, Rayner HC (2007). Dialysis versus conservative management of elderly patients with advanced chronic kidney disease. *Nat Clin Pract Nephrol*, **3**(9), 480–1.

16 De Biase V, Tobaldini O, Boaretti C, et al. (2008) Prolonged conservative treatment for frail elderly patients with end-stage renal disease: the Verona experience. *Nephrol Dialy Transplant*, **23**(4), 1313–17.

17 Wong CF, McCarthy M, Howse MLP, et al. (2007). Factors affecting survival in advanced chronic kidney disease patients who choose not to accept dialysis. *Ren Failure*, **29**, 653–9.

18 Chandna SM, Schulz J, Lawrence C, et al. (1999). Is there a rationale for rationing chronic dialysis? A hospital based cohort study of factors affecting survival and morbidity. *BMJ*, **318**(7178), 217–23.

19 Jablonski A (2004). The illness trajectory of end-stage renal disease dialysis patients. *Res Theory Nurs Pract*, **18**(1), 51–72.

20 Holley JL (2007). Palliative care in end-stage renal disease: illness trajectories, communication, and hospice use. *Adv Chr Kidney Dis*, **14**(4), 402–8.

21 Davison SN (2006). Facilitating advance care planning for patients with end-stage renal disease: the patient perspective. *Clin J Am Soc Nephrol*, **1**(5), 1023–8.

22 Murray SA, Sheikh A (2008). Palliative Care Beyond Cancer: Care for all at the end of life. *BMJ*, **336**(7650), 958–9.

23 Murray SA, Kendall M, Boyd K, et al. (2005). Illness trajectories and palliative care. *BMJ*, **330**(7498), 1007–11.

24 Davison SN, Simpson C (2006). Hope and advance care planning in patients with end stage renal disease: Qualitative interview study. *BMJ*, **333**(7574), 886–9.

25 Steinhauser KE, Christakis NA, Clipp EC, et al. (2001). Preparing for the end of life: preferences of patients, families, physicians, and other care providers. *J Pain Symptom Manage*, **22**(3), 727–37.

26 Steinhauser KE, Christakis NA, Clipp EC, et al. (2000). Factors considered important at the end of life by patients, family, physicians, and other care providers. *JAMA*, **284**(19), 2476–82.

27 Glaser B, Strauss A (1968). *Time for dying.* Aldine, Chicago, USA.

28 Lunney JR, Lynn J, Hogan C (2002). Profiles of older medicare decedents. *J Am Geriatr Soc*, **50**(6), 1108–12.

29 Lunney JR, Lynn J, Foley DJ, et al. (2003). Patterns of functional decline at the end of life. *JAMA*, **289**(18), 2387–92.

30 Williams B, McDaid L, Walker R, et al. (2002). Maximum Conservative Mangement of End Stage Renal Failure; What can patients and their families expect? The Renal Association, UK – Oct 2002 conference, RCP, London. Available at: www.renal.org/pages/pages/meetings/abstracts/abstracts-2002-4.php Accessed 20th April 2009.

31 Murtagh FEM (2009). Understanding and improving quality of care for people with conservatively-managed Stage 5 Chronic Kidney Disease – the course of symptoms and other concerns over time. PhD thesis. King's College London, UK.

32 Department of Health (2008). *End of Life Care Strategy.* Department of Health, London, UK.

33 Murtagh FEM, Addington-Hall JM, Edmonds PM, et al. (2007). Symptoms in advanced renal disease: a cross-sectional survey of symptom prevalence in stage 5 chronic kidney disease managed without dialysis. *J Palliat Med*, **10**(6), 1266–76.

34 Noble H, Kelly D, Rawlings-Anderson K, et al. (2007). A concept analysis of renal supportive care: the changing world of nephrology. *J Adv Nurs*, **59**(6), 644–53.

35 Noble H, Meyer J, Bridges J, et al. (2008). Patient experience of dialysis refusal or withdrawal–a review of the literature. *J Ren Care*, **34**(2), 94–100.

36 Low J, Smith G, Burns A, et al. (2008). The impact of end stage kidney disease on close persons: a literature review. *Nephrol Dialy Transplant Plus*, **2**, 67–79.

37 Ashby M, Op't HC, Kellehear A, et al. (2005). Renal dialysis abatement: Lessons from a social study. *Palliat Med*, **19**(5), 389–96.

38 Murphy EL, Murtagh FEM, Carey I, et al. (2009). Understanding symptoms in patients with advanced chronic kidney disease managed without dialysis: use of a short patient-completed assessment tool. *Nephron Clin Pract*, **111**(1), c74–c80.

39 Bailie GR, Mason NA, Bragg-Gresham JL, et al. (2004). Analgesic prescription patterns among hemodialysis patients in the DOPPS: potential for underprescription. *Kidney Int*, **65**(6), 2419–25.

40 Weisbord SD, Fried L, Mor MK, et al. (2007). Renal provider recognition of symptoms in patients on maintenance hemodialysis. *Clinl J Am Soc Nephrologists*, **2**, 960–7.

41 Gunda S, Smith S, Thomas M (2004). National Survey of Palliative Care in End-Stage Renal Disease in the United Kingdom. *Nephrol Dialy Transplant*, **20**, 392–5.

42 National Institute for Clinical Excellence (2004). Improving Supportive and Palliative Care for Adults with Cancer. National Institute for Clinical Excellence, London, UK.

43 Holley JL (2003). Advance care planning in elderly chronic dialysis patients. *Int Urol & Nephrol*, **35**(4), 565–8.

44 Hines SC, Glover JJ, Babrow AS, et al. (2001). Improving advance care planning by accommodating family preferences. *J Palliat Med*, **4**(4), 481–9.

45 Noble H, Meyer J, Bridges J, et al. (2008). Patient experience of dialysis refusal or withdrawal–a review of the literature. *J Ren Care*, **34**(2), 94–100.

46 Noble H, Meyer J, Bridges J, et al. (2009). Reasons renal patients give for deciding not to dialyze: a prospective qualitative interview study. *Dialy & Transplant*, **38**(3), 82–9.

47 Hines SC, Babrow AS, Badzek L, et al. (2001). From coping with life to coping with death: problematic integration for the seriously ill elderly. *Health Commun*, **13**(3), 327–42.

48 Singer PA, Martin DK, Lavery JV, et al. (1998). Reconceptualizing advance care planning from the patient's perspective. *Arch Intern Med*, **158**(8), 879–84.

49 Fried TR, O'Leary J, Van NP, et al. (2007). Inconsistency over time in the preferences of older persons with advanced illness for life-sustaining treatment. *J Am Geriatr Soc*, **55**(7), 1007–14.

50 Davison SN, Torgunrud C (2007). The creation of an advance care planning process for patients with ESRD. *Am J Kidney Dis*, **49**(1), 27–36.

51 Solano JP, Gomes B, Higginson IJ (2006). A comparison of symptom prevalence in far advanced cancer, AIDS, heart disease, chronic obstructive pulmonary disease and renal disease. *J Pain Symp Mgt*, **31**(1), 58–69.

52 Kurella M, Covinsky KE, Collins AJ, et al. (2007). Octogenarians and nonagenarians starting dialysis in the United States. *Ann Intern Med*, **146**(3), 177–83.

53 National Council for Hospice and Specialist Palliative Care Services. (2001). What do we mean by palliative care? National Council for Hospice and Specialist Palliative Care Services, London, UK.

54 Murtagh FEM, Higginson IJ (2007). Death from renal failure eighty years on: how far have we come? *J Palliat Med*, **10**(6), 1236–8.

55 Burgess E (1999). Conservative treatment to slow deterioration of renal function: evidence-based recommendations. *Kidney Int*, **S70** (55), S17–S25.

Chapter 14

End-stage renal disease in the older person

Lina Johansson and Edwina A Brown

14.1 Introduction

The proportion of older people within the UK is growing with those older than 80 being the fastest-growing age group comprising 4.5% of the total population within England and Wales.[1] The proportion of older people with end-stage renal disease (ESRD) is also increasing. Managing renal disease on the background of old age brings with it additional challenges. Old age often comes with multiple co-morbidities in addition to change in social circumstances leading to potential depression from bereavement, loss of independence, and social isolation. Loss of function is a reality for those who are older, with 75–80% people ≥60 years having a degree of visual or hearing impairment within the general population.[2] A total of 95% of older haemodialysis patients have been found to have some functional impairment in relation to activities of daily living.[3] Coping with a life with ESRD can therefore significantly add to the burden of ageing.

14.2 The ageing dialysis population

Prior to the 1970s, chronic dialysis was a treatment for the young and was rarely used for anyone above the age of 50.[4] Since then, there has been a dramatic increase in the availability of dialysis with greater referral and acceptance of older people onto dialysis. This is because older people are faring better on dialysis. Reflecting on recent years from 1999 to 2006, the 1-year survival on dialysis (after 90 days) of adults ≥65 years improved from 66% to 79%.[5,6] Nearly one-half of the UK dialysis population is aged ≥65 years having increased from 41% to 48% between 1998 and 2006. The latest figures from 2007 show that 50% of those starting dialysis are aged 65 years and older.[7] This trend also applies to the very elderly; in the US, the rate of octogenarians and nonagenarians starting dialysis has increased by 57% (accounting for population growth) from 1996 to 2003.[8] Examples even include the apparently successful start of a centenarian.[9] Age, appropriately, is no longer a barrier to starting dialysis.

14.3 Who is "old"?

The definition of "old" from the Oxford dictionary is "having lived a long time; no longer young" or "of a specified age". This specified age is commonly based around the arbitrary cut-off point of 65 years and above. Within developed countries, old age is dictated by the eligibility for retirement and state pension. Within health-related, and in the renal literature, old age is usually defined between 60 and 70 years and older. Chronological age – although practical – does not reflect an individual's mental and physical response to ageing and, therefore, fails to identify those who are truly vulnerable and who would benefit from less aggressive interventions or those who are robust enough to cope with the consequences of active treatment. An alternative would be to qualify ageing by identifying criteria for those who age successfully. Thus, a biomedical definition of successful ageing is where the individual is relatively free from disease and its risk factors and maintains physical and cognitive functioning and engagement with life.[10] This definition qualified 19% of 867 community-dwelling elderly individuals in the US as having aged successfully.[11] Yet, 50% of the same population rated themselves as having aged successfully despite the presence of chronic illness and functional impairment. This definition, therefore, also fails to recognize the full array of factors (including psychosocial factors) that are involved in ageing.

14.4 Frailty as a measure of ageing

Frailty is a more sensitive indicator of the physical and mental changes associated with advancing age. One definition of frailty is when three of the following five features are present: weight loss (unintentional weight loss of at least 5% of previous year's body weight), weakness (determined by grip strength), slow walking speed, low physical activity, and self-reported exhaustion, all of which are susceptible to decline in illness and age.[12] Using this definition, 7% of community-dwelling elderly in the US have been identified as frail with a high risk of falls, disability, morbidity, and mortality.[12] Although loss of function is a pertinent feature, the concept of frailty has evolved to a syndrome involving the decline of multiple systems, where physiological instability leaves the individual at risk of loss of, or further deterioration in function when exposed to perceived minor stressors, such as cold weather.[13] Depression has also been found to be associated with frailty in large population studies.[14] More recently, it has been shown that cognition – when added to the assessment of frailty – improves its predictive power for some adverse outcomes, such as mortality.[15]

14.5 Frailty in end-stage renal disease

Frailty has been shown to be endemic in all age groups of those on dialysis. Prevalence of frailty increased with age in a dialysis population ($n = 2275$) where 44% of those <40 years, 61% of those in the age range between 40 and 50 years and 78.8% ≥80 years met the study criteria for frailty. Frail patients had over 3 times the risk of mortality within their first year of dialysis compared to the non-frail. In this study, frailty carries a greater hazard ratio of 1-year mortality (hazard ratio (HR): 2.24) than age alone (HR: 1.03) and was associated with increased risk for hospitalizations. [16] Reversing or preventing frailty may, therefore, improve outcomes. Various interventions have been used in dialysis patients but the effect on preventing frailty is not known. In the general population, The Health, Aging and Body Composition study followed 2964 participants in the age range 70–79 years for 5 years. Those who were sedentary compared to those who were engaging in exercise activities were more susceptible to frailty.[17] Therefore, targeting any of the components of frailty such as physical strength, nutrition, or indeed depression could prevent or delay the onset of frailty in older people with ESRD.

14.6 Physical function

Decline in physical function is a feature of normal ageing. Prospective observations have shown that around one-half of community-dwelling people aged >70 will need assistance with some daily activities over a 5-year period.[18] There is a remarkable lack of comparative literature in the older dialysis population.

14.6.1 Physical function in end-stage renal disease

The largest study of physical function in older patients on dialysis gives only cross-sectional data from a single Canadian dialysis centre.[3] Of a total of 168 patients on haemodialysis who were older than 65 years, only 5% were fully independent and had no functional impairment of activity; 95% required assistance with household tasks (e.g. shopping, cleaning, transport); and 52% needed additional support with at least one aspect of personal care (bathing, walking, transferring from bed to chair, and/or dressing). Older people are also at risk of falls which are well recognized to predict functional decline, need for hospitalization, and eventual institutional care. In a longitudinal study of 162 haemodialysis patients over 65 years of age followed-up, on average, for almost a year, 47% had a fall at a rate of 1.60 falls/person-year of follow-up.[19] Injuries occurred in 19% of falls and 41 patients had multiple falls. These rates are higher than in the general population where a similar study has found a fall rate of 30%.[20] One of the main determinants of functional disability in non-dialysis populations is acute hospitalization. Both in the UK and US, older patients will be hospitalized, on average, twice a year.[21,22] In a recent pilot study of 35 older dialysis patients, three-quarters experienced a decline in personal functional independence in association with hospitalization.[23]

The fact that these studies are all very recent and have all been done by the same investigator group demonstrate the general unawareness by the nephrology community of the importance of assessing physical function in the management of older patients with ESRD. Functional independence seems to be the exception. Given the strong relationship between disability and outcomes such as hospitalization and mortality, assessment of physical performance, awareness of level of dependence, and routine elderly care management such as falls-prevention procedures will minimize complications and hospitalization. It will also enhance realistic care planning with patients, families, and caregivers.

14.7 Nutrition

14.7.1 Normal ageing and body composition

Normal ageing is associated with changes in body composition with an increase in fat stores (until at least the age of 65–70) and decrease in lean body mass potentially leading to sarcopaenia (loss of muscle mass).[24] This phenomenon is seen principally in men[25] due to hormonal alterations associated with ageing, such as a decline in testosterone.[26] In a community-dwelling elderly population, 22.6% of women and 26.8% of men had sarcopaenia.[27] Normal ageing, contrary to popular belief, does not appear to be associated with significant body-weight loss. A prospective study observing a healthy population of older white men and women (65–89 years) for 6 years found that weight changes – although mostly losses – were minimal.[28] An unintentional weight loss of between 5% and 10% over 6 months is therefore considered to be clinically significant.

14.7.2 End-stage renal disease and body composition in older people

Fried et al. (2007) found in a prospective cohort study of older people that impaired kidney function was independently associated with a loss of lean body mass in men, but not in women.[29] Protein malnutrition and reduced muscle mass is a common feature in the haemodialysis population, especially in older people. Old age was found to be associated with lower muscle protein stores of 128 HD patients.[30] The ratio of observed/expected lean body mass was found to be less than 1.0 in 80% of 7123 haemodialysis patients from the French National Cooperative Study.[31] The causes for this loss of lean body mass are multiple and related to catabolic factors prevalent in those on haemodialysis and, in particular, those who are older: acidosis, haemodialysis treatment, inflammation, decrease in physical activity, as well as a decrease in nutritional intake. Raised inflammatory markers have been shown to be a determinant of muscle atrophy in 486 haemodialysis incident and prevalent patients between 18 and 70 years of age.[32]

14.7.3 End-stage renal disease and malnutrition in older people

Malnutrition is common in dialysis patients, and appears to worsen with age. Cianciaruso (1995) found increasing levels of malnutrition in haemodialysis patients with increasing age (51% in the ≥65-year age group) using well-validated techniques of nutritional assessment.[33] Another large study of 761 haemodialysis patients found that age was a strong predictor of malnutrition as was the co-morbidity index.[34] The association of malnutrition with age and co-morbidity could be due to the link among malnutrition, inflammation, and atherosclerosis (MIA). Stenvinkel (1999) demonstrated that malnourished haemodialysis patients had higher C-reactive protein levels, elevated calculated intima–media area, and a higher prevalence of carotid plaques compared to those who were well nourished.[34] Those who were carotid plaque free were significantly younger than those who had plaques suggesting that age is a strong factor in the MIA syndrome due to its correlation with cardiovascular disease. There are, however, several other factors that enhance the vulnerability of the older person with ESRD to malnutrition. The Haemodialysis study (HEMO) found the calorie and protein intake in older patients to be less than those younger than 50 years.[35] This could be due to changes in smell and taste found in the older person which could contribute to anorexia as these are exacerbated in uraemia.[36] The dialysis commitment can lead to missing of meals due to time away from home (often exacerbated by hospital transport facilities). Tiredness and time to recover post haemodialysis treatment is reported to be between 375 and 460 min, making food preparation difficult.[37] The complexity of the renal therapeutic diet and fluid restrictions can also act as a deterrent to adequate nutritional intake. The role of social support should not be underestimated in this group, for example, calorie intake was shown to improve in homebound older people who ate in the presence of others.[38]

14.8 Depression

14.8.1 Depression in the older person with end-stage renal disease

As discussed in Chapter 6, depression is often undiagnosed in renal failure due to the similarity of the symptoms of uraemia and the somatic aspects of depression. The risk factors for depression are multi-factorial in older people with or without renal failure. These can be grouped into three broad categories: (1) physical illness – an inverse correlation was found between functionality and depression in an older haemodialysis population;[39,40] (2) social factors such as social isolation, bereavement, loneliness, and stressful life events which can come in the form of an acute event such as relocation or chronic such as caring for a relative; and (3) mental illness which can include a family history of depression, cognitive impairment, and dementia. Older patients with renal failure are already at risk of depression due to the presence of a chronic illness. This, compounded with the risk of experiencing loss or loneliness or mental illness such as cognitive impairment (see later sections), makes the elderly with ESRD particularly vulnerable to depression. Tyrrell et al. found that 61% of 51 haemodialysis patients 70 years or older screened positive for depression[41] compared to depressive symptoms being found in only 15% of the general community-dwelling elderly.[42]

14.8.2 Cultivating the awareness of depression

The psychological symptoms of depression such as feelings of hopelessness are not always obvious and are often accepted as a consequence of living a life with renal disease. Under-diagnosis can also be related to poor staff training in recognizing the signs and symptoms of depression in the context of a chronic illness. In addition, patients themselves, especially older individuals, can be reluctant to be stigmatised with suffering from a mental health condition in addition to their current health burden and therefore can be resistant to recognizing and accepting treatment.[42] Depression in the elderly is associated with a decrease in functionality, reduced quality of life, increased mortality, increased demands on carers, and increased usage of services.[43] Diagnosis and management of depression are discussed further in Chapters 6 and 9.

14.9 Cognitive function

14.9.1 Cognitive function in end-stage renal disease

Cognitive dysfunction is another condition that is much more common in those with renal failure than the general population yet remains under-recognized. It is well known that cognition declines with age.[44] It also appears to be related to renal function. In a 4-year longitudinal cohort of over 3000 community-dwelling elderly in the US, individuals with an estimated glomerular filtration rate (eGFR) of <45ml/min at baseline had an odds ratio of 2.86 of developing cognitive impairment at follow-up as compared to those with an eGFR of >60ml/min.[45]

14.9.2 Prevalence of cognitive dysfunction in older people on dialysis

In the US general population, the prevalence of cognitive impairment (excluding dementia) was found to be 22% in those ≥71 years.[46] The prevalence is far greater in ESRD. Murray et al. (2006) demonstrated in a group of 374 haemodialysis patients aged 55 and older, that 12.7% had normal cognitive function, 13.9% had mild cognitive impairment, 36.1% had moderate impairment, and 37.3% had severe impairment; only 2.9% of this entire dialysis group had a documented history of cognitive impairment.[47] These high prevalence rates of cognitive impairment in older dialysis patients were also found by Tyrrell et al. (2005) in 30–47% (depending on the assessment used) of 51 French patients on peritoneal dialysis and haemodialysis aged 70 or older.[41] Similarly Hain (2008) found that 39.7% of 63 haemodialysis patients (with no diagnosis of cognitive impairment) ≥60 years, had cognitive impairment.[48] The increased prevalence of cognitive impairment in patients with kidney disease is not surprising given their high rate of cardiovascular risk factors and vascular co-morbidities; this is well described in a recent editorial by Weiner.[49] In addition to vascular risk factors, haemodialysis treatment itself could be a further risk factor predisposing to cognitive impairment including hypotension, microembolization, and cerebral oedema.[50] Murray et al. (2007) also investigated acute variation in cognitive function before, during, and following haemodialysis in a group of patients aged 55 or older. It was found that global cognitive function varied over the dialysis procedure with patients performing their best either 1 hour prior to haemodialysis or on the following day.[51] This may be an important factor to consider when delivering education or information to older patients.

14.9.3 Consequences of cognitive dysfunction

Cognitive dysfunction affects memory, decision-making, and ability to plan; so it may impair an individual's ability to make decisions and adjust to the increased demands of a life-threatening disease, such as ESRD.[52] The Dialysis Outcomes and Practice Patterns Study (DOPPS) has shown that cognitive impairment and dementia are associated with an increased risk of death.[53] In the general population, those with mild cognitive impairment are 5–10 times more likely to develop dementia,[54] but the appropriate longitudinal studies have not been done in the dialysis population.

14.10 **Dialysis modality and the elderly**

Dialysis is often a lifelong treatment in the elderly due to the reduced suitability for transplantation because of the presence of multiple co-morbidities. As discussed above, age is not a barrier to dialysis and should not be a barrier to either haemodialysis or peritoneal dialysis. Frailty, however, could be seen as a barrier to peritoneal dialysis due to the resilience needed to cope with the treatment technicalities, especially in the absence of suitable home support. The more relevant question, therefore, is what is the best form of dialysis for the frail and non-frail elderly patient?

Morbidity and mortality outcomes on peritoneal dialysis and haemodialysis in the elderly are similar,[55] therefore, the modality that offers the best quality of life for the individual older person should be the modality of choice, in the absence of medical contraindications to either treatment. Currently within the UK, most elderly patients are on haemodialysis, with the proportion of older patients on peritoneal dialysis diminishing. In 2001, 25% of patients aged ≥65 years in England and Wales were on peritoneal dialysis compared to only 15.9% in 2007.[5,6] This dramatic reduction in the usage of peritoneal dialysis could be due to the perception within nephrology teams that peritoneal dialysis is only suitable for the younger patient. In contrast, in France peritoneal dialysis is extensively and successfully used predominantly in older people, with 55% of the peritoneal dialysis population being older than 70 years. Assisted peritoneal dialysis is strongly supported by the French government with community nurses assisting those unable to perform the treatment independently.[56] In the UK, despite the Department of Health encouraging home-based treatments to support people in their own homes.[57], peritoneal dialysis remains in decline as a treatment for older individuals. Often, those patients who are referred late to nephrology are started and maintained on haemodialysis. Dialysis, irrespective of modality, is a challenging treatment that requires considerable adaptation into one's routine and life. Peritoneal dialysis and haemodialysis are vastly different in nature and are likely to appeal to vastly different types of people. Therefore, all older patients opting for dialysis, to maximize their quality of life, should be provided with the opportunity to opt for their modality of choice.

Case study 1: An octogenarian on peritoneal dialysis

Mr A is an 89-year-old British man who opted for peritoneal dialysis and has been on continuous ambulatory peritoneal dialysis (CAPD) (3 exchanges/day) for 5 months. He had a planned start onto dialysis and had no significant co-morbidities apart from arthritis. He lives alone with no family of his own but is very close to his niece and her family and has a wide social network. Mr A feels that dialysis has not interfered with any aspect of his life (such as recreation, social networks, or diet) apart from his health, which he still regards as good. He has no symptoms of depression despite being placed on anti-depressants when he started dialysis (discontinued after 3 months) and has a good nutritional status. This example illustrates that octogenarians can cope well with a life on dialysis and with a self-care modality despite the absence of support at home.

Ethical analysis of case 1

There is a maxim that good ethics starts with good facts. In the case of Mr. A, as the RPA/ASN guideline recommendation #3 states, it is important to estimate prognosis to facilitate informed decisions. Of the four risk factors for dialysis patients independently associated with a poor prognosis, Mr A has only one – his age. His functional and nutritional statuses are good, and he does not have a life-limiting co-morbidity. Although the average octogenarian starting dialysis might only have a year to live,[8] Mr. A's prognosis is much better than the average. Though some may question starting an 89-year old on dialysis, his case illustrates the need to consider patients individually when making decisions to withhold or start dialysis. For all dialysis patients it is appropriate to conduct advance care planning to promote patient self-determination (see Chapter 4), and Mr. A should be encouraged to include his niece in the discussions and to complete an advance directive naming her as his legal agent for medical decision-making when he loses capacity. The only way to be able to be sure to respect his preferences for treatments such as dialysis, cardiopulmonary resuscitation, a feeding tube, and mechanical ventilation in possible future health states such as dementia or stroke is to ask him in advance. Estimate of prognosis and advance care planning are two key components of supportive care for older dialysis patients grounded in the ethical principles of respect for patient autonomy and respect for persons.

14.11 Decision-making

14.11.1 Decision-making in the older person

Increasingly, there is a shift in encouraging patients with chronic conditions to participate in the management of their illness. This involves making decisions about their treatment rather than solely receiving care; this is described in the Department of Health publication "The Expert Patient: a new approach to chronic disease management for the 21st century".[58] As highlighted in several chapters of this book, patients are encouraged to make decisions about future care and care at end of life. If we are to support patients in making their own decisions, the intricacies of decision-making need to be understood.

14.11.2 Decision-making styles

The mechanics of decision-making are often unconscious and are unrecognized by the healthcare team facilitating the decision-making process by providing information or support. Statements such as "if I were you, I would opt for X treatment" can be viewed by the patient as a convincing statement especially when delivered by a healthcare professional, yet the logic that it is based on is flawed. The healthcare professional is not the patient and therefore cannot know what it is like to be that individual. The patient's life experience of renal disease may also taint their decision-making. For example, a patient may have known someone who had a negative experience with dialysis and therefore wants to avoid that situation. This decision-making is heuristic in style, i.e. it is primarily based on emotions or experiences rather than systematically assessing and weighing the information available and therefore uses a reduced cognitive processing load.

14.11.3 How do older people make decisions?

Comparisons between the decision-making skills of older and younger people have been carried out in the general population. As an example, Finucane et al. (2002) studied 253 older people (mean age: 75 years, range: 65–94 years) and 239 younger adults (mean age: 40 years, range: 18–64 years). Of the comprehension tasks given, older adults made more errors than the younger group, yet both groups had more difficulty understanding the information as the complexity of the problem increased. In the same study, older adults appeared to favour delegating responsibility for decision-making, e.g. preferring not to be involved in choosing a Medicare health plan compared to younger people. Older people also thought themselves to be less analytical when rating their decision-making styles.[59] This is supported by Berg et al. (1999) who found that older people sought less information when exploring the solution to a problem.[60] Despite this, older people have been shown to be able to adapt to an environment that encouraged information intensive strategies to be used[61] and were able to accurately assess information when the environment required set decisions to be made.[62] Time of day also influences how older people make decisions, with early morning being best suited for detailed processing as opposed to the afternoon or evening.[63] Age-related changes in cognition could explain why older people tend to employ streamlined decision-making strategies. Equally, they could be drawing on their knowledge and life experience to compensate for changes in cognition[63] and using more selective and rationalized strategies to collate information to make a decision.

Cognition is not the only aspect that plays a role in the decision-making process. As already discussed, older people tend to relate more to emotional than factual information. This is demonstrated by Williams and Drolet (2005) who showed that older people preferred and recalled more emotional information compared to younger people who preferred fact based information.[64] This could suggest that older patients attempting to make decisions could be susceptible to more heuristic and emotional decision-making styles. It, however, has also been shown that although older people more readily opted for heuristic style decision-making, this could be minimized when justifications for their decisions were solicited.[65] "Framing" refers to choice alterations dependent on the language used. The same study found that older people were more vulnerable to framing than younger adults. This framing effect also disappeared when the older people were required to provide explanations for their choices.

14.11.4 Supporting the older patient in making decisions

As discussed, several factors play a role in decision making in older people and these are different from those who are younger. By encouraging systematic assessment of the information compared to a heuristic decision-making, the patient may be enabled to determine the treatment that is best suited to them. Heuristic decision-making is comparatively effortless and can usually be reached faster yet negates the realities that the patient may encounter once on a specified treatment. In order to encourage systematic processing, the information presented should be readable, balanced, and non-biased with the avoidance of framing and emotional information. An analysis of leaflets used by 32 units in the UK found that 90% of them were of a readability that was rated as "fairly difficult", "difficult", "very difficult", or "extremely difficult". As a comparative measure, "difficult" is defined as the ability required to read a Life Insurance Policy.[66] This illustrates that the vast majority of leaflets within renal units are not supporting the patient in making decisions. This is particularly important for older patients who often have inadequate or marginal health literacy.[67]

14.12 Summary

Gerontological issues feature increasingly within the care of the renal patient. The importance of training physicians in geriatric nephrology is strongly supported by the American Society of Nephrology (ASN) Geriatrics Task Force who have developed a comprehensive and accessible online Geriatric Nephrology Curriculum.[68] Awareness of issues magnified in geriatric nephrology such as frailty, malnutrition, depression, and cognitive dysfunction will help alert the nephrology team to instigate appropriate management. In chronic disease, patients are encouraged to make decisions about their treatments that are often complex. This complexity is exacerbated when cognitive dysfunction is present. Creating a supportive environment is paramount to support older people to manage the day-to-day management decisions of chronic disease as well as the larger life-changing decisions that are often required in ESRD.

References

1 Office for National Statistics. National Statistics Online: latest on ageing. 21/08/2008. http://www.statistics.gov.uk/cci/nugget.asp?ID=949 Accessed on 15th June 2009.

2 Young H, Grundy E, Jitlal M (2006). Care providers, care receivers: A longitudinal perspective. Joseph Rowntree Foundation.

3 Cook WL, Jassal SV (2008). Functional dependencies among the elderly on hemodialysis. *Kidney Int*, **73**(11), 1289–95.

4 Epstein M (1996). Aging and the kidney. *J Am Soc Nephrol*, **7**(8), 1106–22.

5 The Renal Association (2002). UK Renal Registry Report 2001.

6 The Renal Association (2009). The Renal Registry Report 2008.

7 The Renal Association (2008). UK Renal Registry Report 2007.

8 Kurella M, Covinsky KE, Collins AJ, et al. (2007). Octogenarians and nonagenarians starting dialysis in the United States. *Ann Intern Med*, **146**(3), 177–83.

9 Dharmarajan TS, Kaul N, Russell RO (2004). How old is too old to start dialysis? *J Am Geriatrics Soc*, **52**(2), 325–7.

10 Rowe JW, Kahn RL (1997). Successful aging. *Gerontologist*, **37**(4), 433–40.

11 Strawbridge WJ, Wallhagen MI, Cohen RD (2002). Successful aging and well-being: self-rated compared with Rowe and Kahn. *Gerontologist*, **42**(6), 727–33.

12 Fried LP, Tangen CM, Walston J, et al. (2001). Frailty in older adults: Evidence for a phenotype. *J Gerontol A Biol Sci Med Sc*, **56**(3), M146–56.

13 Campbell AJ, Buchner DM (1997). Unstable disability and the fluctuations of frailty. *Age Ageing*, **26**(4), 315–18.

14 Woods NF, LaCroix AZ, Gray SL, et al. (2005). Frailty: emergence and consequences in women aged 65 and older in the Women's Health Initiative Observational Study. *J Am Geriatr Soc*, **53**(8), 1321–30.

15 Avila-Funes JA, Amieva H, Barberger-Gateau P, et al. (2009). Cognitive impairment improves the predictive validity of the phenotype of frailty for adverse health outcomes: the three-city study. *J Am Geriatr Soc*, **57**(3), 453–61.

16 Johansen KL, Chertow GM, Jin C, et al. (2007). Significance of frailty among dialysis patients. *J Am Soc Nephrol*, **18**, 2960–7.

17 Peterson MJ, Giuliani C, Morey MC, et al. (2009). Physical activity as a preventative factor for frailty: the health, aging, and body composition study. *J Gerontol A Biol Sci Med Sci*, **64**(1), 61–8.

18 Gallagher D, Ruts E, Visser M, et al. (2000). Weight stability masks sarcopenia in elderly men and women. *Am J Physiol Endocrinol Metab*, **279**(2), E366–75.

19 Cook WL, Tomlinson G, Donaldson M, et al. (2006). Falls and fall-related injuries in older dialysis patients. *Clin J Am Soc Nephrol*, **1**(6), 1197–204.

20 Tinetti ME, Speechley M, Ginter SF (1988). Risk factors for falls among elderly persons living in the community. *N Engl J Med*, **319**(26), 1701–7.

21 U.S. Renal Data System (2006). USRDS 2006 Annual Data Report: Atlas of End-Stage Renal Disease in the United States, National Institutes of Health, National Institute of Diabetes and Digestive and Kidney Diseases, Bethesda, MD.

22 Lamping DL, Constantinovici N, Roderick P, et al. (2000). Clinical outcomes, quality of life, and costs in the North Thames Dialysis Study of elderly people on dialysis: a prospective cohort study. *Lancet*, **356**(9241), 1543–50.

23 Lo D, Chiu E, Jassal SV (2008). A prospective pilot study to measure changes in functional status associated with hospitalization in elderly dialysis-dependent patients. *Am J Kidney Dis*, **52**(5), 956–61.

24 Baumgartner RN, Stauber PM, McHugh D, et al. (1995). Cross-sectional age differences in body composition in persons 60+ years of age. *J Gerontol A Biol Sci Med Sci*, **50**(6), M307–16.

25 Gallagher D, Ruts E, Visser M, et al. (2000). Weight stability masks sarcopenia in elderly men and women. *Am J Physiol-Endocrin Metab*, **279**(2), E366–75.

26 Morley JE, Kim MJ, Haren MT (2005). Frailty and hormones. *Rev Endocr Metab Disord*, **6**(2), 101–8.

27 Iannuzzi-Sucich M, Prestwood KM, Kenny AM (2002). Prevalence of sarcopenia and predictors of skeletal muscle mass in healthy, older men and women. *J Gerontol A Biol Sci Med Sci*, **57**(12), M772–7.

28 Chumlea WC, Garry PJ, Hunt WC, et al. (1988). Distributions of Serial Changes in Stature and Weight in A Healthy Elderly Population. *Hum Biol*, **60**(6), 917–25.

29 Fried LF, Boudreau R, Lee JS, et al. (2007). Kidney function as a predictor of loss of lean mass in older adults: Health, aging and body composition study. *J Am Geri Soc*, **55**(10), 1578–84.

30 Qureshi AR, Alvestrand A, Danielsson A, et al. (1998). Factors predicting malnutrition in hemodialysis patients: a cross-sectional study. *Kidney Int*, **53**(3), 773–82.

31 Aparicio M, Cano N, Chauveau P, et al. (1999). Nutritional status of haemodialysis patients: a French national cooperative study. French Study Group for Nutrition in Dialysis. *Nephrol Dialy Transplant*, **14**(7), 1679–86.

32 Carrero JJ, Chmielewski M, Axelsson J, et al. (2008). Muscle atrophy, inflammation and clinical outcome in incident and prevalent dialysis patients. *Clin Nutr*, **27**(4), 557–64.

33 Cianciaruso B, Brunori G, Kopple JD, et al. (1995). Cross-sectional comparison of malnutrition in continuous ambulatory peritoneal dialysis and hemodialysis patients. *Am J Kidney Dis*, **26**(3), 475–86.

34 Stenvinkel P, Heimburger O, Paultre F, et al. (1999). Strong association between malnutrition, inflammation, and atherosclerosis in chronic renal failure. *Kidney Int*, **55**(5), 1899–911.

35 Burrowes JD, Cockram DB, Dwyer JT, et al. (2002). Cross-sectional relationship between dietary protein and energy intake, nutritional status, functional status, and comorbidity in older versus younger hemodialysis patients. *J Ren Nutr*, **12**(2), 87–95.

36 Middleton RA, lman-Farinelli MA. (1999). Taste sensitivity is altered in patients with chronic renal failure receiving continuous ambulatory peritoneal dialysis. *J Nutr*, **129**(1), 122–5.

37 Lindsay RM, Heidenheim PA, Nesrallah G, et al. (2006). Daily Hemodialysis Study Group London Health Sciences Centre. Minutes to recovery after a hemodialysis session: a simple health-related quality of life question that is reliable, valid, and sensitive to change. *Clin J Am Soc Nephrol*, **1**(5), 952–9.

38 Locher JL, Robinson CO, Roth DL, et al. (2005). The effect of the presence of others on caloric intake in homebound older adults. *J Gerontol A Biol Sci Med Sci*, **60**(11), 1475–8.

39 Altintepe L, Levendoglu F, Okudan N, et al. (2006). Physical disability, psychological status, and health-related quality of life in older hemodialysis patients and age-matched controls. *Hemodialysis Int*, **10**(3), 260–6.

40 Kutner NG, Brogan D, Dallas Hall W, et al. (2000). Functional impairment, depression, and life satisfaction among older hemodialysis patients and age-matched controls: A prospective study. *Arch Phy Med Rehab*, **81**(4), 453–9.

41 Tyrrell J, Paturel L, Cadec B, et al. (2005). Older patients undergoing dialysis treatment: cognitive functioning, depressive mood and health-related quality of life. *Aging Ment Health*, **9**(4), 374–9.

42 Mulsant BH, Ganguli M (1999). Epidemiology and diagnosis of depression in late life. *J Clin Psych*, **60** Suppl 20, 9–15.

43 Charney DS, Reynolds CF, III, Lewis L, et al. (2003). Depression and Bipolar Support Alliance consensus statement on the unmet needs in diagnosis and treatment of mood disorders in late life. *Arch Gen Psych*, **60**(7), 664–72.

44 Tombaugh TN (2004). Trail Making Test A and B: normative data stratified by age and education. *Arch Clin Neuropsychol*, **19**(2), 203–14.

45 Kurella M, Chertow GM, Fried LF, et al. (2005) Chronic kidney disease and cognitive impairment in the elderly: the health, aging, and body composition study. *J Am Soc Nephrol*, **16**(7), 2127–33.

46 Plassman BL, Langa KM, Fisher GG, et al. (2008). Prevalence of cognitive impairment without dementia in the United States. *Ann Intern Med*, **148**(6), 427–34.

47 Murray AM, Tupper DE, Knopman DS, et al. (2006). Cognitive impairment in hemodialysis patients is common. *Neurology*, **67**(2), 216–23.

48 Hain DJ (2008). Cognitive function and adherence of older adults undergoing hemodialysis. *Nephrol Nurs J*, **35**(1), 23–9.

49 Weiner DE (2008). The cognition-kidney disease connection: lessons from population-based studies in the United States. *Am J Kidney Dis*, **52**(2), 201–4.

50 Madero M, Gul A, Sarnak MJ (2008). Cognitive function in chronic kidney disease. *Semin Dial*, **21**(1), 29–37.

51 Murray AM, Pederson SL, Tupper DE, et al. (2007). Acute variation in cognitive function in hemodialysis patients: a cohort study with repeated measures. *Am J Kidney Dis*, **50**(2), 270–8.

52 Pereira AA, Weiner DE, Scott T, et al. (2005). Cognitive function in dialysis patients. *Am J Kidney Dis*, **45**(3), 448–62.

53 Kurella M, Mapes DL, Port FK, et al. (2006). Correlates and outcomes of dementia among dialysis patients: the Dialysis Outcomes and Practice Patterns Study. *Nephrol Dial Transplant*, **21**(9), 2543–8.

54 Petersen RC, Doody R, Kurz A, et al. (2001). Current concepts in mild cognitive impairment. *Arch Neurol*, **58**(12), 1985–92.

55 Harris SA, Lamping DL, Brown EA, et al. (2002). Clinical outcomes and quality of life in elderly patients on peritoneal dialysis versus hemodialysis. *Perit Dial Int*, **22**(4), 463–70.

56 Verger C, Ryckelynck JP, Duman M, et al. (2006). French peritoneal dialysis registry (RDPLF): outline and main results. *Kidney Int Suppl*, **103**, S12–20.

57 Department of Health (2006). Our health, our care, our say: a new direction for community services. 30/06/2006.

58 Department of Health (2001). The expert patient: A new approach to chronic disease management for the 21st century. 14/09/2001.

59 Finucane ML, Slovic P, Hibbard JH, et al. (2002). Aging and decision-making competence: an analysis of comprehension and consistency skills in older versus younger adults considering health-plan options. *J Behav Deci Making*, **15**, 141–64.

60 Berg CA, Meegan SP, Klaczynski P (1999). Age and experiential differences in strategy generation and information requests for solving everyday problems. International *J Behav Dev*, **23**, 615–39.

61 Mata R, Schooler LJ, Rieskamp J (2007). The aging decision maker: Cognitive aging and the adaptive selection of decision strategies. *Psychol Aging*, **22**(4), 796–810.

62 Multhaup KS (1995). Aging, source, and decision criteria - when false fame errors do and do not occur. *Psychol Aging*, **10**(3), 492–7.

63 Yoon C (1997). Age differences in consumers' processing strategies: An investigation of moderating influences. *J Consumer Res*, **24**(3), 329–42.

64 Williams P, Drolet A (2005). Age-related differences in responses to emotional advertisements. *J Consumer Res*, **32**(3), 343–54.

65 Kim S, Goldstein D, Hasher L, et al. (2005). Framing effects in younger and older adults. *J Gerontol B Psychol Sci Soc Sci*, **60**(4), 215–18.

66 Winterbottom A, Conner M, Mooney A, et al. (2007). Evaluating the quality of patient leaflets about renal replacement therapy across UK renal units. *Nephrol Dialy Transplant*, **22**(8), 2291–6.

67 Gazmararian JA, Baker DW, Williams MV, et al. (1999). Health literacy among Medicare enrollees in a managed care organization. *JAMA*, **281**(6), 545–51.

68 Online Geriatric Nephrology Curriculum (2009). http://www.asn-online.org/education_and_meetings/geriatrics/ Accessed on 15th June 2009.

Chapter 15

Death and end-of-life care in advanced kidney disease

Ken Farrington and E Joanna Chambers

15.1 Introduction

In the past 50 years, renal replacement therapy (RRT) – by means of dialysis and kidney transplantation – has revolutionized the outlook for patients with advanced kidney disease. Millions of people worldwide have been sustained on these therapies, who would formerly have died prematurely. However, we need to recognize that these therapies are imperfect. In particular, the degree of functional renal replacement offered by dialysis is far from complete, with patients tending to be maintained, often for many years, in a persistently uraemic state. As a result, patients on dialysis have a high morbidity and mortality compared with non-uraemic age-matched peers.

In addition, dialysis is a demanding and invasive treatment. Older patients constitute the majority of patients on dialysis programmes, the median age of patients starting RRT in the United Kingdom (UK) in 2005 was 65 years,[1] and the prevalence of both non-renal co-morbidity and dependency increases with age. Coping with the demands of dialysis may be difficult for ageing, increasingly dependent patients, especially in the context of other co-morbidities. Some patients in these circumstances choose not to commence dialysis, opting for a conservative approach. Others who are already on dialysis may consider withdrawing from the treatment. In such situations, it is vitally important to recognize that end of life is approaching, so that high-quality supportive and palliative care can be planned for the individual patient and their carers.

Recently, important policy documents in the UK have addressed these issues. The National Service Framework for Renal Service[2] put forward key quality requirements for end-of-life care, to support people with established renal failure to live out the remainder of their lives as fully as possible, and to die with dignity. The National End of Life Care (EOL) Strategy – promoting high-quality care for all adults at the end of life[3] aims to ensure that all adults – irrespective of their age, place of care, or condition – are able to receive high-quality care at the end of life. Guidelines on the appropriate initiation and withdrawal of dialysis in the US[4] may have had an impact on practice in this area.[5] This chapter will discuss end-of-life issues as they relate to patients with advanced kidney failure. It focusses mainly on those patients whose kidney failure is being treated by dialysis or by conservative means.

15.2 The renal replacement therapy clinical pathway

What distinguishes the management of patients with advanced renal disease from that of patients with advanced chronic disease of other organs is the capacity to maintain life in the complete absence of kidney function – for years or decades – by the resourceful use of the variety of interdependent technologies, which constitute RRT (Fig. 15.1).

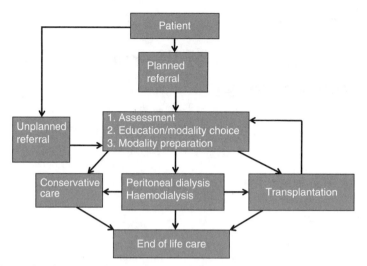

Fig. 15.1 The renal replacement therapy clinical pathway.

Patients with progressive kidney failure, who are referred to renal services in a timely fashion, undergo multi-disciplinary assessment and education in preparation for their selected treatment modality. Such choices emerge from the interplay of patient preference tempered by clinical and social imperatives. Potential transplant recipients need to be free from major extra-renal co-morbidities, whilst – for the frail and dependent – haemodialysis (HD) may be the only practicable renal replacement option, and some such patients may choose to forego dialysis, opting for a conservative approach. For many patients though, the modalities are complementary. A patient may begin on peritoneal dialysis (PD), go on to receive a transplant, and subsequently, perhaps many years later when the transplant has failed, return to HD. Physical deterioration and death can occur at any of these stages, though more commonly and more predictably in patients on the dialysis and conservative parts of the pathway than in transplanted patients. Clearly, end-of-life care is an important element of the pathway.

15.3 Characteristics of the advanced renal failure population

At the end of 2006 there were almost 44 000 patients on RRT in the UK,[6] 45% of whom had a functioning transplant. A similar proportion was on HD, mainly centre-based, the remainder being on PD. The equivalent numbers in the USA were much higher, with over half a million people on RRT, 70% of whom were on dialysis.[7] HD patients were older (median age in UK patients 65 years) than those on PD (59.9 years) and those with transplants (49.9 years). Diabetes as a primary renal diagnosis was present in 20% of UK patients starting on RRT (45% in the USA). More than 50% of incident UK patients had one or more co-morbidities,[8] and one-third were significantly dependent.[9] Those commencing HD had significantly more co-morbidities than those commencing PD.[8] These and other factors relating to the dialysis process itself, contribute to the high mortality amongst dialysis patients, which with a median survival <5 years,[9] is worse than that in many cancers. The expected remaining life years of a dialysis patient in the age range 65–69 years is only 3.9 years compared with 17.2 years for an age-matched person in the general population.[7] The proportion of patients on conservative management programmes is less well known, but may constitute about 15% of the population with advanced kidney failure attending specialist centres.[10] These patients are older, more dependent, and have more co-morbidities than those opting for dialysis.[9] Their survival is poorer, though may not be significantly different from that of dialysis patients with similar co-morbidity and dependency.[10,11]

15.4 **Key elements in the renal end-of-life care pathway**

The UK National End of Life Care Strategy[3] identifies the key clinical elements of end-of-life care as:

1 Discussions as end of life approaches

2 Assessment, planning, and review of care needs

3 Coordination and delivery of high-quality patient-centred care

4 Delivery of high-quality services in different settings

5 Care in the last days of life

6 Care after death.

The strategy also recognizes the need to raise public and professional awareness of end-of-life issues, to enhance their profile in the training and continuing professional development of healthcare workers, to encourage research to inform the evidence base and to establish a platform for clinical audit and quality assurance, and to engage with commissioners.

It is our intention in this chapter to focus on those elements in the end-of-life strategy which relate directly to the delivery of clinical care, and in particular on those areas in which patients with advanced kidney disease may have special problems or needs. The major factor in this is the potential of RRT as a life-sustaining treatment and, once this has been embarked on, the patient's continuing dependence on it. Two groups of patients emerge for particular consideration. The first is of those patients, at or approaching "end-stage", who choose to forego dialysis and opt for conservative management. The second is of those patients who may have been on dialysis for years but are struggling to cope because of progressive co-morbidity and dependency or because of a sudden deterioration in their health due, for instance, to a stroke. The desire not to be a burden can be a major factor in a patient's decision to withdraw. In such situations withdrawal from dialysis may be an option – a situation which usually leads to death in a few days or weeks. Both these groups of patients clearly have particular supportive care and end-of-life care needs.

15.5 **Illness trajectories in advanced kidney failure**

In palliative care practice, it is well-recognized that there may be characteristic patterns of functional deterioration towards the end of life.[12] These are referred to as illness trajectories (Fig.15.2). Four general patterns have been described: sudden death usually due to cardiac dysrhythmia (panel A), rapid intractable decline such as that associated with a terminal malignancy (Panel B), slow deterioration punctuated by abrupt, partially reversible troughs – such as might occur in patients with severe single-organ failure, e.g. heart failure (panel C) – and gradual insidious decline such a might occur in the elderly and generally frail (panel D). Although there is little or no published data, the position would appear to be more complex in patients with advanced kidney failure,[12] partly due to the contribution of dialysis, and partly due to the high prevalence of extra-renal co-morbidity. In dialysis patients all four of these general patterns may occur – in pure form or in combinations. The trajectories may be a little more predictable in those patients managed conservatively.

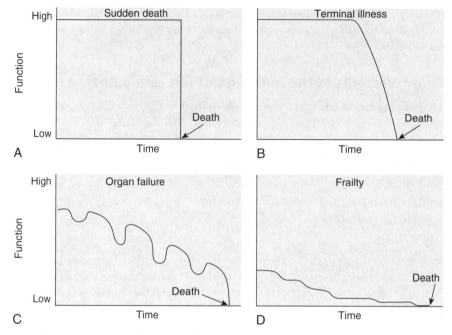

Fig. 15.2 Illness trajectories at the end of life.

15.6 **Diagnosing impending death**

Diagnosing dying is important because it enables a change of emphasis and a change of goals of care from cure and prolongation of life to relief of symptoms, maintenance of comfort, and attention to psychological, social, and spiritual concerns. Clinicians can be uneasy about this, especially if any hope of improvement remains, and more so if a definitive diagnosis is lacking. Generally though, when recovery is uncertain it is better to discuss this rather than leaving the patient and family in false hope.[14] The introduction of good symptom control and psychosocial support for patient and family at this time – involving collaboration with local palliative care services where needed – will not shorten life but may enhance quality of life, whatever may be the outcome for the patient.

In patients with advanced kidney failure who have opted for conservative management, the process of assessment and care planning needs to begin with the decision to forego dialysis, although even within this group the prognosis may vary widely. In dialysis patients, the complexity of illness trajectories adds additional layers of difficulty. In the palliative care field there are triggers[15] which give clues as to whether a supportive or palliative approach is the most appropriate at present, although again there are difficulties in translating these into the dialysis setting. The use of the "surprise question" has been advocated. "Would you be surprised if your patient were to die in next 6–12 months?" The only study which looked prospectively at this question in dialysis patients found that experienced nurse practitioners classified 34 (23%) of 147 dialysis patients in the "no" they would not be surprised group. This group had a 1-year mortality of 29.4% compared with 10.6% for those in the "yes" group; the odds of dying within 1 year for the patients in the "no" group was 3.5 times higher than the "yes" group.[16] Clearly, there are patients with advanced kidney disease with a palpable need for supportive/palliative care and those making a clear informed choice for the focus of care to be 'comfort' rather than 'curative' provide an obvious trigger; so may clinical indicators such as progressive co-morbidity, declining functional status, general physical decline, or the sudden occurrence of a catastrophic event, such as a severe stroke. Other clinical indicators include significant weight loss (>10% over 6 months) and severe hypoalbuminaemia (serum albumin: <25 g/litre), although reversible problems such as inadequate dialysis and intercurrent infections may need to be excluded.

In the dialysis setting, the nursing team play a crucial role in identifying patients approaching end of life. Haemodialysis patients attend for thrice-weekly treatments often for many years. Dialysis nurses – who are intimately involved in the delivery of these treatments – are well-placed to observe changes in the physical, mental, and spiritual status of patients, and to raise these issues with the patients and discuss their concerns within the wider multi-disciplinary team. Units should consider the creation of a "Cause for Concern" register of such patients to facilitate care planning and communication. It is also important that clinical staff at the "front-line" require training in the recognition of the approaching end-of-life phase, and in communication skills to allow them to broach issues with patients, carers, and with other health professionals. The use of regular assessment tools such as the modified Edmonton symptom assessment system[17] or the dialysis symptom index[18] which look at physical and social well-being as well as quality of life may alert clinical staff to changes in the patient's health status and prompt further discussions.

15.7 Starting the conversation: pre-contemplation, contemplation, and action

Starting the conversation concerning end-of-life issues with patients and carers requires well-developed judgement and good communication. Since the subject of the discussion is preparation for death, extreme sensitivity and skill are required. Most patients wish to discuss these issues, but some do not.[19] There is no evidence that engaging in end-of-life discussions will destroy hope; patients view this as an integral component of quality care.[20] Clinicians need to be sensitive to patients' cues and to consider this aspect of care as a process, not an event. Patients have reported that their verbal cues about having 'had enough' or being 'too old and too tired' were often not picked up.[21] In general, clinicians are poorly trained and ill-equipped to deal with end-of-life issues. As a result, patients hesitate to engage, feeling that clinicians are trying to avoid the issue.[22] Holley outlines three stages of patient readiness: pre-contemplation, contemplation, and action.[22] The better the clinician–patient relationship, the better the clinician can establish the patient's stage of readiness, and that of family and carers. It is important to establish a shared view among the clinical team, the patient, and the family and carers, of the patient's current situation and likely prognosis. Sometimes, it may take some time to establish this harmony, but achieving it is necessary before moving on to develop care plans. This process involves the whole of the multi-disciplinary team, including physicians, nurses, social workers, and counsellors. The person taking the lead role in the discussions with an individual patient will vary, and should take into account previous relationships with the patient and family. It is important that the team has a uniform and coherent view relating to issues involving individual patients, so good communication within the team is paramount.

Some patients who withdraw from dialysis are cognitively impaired, and lack the capacity to make the decision to stop dialysis. In these circumstances in the UK, clinicians must act in that person's best interests taking into account any previous recorded wishes and the views of those close to them in line with the UK Mental Capacity Act 2005.[23] Conflict may arise where the views of the family differ from those of the medical team, particularly if there are different views within the family.

There are cultural differences in the way patients respond to the need for end-of-life care. US data suggests that non-white racial or ethnic groups were generally less likely to support end-of-life planning. Blacks consistently preferred continued use of life support (including dialysis) and Asians and Hispanics were more likely to make family-centred end-of-life decisions.[24]

15.8 Involving and supporting carers

The enormous contribution family carers make to the end-of-life care of an individual needs to be formally acknowledged. Most play their part willingly and with love, but often go unrecognized. To be able to support them, it is necessary to understand their needs – both those common to all carers and those particular to the situation the individual carers find themselves in. Carers need information just as much as patients do, on what is likely to happen and on who is there to support them in a crisis, particularly if they are caring at home. Time scales may be difficult to predict, even for patients withdrawing from dialysis, but it is important for the carer to able to gauge how long they will be able to sustain a certain level of commitment, especially if juggling work and family commitments too. Information about local statutory services and other support organizations should be available as it can be invaluable.

Professional carers should take as much pride in the care of those who are dying as in the care of their other renal patients. A climate of support within the team with recognition of the importance of this aspect of their work will contribute to the well-being of staff, many of whom may have known the patient over many years. Renal teams need to acknowledge that professional carers will need to say goodbye to patients well known to them and may also need to grieve in order to enable them to continue to gain satisfaction in their work and to support those most close to dying patients.

15.9 What is a good death?

There can be no easy definition of what constitutes a good death. What is perceived as quality care at the end of life is highly personal. It should be achieved through a process of shared decision-making and clear communication which acknowledges the values and preferences of individual patients and their familes.[25] In general, studies have shown that patients, families, and healthcare professionals place great value on good pain and symptom management, clear decision-making, preparation for death, achieving a sense of completion, being able to contribute to others, and being treated as a "whole person".[25,25] In a related approach, Singer et al.[27] used qualitative interviews in 126 patients – 48 of whom were on dialysis – to identify and describe elements of quality end-of-life care from the patient's perspective. Five domains were identified: receiving adequate pain and symptom management, avoiding inappropriate prolongation of dying, achieving a sense of control, relieving burden on loved ones, and strengthening relationships with loved ones. This framework can guide the development of end-of-life services and also help clinicians when planning individual care. Using Patrick's definition of quality of death and dying as "the degree to which a person's preferences for dying and the moment of death agree with observations of how the person actually died, as reported by others"[28] clinicians can evaluate the quality of service provided. Table 15.1 shows a comparison of the domains found to be important in the studies cited.

15.10 Assessment, care planning, and review

Planning care in the end-of-life phase is vital to achieving a "good death". Clinicians should assume the responsibility for initiating care planning and help guide patients and their families

Table 15.1 A comparison of domains of importance in end-of-life care

Singer[26]	Steinhauser[24]		Patrick[27]	
	Multi-disciplinary group	Patients	Domains	Specific issues (selected)
Pain and symptom management	Pain and symptom management		Symptoms and personal care	
Avoidance of inappropriate dying	Decisions about treatment preferences		Treatment preferences	Avoidance of ventilator or dialysis
Achieving a sense of control	Being treated as a whole person	Mentally aware	Whole person concerns	Having control over what is going on around you
				Being able to laugh, smile, be touched and hugged
Relieving burden		Not being a burden	Preparation for death	Avoiding strain on loved ones
Strengthening relationships		Helping others	Family	Spending time with spouse, children, friends, pets, alone
	Preparation for death	Having funeral arrangements planned	Preparation for death	
	Sense of completion	Coming to peace with God		Feeling at peace with dying Having a spiritual service or ceremony before death
			Moment of death	Dying in one's place of choice Having desired people present at death

through the process.[29] Patients vary in their desire for information and their involvement in medical decision-making, so the process and the care plan itself should be tailored to individual patient preferences.

End-of-life care planning in the renal setting is not well developed in many renal centres, but the scope of such care plans has been well outlined in the End of Life Strategy[3] which provides a firm basis for their development. Much more needs to be developed in the renal unit setting to ensure improvements in the quality of end-of-life care. The initiation of new end-of-life care roles for renal professionals, including those of clinical lead and key-workers could promote initiatives to ensure enhanced staff awareness and training with consolidation of links with community palliative care and patient transport services, joint working with palliative care services, and the creation of local frameworks to ensure the delivery of appropriate care for people in the dying phase of their illness and after death. Clinicians may utilize end-of-life tools such as Preferred Priorities of Care (PPC)[30] or The Liverpool Care Pathway for the Dying. Hospices and specialist palliative care services need to be fully integrated in the strategic planning for end-of-life care services for patients with advanced kidney disease, acting as an expert resource within renal units as well as offering day care and community outreach teams, with the ability to admit those with specialist care needs for complex pain and symptom control. There is a major role for palliative care services in supporting the palliative care education and training of renal professionals.

The care plan should be drawn up by a team-member competent in assessment processes with knowledge of local service providers, referral criteria, and support services and with access to multi-disciplinary input which should include social workers, counsellors, and palliative care specialists. It should record patient's preferences, perhaps with reference to the PPC document.[30] The plan should be regularly updated and reviewed as the patient's condition changes, recording on-going assessments, the outcome of multi-disciplinary team meetings, and communication with primary care and palliative care services. The plan should include details of nominated renal Key-Worker, and be available to all who have a legitimate reason for access, including out-of-hours and emergency/urgent care services.

Coordination of care across boundaries is vital to ensure good end-of-life care, and the patient's renal key-worker should play a major role in facilitating this. A register of patients within renal units with end-of-life care needs might be considered. Renal patients (CKD 4 & 5) with end-of-life care needs should also be entered on to primary-care supportive-care registers set up by those using the Gold Standard Framework with consequent regular discussion at primary healthcare meetings. Rapid access to end-of-life care is also important to prevent inappropriate default "cure-centred" care being administered in the event of a sudden deterioration in patient on dialysis. Fast-track discharge-planning with availability of sufficient community services, including responsive patient-transport services, would provide the hospitalized patient with minimal residual renal function – who has withdrawn from dialysis – the option of dying at home.

15.11 Prognosis

"How long will I last" is a vitally important piece of information for a patient contemplating withdrawal from dialysis. It is also important for family and carers, and for health professionals and members of voluntary services who are all involved in planning the patients care. The major factor determining prognosis in these circumstances is the degree of residual renal function the patient has. This is not formally measured in most renal units, since it involves interdialytic urine collections. If the patient has been on dialysis for many years, it is likely that the residual function is minimal. In others, an estimate can be gained from perusing records of the patient's interdialytic weight gains; the higher these are, the lower the urine output is likely to be. Finally, asking the patient or carer to estimate their urine output may be helpful. A patient with minimal residual renal function is likely to survive no longer than a week or 10 days.[31] Patients with significant residual function (even 3–4% of normal function) can survive for weeks or even months, in the absence of other life-threatening co-morbidity. Clearly, there are major differences in the approach to end-of-life care in these two settings and careful attention to detail is required for effective planning of care.

Prognosis in conservatively managed patients is more difficult still, and depends again on the degree of residual function the patient has when the decision is taken to adopt a conservative approach, together with the severity of their non-renal co-morbidity. It is easier in these circumstances to generate serial estimated glomerular filtration rate (eGFR) levels from serum creatinine measurements, and to estimate the rate of decline of renal function. However, it is difficult to estimate at what level of residual renal function a patient will become ill since there is much inter-individual variation. In addition, patients opting for conservative management very frequently have severe extra-renal co-morbidity and death before end-stage (CKD 5) is common. In one study the median survival of conservatively managed patients commencing with a mean Cockcroft–Gault creatinine clearance of 8.9 ml/min was 6.3 months.[10] In another study,[13] 1- and 2-year survivals were 68% and 47%, respectively, from the time a patients reached an eGFR of 15 ml/min/1.73 m^2. Survival was considerably lower in those with high co-morbidity.

15.12 **Modes of dying in advanced kidney failure**

There are three "final common pathways" by which death occurs in patients with advanced kidney disease, uncomplicated by extra-renal co-morbidity. These are volume overload, "uraemia", and hyperkalaemia, although overlaps are common. Volume overload can cause intractable breathlessness, and uncomfortable peripheral oedema. This is commoner in patients with minimal residual function in whom diuretics are useless. Breathlessness is a difficult symptom to treat (see below) and efforts should be made to prevent fluid accumulation by ensuring the patient is at their "dry weight" prior to dialysis withdrawal, and by encouraging continued salt restriction and care with fluid intake. If the patient has residual renal function, high-dose diuretics can be helpful. "Uraemia" is a term used to mean increasing symptoms of anorexia, nausea, and lethargy due to the accumulation of toxins; little can be done to prevent this. The mode of death in hyperkalaemia can be sudden due to cardiac dysrhythmia. This mode may be the most preferable, to the patient once he or she has completed any end-of-life business and said his or her goodbyes, although death by this mode tends to be unpredictable and it is thus less likely that a close relative will be able to be present at the moment of death, if they had so wished. Generally, attempts to prevent potassium accumulation after dialysis withdrawal are not indicated.

15.13 **Care in the last days**

15.13.1 **Treating difficult symptoms**

Patients on dialysis experience multiple symptoms,[32–34] see Chapter 7 for the most common. The burden of symptoms is likely to be higher in those coming towards the end of life and although dialysis-related symptoms may ease after dialysis withdrawal, those related to co-morbid conditions are likely to continue and those associated with uraemia and fluid overload may worsen. Many patients withdraw from dialysis, in part, due to their symptom burden.[35]

Only two studies have looked at symptoms following withdrawal from dialysis.[31,36] These indicate that pain, agitation, myoclonus, dyspnoea, nausea, and fatigue were prominent right up to the last 24 h of life with one-quarter of patients described as having unrelieved suffering,[37] although Cohen's study states that most patients were considered to have died well.

Symptom prevalence is high in conservatively managed patients and comparable to that in advanced cancer populations, albeit with a distinctive prevalence and severity pattern,[38] with fatigue, shortness of breath, and restless legs being more prominent in those with kidney failure. Prescribing in anticipation of common symptoms at the end of life and attention to route of administration aiming to use the easiest and least invasive are important management concerns.

Pain may not be a major feature of dying following dialysis withdrawal, but, when already present, it is likely to continue. In addition to this, reduced mobility may provoke joint stiffness and skin pressure. Family questionnaires after death show that 73% of patients had pain in the last week, and that in 36%, it was severe.[37] Fear of a pain is a major concern for patients and families, and acknowledging this aids management. Those in pain need regular analgesia in line with the principles of the World Health Organization (WHO) analgesic ladder (Chapter 8). Those without pain need rapid access to analgesia should it occur. If drugs cannot be given orally and the pain is mild, rectal paracetamol and non-steroidal anti-inflammatory drugs (NSAIDs) may be highly effective, if acceptable to the patient. Where pain is more severe and parenteral treatment is required, the subcutaneous route is the least painful – used either intermittently through a butterfly needle retained *in situ* or by continuous infusion with a syringe driver. The Guidelines for Liverpool Care Pathway prescribing in advanced kidney disease[39] is a valuable resource and more detailed guidelines are appended pp. 293–96. The recommended strong opioids for subcutaneous use are fentanyl or alfentanil. Unpleasant toxicity – with myoclonus, hallucinations, and agitation – can result from the metabolites of morphine. When time is short, recovery from such toxicity is unlikely. The pain of uraemic pericarditis and of the acutely rejected kidney may be relieved by steroids.

Shortness of breath is common in the last days, whatever the cause of dying. It is more common in advanced kidney disease because of fluid overload and acidosis. General measures – such as ensuring a comfortable position, fanning with cool air, administering oxygen, and the reassuring presence of family or staff – are often helpful. Strong opioids, in doses 50–100% of those needed for analgesia, can be given as needed. Benzodiazepine such as midazolam, given subcutaneously – separately or with opioids – may help, particularly when there is accompanying agitation, distress, or panic. In these circumstances, sublingual lorazepam may foster a sense of control. Exceptionally severe breathlessness due to fluid overload may be improved by isolated ultrafiltration.

Retained secretions may cause distress, particularly in those close to the patient. Management depends on anticipation; anti-secretory drugs such as hyoscine butylbromide, hyoscine hydrobromide, and glycopyrronium – each given by subcutaneous injection or infusion – reduce further production but cannot dry secretions that are already present. Hyoscine butylbromide does not cross the blood–brain barrier, so causes less sedation and paradoxical agitation than the hydrobromide.

Terminal restlessness and agitation occurs in a high proportion of all terminal illnesses, but particularly so in uraemia. Psychological and spiritual issues, physical causes such as pain, potential drug toxicities, and environmental issues compromising cognition must all be dealt with before resorting to drug treatment. Twitching, myoclonus, and anxiety usually responds to sedation with benzodiazepines such as midazolam – see appendix guidelines. Confusion, delirium, and hallucinations are better managed with antipsychotics such as haloperidol. Monitoring the effect of a stat dose may facilitate dose finding for subsequent continuous subcutaneous infusion, if required.

Nausea and vomiting controlled by an antiemetic prior to the terminal phase should be managed by continuous infusion of the same agent (for antiemetics that can be given subcutaneously see appendix p. 295 and Chapters 7 and 8) if the patient becomes unable to swallow. For those not previously on an antiemetic, haloperidol, as required, is usually effective for nausea associated with uraemia. Subcutaneous low-dose levomepromazine is a good second line drug.

Other symptoms of progressive uraemia include thirst, itching, convulsions, and hiccoughs. Thirst can frequently be relieved by good mouth-care, review of medication, ice chips, and liberation of oral intake, provided this will not exacerbate breathlessness. Saliva substitutes are sometimes helpful. Liberal moisturizing of the skin and antihistamines may help itch, though this is a difficult symptom to treat. Midazolam in a syringe driver is non-invasive and usually sufficient to control twitching and prevent fits. Hiccoughs, although uncommon terminally, can be very distressing; metoclopramide and haloperidol may be of benefit.

For drugs and dose modifications see guidelines Appendix p. 295 and 296.

15.13.2 Avoidance of prolongation of dying and achieving a sense of control

A consistent finding from studies of patients wishes around end-of-life care, including those on dialysis, is that they do not wish to be subjected to interventions with minimal, if any, potential for benefit.[26] Being allowed to die naturally without attachment to machines when unconscious is an oft-cited example.

Resuscitation status is also important. Staff caring for these patients in hospital need to record this. However, if the patient has not made his or her wishes known but the chance of resuscitation being successful is infinitesimal, there is no need to discuss this with the patient – just as one would not initiate discussion about any other futile treatment. A more sensitive way of wording such decisions is to talk of allowing natural death.

With the avoidance of prolongation of life comes achieving a sense of control. This sense of control also encompasses choices about the setting in which the patient is cared for, about who is around them, as well as shared decision-making about drug management. The use of tools, such as the PPC the UK,[30] can help people state their preferences for place of care and place of death and contribute to their sense of control

15.13.3 Relieving the burden and strengthening relationships

It is important to enable a patient to achieve a sense of peace and completion at the end of their life, so that they are not worrying about those who may have been caring for them in the previous period. Relief from that sense of being a burden may help strengthen their relationships with loved ones. The place in which an individual feels most at ease and therefore able to strengthen relationships will vary. For some it is the familiar hospital ward, with staff who are well known to them, which is most appropriate. For others it is the environment of the hospice, and for yet others the familiarity of home. It may be of great comfort to the carer, if it has been possible to spend precious time with their loved one before he or she died. Spiritual care should be an integral part of all clinical care. The need for such care is heightened as the end of life approaches – the time we are most likely to try to make sense of our lives. For those for whom formal religion is an integral part of their living, it will also be an integral part of their dying. All patients being cared for at the end of their lives should have their spiritual and religious needs assessed and responded too.

15.14 Care after death

For family and carers, the days and weeks after death of a loved one can be forbidding, especially for those whose time, strength, and emotions have been consumed in caring for many weeks, months, or years. Continued care after death is important and an integrated approach should be taken. Use of the 'care after death' section of Liverpool Care Pathway or, in primary care and care homes, the Gold Standard Framework after Death Analysis can facilitate improved bereavement care which must be culturally appropriate for the bereaved person. Subsequent use could be made of the VOICES questionnaire to evaluate the carer's experience. The needs of professional carers are often forgotten. Renal physicians and dialysis staff for instance may have known patients for many years or decades, and are also bereaved.

15.15 **Conclusion**

The provision of quality end-of-life care is as important as other aspects of the care of renal patients but with different goals and emphasis. By focussing on what is important to the patient we should aim to enable the person who is dying to achieve comfort and dignity. By doing so, support is given also to the family and the professional staff caring for them. It helps patients and family to see the same level of medical commitment continue through the terminal phase as was present prior to it; what changes is the goal of that care. Staff can then take pride in and gain satisfaction from fulfilling their vocation to 'cure sometimes, to help often, to comfort always".[40]

Case

Alan was 52. He had suffered from diabetes since the age of 10. He developed kidney failure and was referred for consideration of dialysis. He had many other problems. He was partially sighted. He had had amputations of his right leg and of part of his left foot. He had a supportive wife and family. His mobility was severely limited and had extensive social service support. He was very reliant upon his wife, who had given up work to care for him. Alan and his family were supported by the whole renal team in choosing peritoneal dialysis as the most suitable treatment option. The treatment worked well, providing a good quality of life for over 4 years, although during this time he was becoming more and more dependent. He developed severe ulcers on his left leg and underwent a bypass operation to try to improve the blood supply to his leg. Unfortunately, further complications occurred and amputation of his leg was discussed. At this stage Alan, recalling the discussions which had taken place prior to commencement of dialysis, indicated to a member of the peritoneal dialysis team that he wanted to explore the implications of stopping dialysis. Following full discussion, involving his family and various team members, he decided that he wished to have no further surgery and to withdraw from dialysis. At his wish he was referred to a hospice near to his home. He subsequently transferred to the hospice, where he died peacefully 5 days later. His wife and family received bereavement support from the Hospice and Renal Counsellor.

Ethical case analysis

A thorough approach to this patient's care throughout his illness helped him at the end of his life. After the bypass surgery failed to save his left leg, Alan recalled discussions conducted with him prior to the initiation of dialysis. Fortunately, he had been fully informed of his dialysis options as recommended by the RPA/ASN guideline recommendation # 2 on informed consent or refusal. It states, "Physicians should fully inform patients about their diagnosis, prognosis, and all treatment options, including: 1) available dialysis modalities, 2) not starting dialysis and continuing conservative management which should include end-of-life care, 3) a time-limited trial of dialysis, and 4) stopping dialysis and receiving end-of-life care. Choices among options should be made by patients or, if patients lack decision-making capacity, their designated legal agents. Their decisions should be informed and voluntary. The renal care team, in conjunction with the primary care physician, should insure that the patient or legal agent understands the consequences of the decision". Alan remembered option #4 and decided he had reached a point when it was his preferred course of action. The renal care team fully discussed Alan's choice with him and determined that it was informed and voluntary. They honoured his wish to stop dialysis and implemented the RPA/ASN guideline recommendation #9 on palliative care. This recommendation urges that hospice healthcare professionals be involved in managing the medical, psychosocial, and spiritual aspects of end-of-life care for these patients and their families. His family also benefited from the hospice referral because the families of patients enrolled in hospice receive bereavement support after the patient's death.

Appendix

(see next page)

Guidelines for healthcare professionals on the care of patients with established renal failure who are in the last days of life

The aim of treatment is the comfort of the patient and the support of those close to them

Use these guidelines when the whole team, the patient and family agree that the patient is in the last days of his or her life

It is a guide to treatment and practitioners should exercise their own professional judgement according to the clinical situation

It is helpful to have considered the following questions:

- Do the patient, family, and healthcare professionals recognize that the end of life is approaching?
- Has the preferred priorities of care been discussed with patient and family and their wishes recorded?
- Have the patient and family been asked about their cultural, spiritual, and religious needs at this time?
- Have all unnecessary investigations, including blood tests and routine monitoring, e.g. blood pressure (BP), been discontinued?
- Have medications been rationalized; retaining only those needed for symptom control or quality of life?
- Is comfort care, particularly care of mouth and skin, in place?
- **Are the drugs needed for palliation prescribed by route appropriate for the patient's situation and are they available as needed?**

Pain control

For good symptom control prn medication should be prescribed for likely symptoms even when the patient is asymptomatic. All of the drugs listed below should be given subcutaneously (s/c), unless otherwise specified.

PAIN

- **All patients should have a strong opioid prescribed, to be available as needed (prn)**
- **Recommendation: Fentanyl 12.5–25 μg s/c prn up to hourly**
- 1 **Patient in pain: opioid naïve** (see also Box 15.2 for adjuvant drugs)
  - (a) Pain intermittent
    - prescribe fentanyl 12.5 or 25 μg s/c as needed up to hourly

Box 15.1

The patient has a **fentanyl patch**

- If the pain is controlled **continue** with the patch
- If pain is not controlled continue **with patch and** titrate additional analgesia with prn or continuous s/c fentanyl or alfentanil

◆ after 24 h or sooner, review medication, if two or more prn doses needed or if patient still in pain

◆ set up s/c syringe driver (SD) to run over 24 h

◆ starting dose usually fentanyl 100–250 μg/24 h

◆ 25 μg of fentanyl s/c is ≅2 mg s/c morphine or 1.5 mg s/c diamorphine

(b) Pain continuous

◆ give stat dose s/c fentanyl then start continuous s/c infusion in syringe driver with fentanyl

◆ starting dose depends on patient's frailty & severity of pain; 100–250 μg /24 h fentanyl

◆ prescribe prn medication, s/c fentanyl 1/10th of the 24-h dose, this can be given hourly if needed

◆ increase or decrease dose in syringe driver depending on response or side effects

2 **Patient in pain: already on strong opioid** (see Box 15.1 if patient already on a fentanyl patch)

◆ if on other strong opioid convert to dose equivalent of fentanyl; or alfentanil

◆ if >600μg fentanyl/24 h required, see supporting information; contact palliative care team

(a) Opioid responsive pain:

◆ increase present dose by 25–30% or

◆ add up previous day's prn doses and add to the regular dose (but do not include doses used for specific movement related pain, e.g. dressing change or washing)

◆ **AND prescribe prn s/c fentanyl dose at 1/10th 24-h dose hourly – see also above**

(b) Opioid poorly responsive

◆ consider adjuvant; see Box 15.2 or contact local palliative care services

◆ All strong opioids should be monitored carefully, recognizing that pain and the patient's clinical condition often changes rapidly

---

Box 15.2

Adjuvant drugs for specific indications

◆ **bowel colic** – consider hyoscine butylbromide (Buscopan) 20mg s/c stat and up to 240 mg/24 hours

◆ **joint stiffness, pressure sores** – consider oral or rectal paracetamol or NSAID

◆ **neuropathic pain** – consider clonazepam 500 micrograms sc prn or nocte, can be given 12 hourly

◆ **associated anxiety & distress** – midazolam 2.5mg s/c hourly

A combination of midazolam and fentanyl or alfentanil can be very effective in agitated patients who are in pain.

For the symptoms below, all patients should have prn medication prescribed and available

At this stage, the goal is relief of symptoms and the cause of the symptom may not be relevant

Retained respiratory tract secretions

Symptoms absent: Hyoscine butylbromide 20 mg s/c 2-hourly prn

Symptoms present: Hyoscine butylbromide 40–120 mg/24 h s/c via syringe driver (SD) + 20 mg 2-hourly prn up to 240 mg/24 h

Terminal restlessness and agitation

Symptoms absent: Midazolam 2.5 mg s/c up to hourly prn. NB may be cumulative effect

Symptoms present: Midazolam 2.5 mg s/c up to hourly prn. If two or more doses required, consider syringe driver with 10–20 mg/24 h + prn dose

If agitation from hallucinations or disordered thought, use haloperidol at dose below for nausea and vomiting

Nausea and vomiting

Symptoms absent:

1 If already taking effective anti-emetic, e.g. metoclopramide, haloperidol, or levomepromazine, it can be given via SD over24 h

2 If not taking an anti-emetic: prescribe haloperidol 1.5 mg prn 8 hourly or levomepromazine 5 mg s/c prn 8 hourly

Symptoms present:

Start levomepromazine 5 mg s/c prn up to 8 hourly or start 5–10 mg/24 h by continuous s/c infusion, with further two doses of 5 mg s/c /24 h prn

Shortness of breath – The following **may** be helpful whatever the cause:

◆ Positioning the patient – a cool fan on the face – oxygen, if hypoxic and the reassuring presence of family or staff

◆ Strong opioids such as fentanyl, used at half to the full recommended dose for pain; use prn up to hourly or in SD if repeated doses needed

◆ Benzodiazepines, such as midazolam 2.5 mg s/c can be given up to hourly if associated with anxiety or panic attacks

Fluid overload – is less common than might be expected but very distressing if it occurs. Use above guidance for shortness of breath or consider

◆ Sub-lingual nitrates

◆ **If appropriate** consider: high-dose furosemide or ultra filtration for comfort

Supporting information for pain control and other symptom management

◆ Fentanyl and alfentanil are suggested as alternative strong opioids to morphine for patients in renal failure as they have no active metabolites with the potential to cause symptomatic and distressing toxicity such as myoclonic jerks, agitation, and hallucinations.

◆ **In the opioid-naïve patient successful pain relief can be achieved with low doses, e.g. 100–200 μg/ fentanyl/24 h without excess sedation;** s/c fentanyl is about 75 times as potent as s/c morphine so:-

  • 200 μg s/c Fentanyl/24 h is **approximately** equivalent to 30 mg oral or 15 mg s/c morphine/24 h and 4 mg oral hydromorphone/24 h

◆ Alfentanil is 1/4–1/5 as potent as fentanyl, and 10 times as potent as subcut diamorphine or 15 times as potent as s/c morphine. Use when doses of fentanyl exceed 600 μg/24 h as fentanyl less soluble and the volume too great for the syringe driver

◆ Alfentanil is not normally recommended for dose titration as it has a very short duration of action (30–60 min). It is useful for painful procedures or incident pain however, the suggested prn dose for patient on s/c alfentanil would be approx $1/10^{th}$ the 24-h dose

◆ Fentanyl and alfentanil can be mixed with all the common drugs in a syringe driver, though alfentanil and cyclizine may crystallize and so should be avoided

◆ Clonazepam can be given subcutaneously and may provide a useful adjuvant for neuropathic pain. As there is increased sensitivity to benzodiazepines in ESRD, titrate carefully against toxicity, starting with 500 μg/24 h to a maximum of 2 mg/24 h

◆ NSAIDS may worsen renal function, however for patients in the last days of life this may not be relevant and comfort is paramount

◆ The following anti-emetics can be given subcutaneously: metoclopramide; haloperidol,levomepromazine, and cyclizine

  • Maximum recommended dose in renal impairment: metoclopramide = 30 mg/24 h;

◆ Cyclizine is **not**, however, recommended as it may cause hypotension and tachyarrythmias in patients with cardiac disease; in addition, it may aggravate an already dry mouth and crystallizes with hyoscine butyl bromide and alfentanil

◆ Glycopyrronium can be used as an alternative to hyoscine butyl bromide for retained secretions

◆ Single daily s/c dexamethasone at 6–8 mg can be used for uraemic pericarditis or rejection pain

◆ If patient no longer able to take regular anticonvulsant; midazolam in a syringe driver at 10–20 mg/24 h can be used to prevent fits

If uncertain, please contact senior medical, nursing, or pharmacy staff on your team or your local palliative care service

References

1 Farrington K, Rao R, Gilg J, et al. (2007). New adult patients starting renal replacement therapy in the UK in (Chapter 3). *Nephrol Dial Transplant*, **22** Suppl 7, vii11–29.

2 Department of Health (2005). National Service Framework for Renal Services – Part Two: Chronic kidney disease acute renal failure and end of life care. (GENERIC).

3 Department of Health (2008). End of Life Strategy – promoting high quality care for all adults at the end of life.

4 Clinical practice guidelines on shared decision-making in the appropriate initiation of and withdrawal from dialysis for the Renal Physicians Association/American Society of Nephrology Working Group (2000). *J Am Soc Nephrol*, **11**, 2.

5 Holley JL, Davison SN, Moss AH (2007). Nephrologists' changing practices in reported end-of-life decision-making. *Clin J Am Soc Nephrol*, **2**, 107–11.

6 Farrington K, Rao R, Stenkamp R, et al. (2007). All patients receiving renal replacement therapy in the United Kingdom in 2005 (chapter 4). *Nephrol Dial Transplant*, **22** Suppl 7, vii30–50.

7 United States Renal Data Systems Annual Data Report (2008). http://www.usrds.org/2008/pdf/V2_02_.pdf)

8 Tomson C, Udayaraj U, Gilg J, et al. (2007). Comorbidities in UK patients at the start of renal replacement therapy (chapter 6). *Nephrol Dial Transplant*, **22** Suppl 7, vii58–68.

9 Chandna SM, Schulz J, Lawrence C, et al. (1999). Is there a rationale for rationing chronic dialysis? A hospital based cohort study of factors affecting survival and morbidity. *BMJ*, **318**, 217–23.

10 Smith C, Da Silva-Gane M, Chandna S, et al. (2003). Choosing not to dialyse: evaluation of planned non-dialytic management in a cohort of patients with end-stage renal failure. *Nephron Clin Pract*, **95**, c40–6.

11 Murtagh FE, Marsh JE, Donohoe P, et al. (2007). Dialysis or not? A comparative survival study of patients over 75 years with chronic kidney disease stage 5. *Nephrol Dial Transplant*, **22**, 1955–62.

12 Lunney JR, Lynn J, Foley DJ, et al. (2003). Patterns of functional decline at the end of life. *JAMA*, **289**, 2387–92.

13 Murtagh FE, Murphy E, Sheerin NS (2008). llness trajectories: an important concept in the management of kidney failure. *Nephrol Dial Transplant*, **23**, 3746–48.

14 Ellershaw J, Ward C (2003). Care of the dying patient: the last hours or days of life. *BMJ*, **326**, 30–4.

15 Gold Standards Framework (2006). http://www.goldstandardsframework.nhs.uk/gp_contract.php

16 Moss AH, Ganjoo J, Sharma S (2008). Utility of the "Surprise" Question to Identify Dialysis Patients with High Mortality. *Clin J Am Soc Nephrol*, **3**, 1379–84.

17 Davison S, Jhangri G, Johnson J (2006). Longitudinal validation of a modified Edmonton symptom assesment system (ESAS) in haemodialysis patients. *Nephrol Dial Transplant*, **21**, 3189–95.

18 Weisbord SD, Fried LF, Arnold RM, et al. (2004). Development of a Symptom Assessment Instrument for Chronic hemodialysis patients: The Dialysis Symptom Index. *J Pain Symptom manag*, **27**, 226–40.

19 Barnes K, Jones L, Tookman A, et al. (2007). Acceptability of an advance care planning interview schedule: a focus group study. *Palliat Med*, **21**, 23–8.

20 Davison SN, Simpson C (2006). Hope and advance care planning in patients with end stage renal disease: qualitative interview study. *BMJ*, **333**, 886.

21 Russ AJ, Shim JK, Kaufman SR (2007). The value of "life at any cost": talk about stopping kidney dialysis. *Soc Sci Med*, **64**, 2236–47.

22 Holley JL (2007). Palliative care in end-stage renal disease: illness trajectories, communication, and hospice use. *Adv Chr Kidney Dis*, **14**, 402–8.

23 Mental Capacity Act (2005). http://www.dca.gov.uk/menincap/legis.htm

24 Kwak J, Haley WE (2005). Current research findings on end-of-life decision making among racially or ethnically diverse groups. *Gerontologist*, **45**, 634–41.

25 Steinhauser KE, Christakis NA, Clipp EC, et al. (2000). Factors considered important at the end of life by patients, family, physicians, and other care providers. *JAMA*, **284**, 2476–82.

26 Steinhauser KE, Clipp EC, McNeilly M, et al. (2000). In search of a good death: observations of patients, families, and providers. *Ann Intern Med*, **132**, 825–32.

27 Singer PA, Martin DK, Kelner M (1999). Quality end-of-life care: patients' perspectives. *JAMA*, **281**, 163–8.

28 Patrick DL, Engelberg RA, Randall Curtiss J (2001). Evaluating the Quality of Dying and Death. *J Pain Symptom manag*, **22**, 717–26.

29 Davison SN (2006). Facilitating advance care planning for patients with end-stage renal disease: the patient perspective. *Clin J Am Soc Nephrol*, **1**, 1023–8.

30 Preferred Priorities for Care (2007). http://www.endoflifecareforadults.nhs.uk/eolc/CS310.htm .

31 Cohen LM, Germain MJ, Poppel DM, et al. (2000). Dying well after discontinuing the life-support treatment of dialysis. *Arch Intern Med*, **160**, 2513–18.

32 Weisbord SD (2007). Symptoms and their correlates in chronic kidney disease. *Adv Chronic Kidney Dis*, **14**, 319–27.

33 Davison SN, Jhangri GS, Johnson JA (2006). Cross-sectional validity of a modified Edmonton symptom assessment system in dialysis patients: a simple assessment of symptom burden. *Kidney Int*, **69**, 1621–5.

34 Murtagh FE, Addington-Hall J, Higginson IJ (2007). The prevalence of symptoms in end-stage renal disease: a systematic review. *Adv Chr Kidney Dis*, **14**, 82–99.

35 Davison SN (2002). The impact of pain in hemodialysis patients : effects on mood, sleep, daily actvity and the desire to withdear from dialysis. *J Am Soc Nephrol*, **13**, 589A.

36 Chater S, Davison SN, Germain M, et al. (2006). Withdrawal from dialysis: a palliative care perspective. *Clin Nephrol*, **66**, 464–72.

37 Cohen LM, Germain M, Poppel D, et al. (2000). Dialyisis Discontinuation and Palliative Care. *Am J Kidney Dis*, **36**, 140–4.

38 Murtagh FE, Addington-Hall JM, Edmonds PM, et al. (2007). Symptoms in advanced renal disease: a cross-sectional survey of symptom prevalence in stage 5 chronic kidney disease managed without dialysis. *J Palliat Med*, **10**, 1266–76.

39 DH Renal NSF team and Marie Curie Palliative Care Institute (2008). Guidelines for Liverpool Care Pathway prescribing in advanced kidney disease.

40 Anon 16th century French. *Guerir quelquefois, soulager souvent, comforter toujours.*

Index